Transplantation

A COMPANION TO SPECIALIST SURGICAL PRACTICE

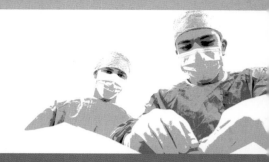

Series Editors
O. James Garden
Simon Paterson-Brown

Transplantation

FIFTH EDITION

Edited by

John L. R. Forsythe
MBBS MD FRCS(Ed) FRCS(Eng) FEBS
Honorary Professor and Consultant Transplant
Surgeon, Transplant Unit,
Royal Infirmary of Edinburgh, UK

Edinburgh   London   New York   Oxford   Philadelphia   St Louis   Sydney   Toronto   2014

SAUNDERS

ELSEVIER

Fifth edition © 2014 Elsevier Limited. All rights reserved.

First edition 1997
Second edition 2001
Third edition 2005
Fourth edition 2009
Fifth edition 2014

ISBN 978-0-7020-4960-6
e-ISBN 978-0-7020-4968-2

British Library Cataloguing in Publication Data
A catalogue record for this book is available from the British Library

Library of Congress Cataloging in Publication Data
A catalog record for this book is available from the Library of Congress

your source for books, journals and multimedia in the health sciences
www.elsevierhealth.com

Working together to grow libraries in developing countries

www.elsevier.com • www.bookaid.org

The Publisher's policy is to use **paper manufactured from sustainable forests**

Printed in China

Commissioning Editor: Laurence Hunter
Development Editor: Lynn Watt
Project Manager: Vinod Kumar Iyyappan
Designer/Design Direction: Miles Hitchen
Illustration Manager: Jennifer Rose
Illustrator: Antbits Ltd

Contents

Contents

Contributors

Murat Akyol, MD, FRCS
Consultant Transplant Surgeon, Royal Infirmary
of Edinburgh; Honorary Clinical Senior Lecturer,
University of Edinburgh, Edinburgh, UK

**John J. Casey, MBChB, PhD, FRCS(Glasg),
FRCS(Ed), FRCS(Gen Surg)**
Consultant Transplant Surgeon and Honorary Clinical
Senior Lecturer, Transplant Unit, Royal Infirmary of
Edinburgh, Edinburgh, UK

**Marc J. Clancy, MA, MBChB, FRCS(Eng), PhD,
FRCS(Gen Surg)**
Consultant Transplant and General Surgeon, Clinical
Lead for Transplantation, Honorary Associate
Clinical Professor; Transplant Unit, Western Infirmary,
Glasgow, UK

John H. Dark, FRCS, FRCP
Professor of Cardiothoracic Surgery, Newcastle
University; The Freeman Hospital, Newcastle upon
Tyne, UK

Philip A. Dyer, PhD, FRCPath
Consultant Clinical Scientist and Professor in
Transplantation Science, Scottish National Blood
Transfusion Service, Royal Infirmary of Edinburgh,
Edinburgh, UK

Peter Friend, MD, FRCS
Professor of Transplantation, Nuffield Department
of Surgical Sciences, University of Oxford; Director,
Oxford Transplant Centre, Oxford, UK

Asif Hasan, MBBS, FRCS(Ed), FRCS(CTh)
Consultant Cardiothoracic Surgeon, Freeman
Hospital, Newcastle upon Tyne, UK

Ann-Margaret Little, BSc, PhD, FRCPath
Consultant Clinical Scientist, Head of Laboratory,
Histocompatibility and Immunogenetics Service,
Gartnavel General Hospital, Glasgow, UK

Roslyn B. Mannon, MD, FASN
Professor of Medicine, Division of Nephrology,
Professor of Surgery, Division of Transplantation,
University of Alabama, Birmingham, AL, USA

Lorna P. Marson, MD, FRCS
Senior Lecturer and Consultant Surgeon in
Transplant Surgery, Transplant Unit, University
of Edinburgh and Royal Infirmary of Edinburgh,
Edinburgh, UK

Shikha Mehta, MD
Assistant Professor of Medicine, University of
Alabama, Birmingham, AL, USA

Camille Nelson Kotton, MD
Clinical Director, Transplant and
Immunocompromised Host Infectious Diseases,
Infectious Diseases Division, Massachusetts
General Hospital/Harvard Medical School,
Boston, MA, USA

John O'Callaghan, MBBS, MRCS
Transplant Registrar, Oxford Transplant Centre,
Churchill Hospital, Oxford, UK

Gabriel C. Oniscu, MD, FRCS
Consultant Transplant Surgeon, Honorary Clinical
Senior Lecturer, Transplant Unit, Royal Infirmary of
Edinburgh, Edinburgh, UK

Rutger J. Ploeg, MD, PhD, FRCS
Professor of Transplant Biology and Honorary
Consultant Surgeon, Nuffield Department of Surgical
Sciences, University of Oxford; Oxford Transplant
Centre, Oxford, UK

Elizabeth A. Pomfret, MD, PhD
Chair, Department of Transplantation and
Hepatobiliary Diseases, Professor of Surgery, Tufts
University School of Medicine, Lahey Clinic Medical
Center, Burlington, MA, USA

James J. Pomposelli, MD, PhD
Associate Professor of Surgery,
Tufts Medical School; Surgical Director of
Transplantation, Lahey Clinic Medical Center,
Burlington, MA, USA

Christopher J. Rudge, CBE, FRCS
Honorary Professor, Queen Mary, University of
London, London, UK

Contributors

Caroline J. Simon, MB BCh, BAO(Hons), BMedSc
Senior Transplant Fellow, Department of
Transplantation and Hepatobiliary Diseases, Lahey
Clinic Medical Center, Burlington, MA, USA

Mary Ann Simpson, PhD
Director of Clinical Research, Transplantation, Lahey
Clinic Medical Center, Burlington, MA, USA

George Tse, MSc, MRCSEd, MBChB, BSc(Hons)
Clinical Research Fellow, Transplantation Surgery,
The University of Edinburgh; MRC Centre for
Inflammation Research, The Queen's Medical
Research Institute, Edinburgh, UK

David Turner, PhD, FRCPath
Consultant Clinical Scientist, Histocompatibility and
Immunogenetics, Scottish National Blood Transfusion
Service,Royal Infirmary of Edinburgh, Edinburgh, UK

Alex T. Vesey, MBChB, MRCS
Registrar in Transplant Surgery, Surgical
Registrar,Department of Renal Transplantation,
Western Infirmary, Glasgow, UK

Gregory Veillette, MD
Clinical Instructor, Department of Surgery, Division
of Transplantation, University of California, San
Francisco, CA, USA

Flavio Vincenti, MD
Clinical Professor of Medicine and Surgery,
Department of Medicine and Surgery, Deborah
Faiman Endowed Chair in Kidney Transplantation,
UCSF Medical Center, San Francisco, CA, USA

David Wojciechowski, DO
Assistant Clinical Professor of Medicine, Medicine-
Nephrology, UCSF San Francisco, CA, USA

Series Editors' preface

It is now some 17 years since the first edition of the *Companion to Specialist Surgical Practice* series was published. We set ourselves the task of meeting the educational needs of surgeons in the later years of specialist surgical training, as well as consultant surgeons in independent practice who wished for contemporary, evidence-based information on the subspecialist areas relevant to their general surgical practice. The series was never intended to replace the large reference surgical textbooks which, although valuable in their own way, struggle to keep pace with changing surgical practice. This Fifth Edition has also had to take due account of the increasing specialisation in 'general' surgery. The rise of minimal access surgery and therapy, and the desire of some subspecialties such as breast and vascular surgery to separate away from 'general surgery', may have proved challenging in some countries, but has also served to emphasise the importance of all surgeons being aware of current developments in their surgical field. As in previous editions, there has been increasing emphasis on evidence-based practice and contributors have endeavoured to provide key recommendations within each chapter. The eBook versions of the textbook have also allowed the technophile improved access to key data and content within each chapter.

We remain indebted to the volume editors and all the contributors of this Fifth Edition. We have endeavoured where possible to bring in new blood to freshen content. We are impressed by the enthusiasm, commitment and hard work that our contributors and editorial team have shown and this has ensured a short turnover between editions while maintaining as accurate and up-to-date content as is possible. We remain grateful for the support and encouragement of Laurence Hunter and Lynn Watt at Elsevier Ltd. We trust that our original vision of delivering an up-to-date affordable text has been met and that readers, whether in training or independent practice, will find this Fifth Edition an invaluable resource.

O. James Garden BSc, MBChB, MD, FRCS(Glas), FRCS(Ed), FRCP(Ed), FRACS(Hon), FRCSC(Hon), FRSE
Regius Professor of Clinical Surgery, Clinical Surgery School of Clinical Sciences, The University of Edinburgh and Honorary Consultant Surgeon, Royal Infirmary of Edinburgh

Simon Paterson-Brown MBBS, MPhil, MS, FRCS(Ed), FRCS(Engl), FCS(HK)
Honorary Senior Lecturer, Clinical Surgery School of Clinical Sciences, The University of Edinburgh and Consultant General and Upper Gastrointestinal Surgeon, Royal Infirmary of Edinburgh

Editor's preface

Although part of a surgical series, this volume is not just for surgeons. It is for all those who play an important role in the transplant procedure. Thus, it has been designed to interest nursing staff who care for organ failure patients, transplant coordinators, theatre staff, immunology laboratory staff, paramedical personnel, physicians and surgeons. Modern techniques in transplantation and new forms of immunosuppression, emphasised throughout this volume, have increased the complexity of clinical and ethical dilemmas which face the whole team caring for the transplant patient. Appropriate response to such dilemmas is required to ensure the continued success of transplantation medicine.

As in previous editions of this volume, this is less of a new edition and more a new book. For many chapters a new author has been commissioned, therefore giving a different view on a subject whilst bringing the factual information up to date. In other chapters the authors from the previous editions have been retained but the brief has been to write chapters in a slightly different way, emphasising newer techniques or dilemmas in transplantation.

It has often been said that transplant medicine is the best example of multidisciplinary team care and this fact makes the specialty both challenging and rewarding. I hope that all members of that team find something in this new book that helps in the care of their patients.

John L.R. Forsythe
Edinburgh

Evidence-based practice in surgery

Critical appraisal for developing evidence-based practice can be obtained from a number of sources, the most reliable being randomised controlled clinical trials, systematic literature reviews, meta-analyses and observational studies. For practical purposes three grades of evidence can be used, analogous to the levels of 'proof' required in a court of law:

1. **Beyond all reasonable doubt.** Such evidence is likely to have arisen from high-quality randomised controlled trials, systematic reviews or high-quality synthesised evidence such as decision analysis, cost-effectiveness analysis or large observational datasets. The studies need to be directly applicable to the population of concern and have clear results. The grade is analogous to burden of proof within a criminal court and may be thought of as corresponding to the usual standard of 'proof' within the medical literature (i.e. $P<0.05$).

2. **On the balance of probabilities.** In many cases a high-quality review of literature may fail to reach firm conclusions due to conflicting or inconclusive results, trials of poor methodological quality or the lack of evidence in the population to which the guidelines apply. In such cases it may still be possible to make a statement as to the best treatment on the 'balance of probabilities'. This is analogous to the decision in a civil court where all the available evidence will be weighed up and the verdict will depend upon the balance of probabilities.

3. **Not proven.** Insufficient evidence upon which to base a decision, or contradictory evidence.

Depending on the information available, three grades of recommendation can be used:

a. Strong recommendation, which should be followed unless there are compelling reasons to act otherwise.

b. A recommendation based on evidence of effectiveness, but where there may be other factors to take into account in decision-making, for example the user of the guidelines may be expected to take into account patient preferences, local facilities, local audit results or available resources.

c. A recommendation made where there is no adequate evidence as to the most effective practice, although there may be reasons for making a recommendation in order to minimise cost or reduce the chance of error through a locally agreed protocol.

> ✔✔ Evidence where a conclusion can be reached 'beyond all reasonable doubt' and therefore where a strong recommendation can be given.
> This will normally be based on evidence levels:
> • Ia. Meta-analysis of randomised controlled trials
> • Ib. Evidence from at least one randomised controlled trial
> • IIa. Evidence from at least one controlled study without randomisation
> • IIb. Evidence from at least one other type of quasi-experimental study.

> ✔ Evidence where a conclusion might be reached 'on the balance of probabilities' and where there may be other factors involved which influence the recommendation given. This will normally be based on less conclusive evidence than that represented by the double tick icons:
> • III. Evidence from non-experimental descriptive studies, such as comparative studies and case–control studies
> • IV. Evidence from expert committee reports or opinions or clinical experience of respected authorities, or both.

Evidence which is associated with either a **strong recommendation** or **expert opinion** is highlighted in the text in panels such as those shown above, and is distinguished by either a double or single tick icon, respectively. The references associated with double-tick evidence are highlighted in the reference lists at the end of each chapter along with a short summary of the paper's conclusions where applicable.

The reader is referred to Chapter 1, 'Evidence-based practice in surgery' in the volume, *Core Topics in General and Emergency Surgery* of this series, for a more detailed description of this topic.

1

Controversies in the ethics of organ transplantation

Marc J. Clancy
Alex T. Vesey

Introduction

- Clinical transplantation remains a relatively young field, yet it has created considerable ethical debate. Development of clinical programmes has required the rapid parallel development of ethical frameworks to justify the steps taken in the name of patient benefit.
- In many ways, the rate of technological advance has exceeded the development of the ethical, cultural and legal framework within which transplantation takes place. This has resulted in a variety of fascinating ethical debates but also represents a barrier to fully realising the potential of transplantation.
- All transplant professionals have a responsibility to be aware of the many ethical issues that surround transplantation and organ donation. It is also desirable for such professionals to be familiar with the terminology used to describe and discuss the ethics of transplantation.
- Good ethical practice should always be integral to efforts made to advance the science of transplantation. Interaction with stakeholders, lawmakers and those who determine public policy will be essential to the development of optimal future programmes.

Key terminology

Fundamental principles of bioethics

Beneficence Doing good for the patient must be the central moral objective for all healthcare staff.

Non-maleficence All effort must be made to avoid causing harm or distress to patients and their families. A central principle in organ donation is that donors are by definition 'harmed' in order to facilitate donation. This harm must be weighed up against the good that results from transplantation.

Autonomy The patient's autonomy must be respected. The individual has a (near) absolute right to determine their own fate – including that of their organs after death.

Justice Healthcare professionals should strive to seek fairness. Particularly relevant to transplantation where multiple conflicts of interest exist between various stakeholder groups.

Other terms

Deontology From the Greek 'deon' meaning obligation or duty. The ethical position which judges the morality of an action or belief on its adherence to a rule, e.g. 'do no harm' or 'always strive to save a life'.

Consequentialism Contrasts with deontology; judging the morality of actions according to their consequences.

Utilitarianism The ethical position that the value of a particular course of action is determined by how much 'good' or happiness results, the total 'good' usually referring to the world as a whole.

Altruism In a transplant context, the voluntary wish of the individual to make the 'gift' of donation of their organs (or equivalent) without expectation of reward.

Dignity A complex and difficult term to define but, in this context, one reflecting the unique and precious status of the human being and the ethical requirement not to treat the individual disrespectfully or harmfully in both life and death.

Futility A concept that relates to a patient who has reached a point when there is no realistic prospect of a successful outcome, whatever their medical care.

Equity The concept of fairness/justice often used in connection with the way organs are allocated and utilised. Also applied to access to transplant for different individuals.

Death, organ donation, patient autonomy and the choice to donate

While living donation has been integral to kidney transplantation for decades, deceased donors have always constituted the majority of transplant activity. Death and its diagnosis seemed a simple and easily understandable concept until complex modern intensive methods and care of transplantation forced society to question it in more detail.

If doctors are striving to save the life of a patient, and yet there exists a possibility that the patient must die and donate their organs (so that other patients may be helped), there may be a perceived conflict of interest for the responsible physician. To avoid this, a clear separation between medical care in life and the facilitation of deceased donation has been established. The pivotal component of this is the establishment of death.

When does death occur?

Substantial ethical debate surrounds the exact definition of death and this is reflected in the variability of definition between societies.[1,2]

Standard clinical tests for the certification of death include the absence of circulation, respiration, any response to pain or pupillary response to light. However, these tests require a valid setting and need to be confirmed over a sufficient length of time in order to ensure no reasonable possibility of spontaneous reversal. Brain stem death[3] allowed certification of death based on irreversible loss of brain stem function. This complex and intensively scrutinised mechanism for individuals to be declared legally dead has allowed organ donation even when the donor has a beating heart and viable organs maintained via mechanical ventilation.

The key ethical principle is that donation should proceed only after death has been established and no prospect of spontaneous autoresuscitation exists.[4]

Similarly, the decision to cease attempts at life-preserving treatments should be taken in a manner independent of considerations relating to organ donation and be based purely on the concept of patient benefit.

The idea of brain death remains a focus for ethical debate despite its long enshrinement in law. Initially the term 'brain dead' was applied, yet the demonstration of viable neuronal tissue was cited as a refutation of this as a valid state of death. This led to a change of terminology, with 'brain stem dead' being the currently accepted expression.[5]

The management of patients to facilitate organ donation either through the donation-after-brain stem-death (DBD) pathway or the alternative donation-after-circulatory-death (DCD) pathway remains one of the biggest ethical debating points of 21st century transplantation and intensive care medicine.

Guidance on the determination and diagnosis of death can be found in the Academy of Royal Colleges Code of Practice for the Diagnosis and Confirmation of Death (2008);[6] however, there remains no statutory definition of death in the UK and the working definition, 'the irreversible loss of the capacity for consciousness combined with irreversible loss of the capacity to breathe', put forward by the Department of Health, seems both practicable and socially acceptable. However, further clarification of this definition may be of benefit to all stakeholders.

Futility, the patient's best interests, and the decision to withdraw life-sustaining treatments

In a situation where organ donation may be feasible, what constitutes a potential donor's best interests? Before organ donation and transplantation, it was accepted that when a stage of futility was deemed to have been reached, further life-prolonging interventions were not in a dying patient's best interests. This was observed in the early days of transplantation, when continuing intervention was seen as unethical as these interventions were not designed for the benefit of the potential donor. This debate was particularly fierce around the issue of elective ventilation, with a historical conclusion that this was not an ethically desirable course of action.[7]

However, the nature of futility itself may have been changed by the very existence of the possibility for organ donation. Few citizens in the developed world are unaware that donation of organs after death is a possibility. In the UK, originally through the organ donor card system and more recently through the organ donor register (ODR), the opportunity to document one's wishes relating to organ donation has become increasingly accessible. This *opt-in* system has donor autonomy at its heart. In states like Spain, however, *opt-out* is the legal norm,[8] when the individual must record a wish to opt out of organ donation or it will be assumed that the wish is to go ahead with this action. Other options such as *mandated choice* come somewhere in between, and the desirability and likely effect on donation rates of each system are widely debated.[9] What is certain, though, is that the stated, informed and autonomous wish of a competent, living person to donate their organs can be regarded as a form of mandate to advance organ donation, even if this action may include interventions traditionally considered futile and therefore unethical.

In this context, what we mean by 'best interests' is less clear-cut. Many – including these authors – would regard it as unethical for a medical practitioner to withhold interventions designed to facilitate the successful donation of an individual who had expressed a clear wish to donate. However, this is not a simple argument. In the context of a highly pressured national intensive care service, efforts to facilitate organ donation from the dead or for those who will inevitably become dead may compete directly for human and material resources, in caring for the living. This argument is made doubly complex by the fact that third-party patients whose lives may be saved by the organs of the former group die on a daily basis. This ethical standpoint is dynamic across the healthcare professional spectrum and regular review will be beneficial to the working practices of the health service and to society as a whole.

Donor pain, distress and individuals' rights after death

Invasive but potentially life-saving interventions such as intubation and cardiopulmonary resuscitation have the capacity to cause pain and distress to an individual. Administering measures like these in attempting to save an individual's life is clearly ethically justifiable. But if the measures are contemplated in a patient who is deemed to be irreversibly dying in order to maintain tissue perfusion to facilitate organ donation, the ethics are not so straightforward.

In the UK, the Human Tissue Act (2004) and Human Tissue (Scotland) Act (2006) legally sanction 'the minimum' necessary steps to preserve organs in a state that allows successful donation.[10,11] The principles of non-maleficence and individual dignity suggest that ethically only the least invasive methods and steps should be taken to preserve organs after death. It must be recognised that advancing technology may redefine and perhaps increase the 'minimum' necessary steps. Additionally, the overall process of donation should also respect the individual's right to continuity of care, particularly with reference to access for relatives and communication/explanation of events.

Beyond the isolated concept of elective ventilation, perhaps the central ethical conundrum surrounding deceased donor transplantation is whether facilitation of a stated wish to donate provides ethical justification for interventions that may be considered futile in live-saving terms. The autonomy of the individual who has described a wish to donate would support interventions – even if theoretically painful or undignified – in order to fulfil their stated desire. The widely expressed view that death denies the individual 'rights' in the legal sense is at odds with the way in which we handle an individual's last will and testament, and in purely ethical terms it must be seen as reasonable to go to some lengths to honour an individual's wishes after death.

The conflict between donation and dignity in death

In the context of DBD, organ retrieval occurs in an operating theatre after confirmation of death has been carried out following the performance of brain stem tests.

Hypnotics and muscle relaxant medications are frequently employed. Controlled donation after circulatory death follows a period during which supportive treatments, often mechanical ventilation and inotropic cardiac support, are withdrawn. During this period there is an 'agonal' phase during which respiratory distress, movements consistent with discomfort, etc. may be observed. These findings may be detected whether or not the individual goes on to be an organ donor but this situation is ethically complex. The following considerations are germane and need to be weighed against each other:

- facilitation of the individual's autonomous wish to donate their organs (as discussed above);
- the right (and/or desire) for a dignified death – including the presence of the next of kin;
- the societal responsibility to optimise the quality of the organ donated by the individual's altruism.

Clinical protocols and individual conduct have evolved – and continue to evolve – to reflect a balance between these factors.

Relatives' right to veto the act of organ donation

As noted above, different legislatures across the globe have approached the individual's right to request organ donation by framing laws that are generally based on one of two principles. 'Opt-in' requires that the individual somehow records or comments, during life, that they would wish to be a potential organ donor. The opt-out system assumes that the individual does want to be a donor, given the appropriate circumstances at the time of their death, unless they have specifically opted out of the state organ donation system. Nuances apply in different countries. For instance, in Scotland, which has a slightly different law to the rest of the UK, the Human Tissue (Scotland) Act 2006[11] enshrines the concept of authorisation for donation that does not insist upon full informed consent but accepts that an individual may wish to indicate their advance directive towards organ donation. In such circumstances, the registration of a citizen on an organ donor register has much greater legal force and, at least in theory, carries legal primacy over the wishes of the next of kin. However, over a 5-year period from 2005 to 2010, 7.1% of all cases of potential deceased donation in the UK had a full or partial caveat placed on the organ donation process by relatives. No organ donation/transplant clinician would directly countermand the views of relatives in this difficult situation and it is, of course, quite possible that an individual might have rescinded their views, expressed on something such as an organ donor register, and it would then be expected that the next of kin would be the conduit for such a change of view coming to light. However, the likelihood is that the family member is countermanding the views of their loved one for a whole host of different reasons, including their own understanding of organ retrieval and donation. Even in countries with an opt-out system, it would be highly unusual for donation to proceed in the face of strong objection from a next of kin.[12]

Once again, this aspect of deceased donation brings an ethical tension between individual autonomy (the right of the citizen to decide what happens to their organs following death), non-maleficence to the family who might experience further extreme distress should their views not be taken into account and the utilitarian view that organs should be removed in all such circumstances for the greater benefit of society. Each country has achieved a reasonable compromise based on societal and cultural beliefs but it is acknowledged that such levels of compromise may need to be revisited from time to time as a change in societal view or need for organ donation evolves further.

The paradigm of uncontrolled DCD donation – still with ethical challenges

In any discussion with the general public concerning organ donation, it is commonly assumed that in circumstances where an individual is involved in an accident, is then taken to hospital and attempts are made for resuscitation but that resuscitation is unsuccessful, then the possibility of organ donation may be carried out. However, the truth remains that perhaps the largest group of missed potential organ donors are those who might potentially donate through an uncontrolled donation after circulatory death programme, as occurs in Spain, the Netherlands and parts of the USA.

Uncontrolled DCD donation includes a number of additional components that raise important ethical questions. The majority of this potential donor group either suffer sudden cardiac arrest in the community and are brought into hospital whilst undergoing cardiopulmonary resuscitation or suddenly arrest inside the hospital. This situation evolves far more rapidly than the majority of donations after brain death or controlled donations after circulatory death.

Early approach to the bereaved

The rapid approach to relatives that is required to obtain consent or authorisation is challenging. There is a moral balance to be struck – whilst it is important to respect the autonomy and altruism of a person who may have discussed or documented their wish to donate, it is important to be sensitive to the additional distress that may be caused by approaching newly bereaved next of kin.

The experience and expertise of the UK Specialist Nurse in Organ Donation (SNOD) network is central to the successful negotiation of this difficult situation. Evidence suggests that the approach regarding donation to relatives following death of their loved one is actually most often a comfort and rarely the cause of additional distress.[12,13] This is clearly the case in the Netherlands and Spain, where uncontrolled DCD is well established.[14] The cultural acceptability of this donation pathway in the UK remains to be confirmed on a large scale.

Pre-consent preservation measures

Uncontrolled DCD cannot proceed successfully without employing external preservation measures designed to maintain organ quality. These include external mechanical chest compression, in situ peritoneal cooling or, more recently, in situ perfusion of organs via a femoral cannula.[15] These interventions must be instigated rapidly, frequently before the next of kin can be consulted. The Organ Donor Register provides a valuable resource in the context of uncontrolled DCD. If an individual has documented their desire to donate, pre-consent preservative measures can be ethically justified as the patient's autonomy will have been respected.

If the deceased's wishes were unknown at the time of presentation, it could be argued (less robustly perhaps) that the instigation of pre-consent organ preservation measures protects the right of the individual to donate until the next of kin can be consulted. The legal requirement for 'minimum' preservative steps is equally ethically applicable in this situation and must also be withheld until death is certified.

Preservation measures and the potential to restore cerebral circulation

Ethical concerns exist regarding the potential for preservative measures to restore cerebral circulation. Such restoration can create a grey area in which the status of the potential donor as truly dead may be in question.[16] This returns us to the problem of the definition of death. DBD donors may have excellent cerebral blood supply but are deemed to be unequivocally dead, so cerebral perfusion per se is clearly not ethically incompatible with death and donation. This area of controversy must be further clarified to allow protocols that ensure unambiguity of the state of death and that ensure that ethical concerns regarding cerebral reperfusion are adequately considered. Of course, the problem may be with the preservation method and not the definition of death.

The extremes of deceased donation

In certain societies, the routine use of organs from executed prisoners has been documented.[17] The majority of transplant professionals would regard this as morally highly dubious; less extreme examples of potential donors and their ethical acceptability continue to provoke debate. In certain European societies, assisted suicide is legal and it has been possible for such individuals to become organ donors.[18] Assisted suicide is illegal in the UK but this may not always be the case and changes in law around the care of individuals at the end of life often have significant implications for transplantation.

The term 'persistent vegetative state' (PVS) is a concept that falls outside the current legal definition of brain stem death, yet is a state of such severe cerebral injury that its nature provokes debate around the definition of death. Some would argue that to remove organs from such individuals would constitute murder. Others argue that life is defined by the capability of the individual to interact with the wider world and that, given individuals in a PVS are incapable of this, they should be regarded as dead and therefore as potential deceased donors.[19] These extreme examples are currently the province of the philosophical world. If clinical transplantation has proved anything in its short lifetime, it is that what seems purely abstract and philosophical can very quickly become material to everyday decisions.

Allocation of organs

The concept that the organs of someone who has died can be preserved and transplanted into another person was initially unproblematic in ethical terms. The pioneers of transplantation identified specific recipients on the basis of urgent need and directly allocated a suitable organ when it became available without a specific process. This, despite frequent local objections, was accepted. The current situation could not be more different. Thousands of people wait for an organ from a limited pool of donors. This situation has forced societies to consider how organs should be allocated and to develop ethically and legally approved systems of organ allocation.

This remains an area of substantial controversy. The UK organ allocation systems are subject to regular review, recognising that the parameters must regularly be re-evaluated in the context of society as a whole.

Urgent clinical need remains the most unambiguous parameter and this is accurately reflected in the UK's systems of allocation for liver and heart transplants. In these cases, the potential recipient must be certain to die without a suitable graft and their clinical status defines their priority as 'super urgent' and above all other potential recipients who have more physiological reserve. This category may provoke ethical controversy if applied to slightly less urgent cases, since status may rest on physiological parameters that are modifiable, meaning actions to improve the recipient's clinical status may alter their status score (e.g. MELD/UKELD in liver transplantation) and have implications for priority of transplant allocation.

However, most organs are not allocated in this way. In the case of the most frequently transplanted organ, the kidney, patients are invariable clinically stable and often in receipt of life-preserving treatment in the form of dialysis. Renal transplantation is therefore not immediately life-saving but is life-prolonging and associated with an improved quality of life.

So to which of the several thousand deserving patients on the waiting list should a given kidney be allocated? Clinicians would not agree, nor would there be universal agreement between any section of society or indeed key stakeholders such as the patients on the waiting list.

Many factors must be considered in making the allocation decision, but the key parameters are outlined below.

Benefit (utility)

Organs should be allocated to 'do maximum good' in terms of providing the best outcomes for patients. This may not equate to optimising the outcomes for an individual transplanting centre.

'Maximum good' should refer to the greatest benefit for the whole cohort of patients on the National Transplant Waiting List for that organ and is probably best – if imperfectly defined – in terms of the number and quality of life-years gained for the intended recipient.

This concept has important implications for the decision to list patients or to remove them from the active waiting list. Ethically, it is essential that efforts are made to define a threshold at which transplantation of a given organ ceases to be sufficiently beneficial and that this is regularly applied to all potential recipients. It must be accepted that the level of scientific evidence relevant to this area leaves something to be desired. Furthermore, constant re-evaluation is necessary in the light of a dynamic balance between organ supply and demand and the changing technology of transplantation as a whole, which has forced us to regularly redefine the limits of its benefit.

Fairness (equity)

The first component of fairness in organ allocation must be equity of access to the treatment of transplantation. In the early years of kidney transplantation, closeness of immunological matching had a major impact on graft survival. With advances in immunosuppression and other technologies, this factor became of less immediate clinical significance. Initially, the UK kidney allocation system was heavily influenced by human leucocyte antigen (HLA) matching and the effect of this was to diminish the likelihood of allocation to those individuals with tissue types represented at a lower frequency in the population as a whole, such as ethnic minority groups. This was very reasonably judged to be unacceptable in societal terms and led to changes that increased the influence of waiting time on allocation. There was a consequent redistribution of allocated organs that to some extent addressed the perceived unfairness. However, equity of access is not the only form of fairness that must be considered. Geographical equity has also been identified as a relevant issue, with listing rates showing a degree of variation across the country. Some of the reasons underlying this are unavoidable but it is essential that systemic factors and clinical practices do not prejudice any individual's opportunity to be transplanted if that individual's clinical condition dictates both a need and a suitable potential benefit.

Transparency

The allocation decision is frequently a life and death decision and invariably a decision of life-changing significance for both the recipient and those not receiving the organ in question. On that basis it becomes essential that the process and parameters used in allocation are accessible and clear to all. Adherence to the stated standard should be audited.

Legality

Allocation proceeds within a societal context and must recognise the dynamic legal requirements of that society. For instance, an allocation system that discriminated between individuals based on physical/mental handicap, gender or the ability to pay would probably infringe the law, in addition to any questions of inequity.

Societal mandate

Organ donation and transplantation is reliant on broad public support for its existence. In some cases there is a conflict between the majority societal opinion of what is desirable and what is dictated by law, ethics and clinical need. For instance, research suggests that the majority of society does not support the allocation of organs to convicted criminals. Generally, this is not enacted by those in charge of allocation unless the criminal has objective criteria for not being listed, such as a past history of treatment non-compliance.

Flexibility

Clinical transplantation has come about – and reached its status as mainstream – as a result of pushing the limits of what is acceptable as a medical intervention. In principle it is undesirable to prevent or delay future innovation and advancement, and it is very unlikely that the limits of benefit in transplantation have been reached. Organ allocation must retain a mechanism for responding to advances in science and allow new and potentially more beneficial technologies to bear fruit in patient benefit.

The implications of variable organ quality

Transplantation began by using only highly selected, optimal organs from the very youngest of donors, healthy until time of death. The organs were then rapidly implanted into recipients at a site physically close to the site of donation. As transplantation was shown to be successful, increasing numbers of patients were wait-listed until demand outstripped supply and it became necessary to compromise the parameters by which organs were judged acceptable for transplantation.

This compromise has eventually led to the concept of the 'expanded criteria' donor also called, in the UK, the Higher Risk Donor. A transplant from such a donor still confers a significant benefit but is associated with a relatively poorer graft outcome when compared to a non-ECD organ.

The main parameters that mark out an ECD are age >60 or age <60 with two of the following: donor hypertension, terminal creatinine >1.5 mg/dL or cerebrovascular accident as the stated cause of death.

In the UK, the majority of donors continue to be after brain death. However, this pool appears to be relatively fixed in number within the constraints of the current UK health service. The majority of the increase in deceased organ donors since 2008 has been made up of DCD donors. These accounted for 37% of all UK deceased donors in 2010–11.[20] DCD donors may donate kidney, liver, pancreas, lung and multiple other tissues,[21] although the number of organs donated per donor is less than for DBD. In addition, research is under way in the UK into cardiac donation from DCD donation, which entails the controversial concept of restarting the heart after certification of death.[22]

The observed expansion in deceased donor numbers since 2008 has also comprised in the main older donors, more obese donors and more donors with hypertension. Clearly the 'biological age' of the organs donated is changing in an unfavourable direction for clinical transplantation outcomes. The implication of this is that the risk/benefit profile of any given transplant may vary widely. This variability is not always accurately accounted for in the practices of allocation and consent.

In DBD donation the conditions of retrieval are standardised and well controlled. In DCD donation (in Maastricht category III and even more so in categories II and I) the conditions of donation are much more complicated; the agonal phase is variable and this makes it impossible to predict the subsequent effect on the organs that are retrieved under conditions of hypoperfusion/warm ischaemia.

This makes transplant of an organ following DCD donation more high risk (including intraoperative complexity, postoperative recovery period and long-term outcomes), especially if the organ is transplanted into a high-risk-marginal recipient. This situation presents complex clinical and ethical dilemmas.

Balance of donor and recipient risk

With the increasing use of expanded criteria donors and DCD organs and the willingness to accept progressively older patients with a higher comorbidity for transplantation, the transplant community should perhaps change its focus from the separate donor and recipient risk status towards the concept of the *marginal transplant* instead.

The multiple potential combinations of different donors to varying recipients leads to a wide variety of complex scenarios both in terms of the clinical complexity and in terms of the risks and benefits of the transplant.

Where, for instance, a DCD organ from an older donor is given to a low-risk recipient, an organ with pre-existing damage that may reduce its long-term function and longevity is allocated to a patient with high expectations regarding the function and outcome of the transplant, as well as a longer life expectancy and temporal requirement for organ replacement therapy. In the event of graft loss the recipient may become highly sensitised with antibodies to the donor HLA and is highly likely to need relisting after a relatively short time. The likely sensitisation from the transplant will limit the suitable donor pool and increase waiting time the second time around. Indeed, many patients with a previously failed kidney transplant will never receive a second.

One approach to avoiding this undesirable chain of events might be to not transplant lower risk recipients with DCD or marginal organs. This approach would benefit the patient group in the event of transplantation since they would in all likelihood receive an optimal deceased donor organ with excellent prospects for long-term function and graft survival. This advantage would come at the expense of reducing their overall chance of transplantation, given their pool of potential donors has been restricted.

The optimal donor pool for all other patients on the waiting list would, of course, be reduced as a consequence too. This kind of policy might be seen to disadvantage recipients who are older or more medically 'high risk' and it remains unclear whether this would be ethically acceptable to patients or clinicians.

Under these circumstances where an extended criteria or DCD organ is allocated only to a marginal recipient, the utilitarian argument – that organs with a potential for great longevity achieve only a small fraction of it within these recipients – is postulated by many as an argument in favour of this kind of allocation policy.

However, when viewed in purely ethical terms (especially in terms of equity), patients who are medically 'high risk' with a lower life expectancy than average would have a lower chance of an optimal organ for transplant. Such patients already experience poor life quality because of their illness – is it therefore ethical to treat them as 'second class citizens', deserving less priority in the national allocation scheme, simply because their life expectancy is less? This conundrum is hard to solve and current UK allocation policy has evolved in response by introducing a component of age matching as well as reducing the influence of HLA matching in order to find a better balance between optimal outcomes and access for all individuals. That evolution accepted, the current UK national allocation policy does not reflect in any way the wide variation in kidney quality. DCD kidneys are still, at the time of writing, allocated at local discretion (with availability of patient rankings as if the kidneys were DBD for guidance). Current NHSBT initiatives to make DCD kidneys a similarly 'national' resource will lose this clinician local discretion and may make incorporation of organ quality into allocation more difficult, not less. Furthermore, the current scheme for kidneys does not really reflect another important factor – the patient's autonomy regarding acceptance of an organ with higher risk.

Autonomy and patient choice in allocation

Patients on the waiting list for transplantation have a wide variety of expectations for the outcome of their transplants. This is a function of the severity of their clinical condition and how much they are already suffering in their day-to-day lives. Patients with good life quality may – when counselled in detail – wish to wait for an optimal organ that would improve their life quality and expectancy substantially rather than accept a more marginal graft.

The science of organ evaluation is still advancing but the plethora of so-called 'donor risk indices' remain a relatively crude way of predicting how well and for how long any given organ is likely to work. Additionally, there are many external factors that influence these outcomes, making both counselling and decision-making difficult. Risk indices use multiple parameters and historical outcome measures to predict the outcome of future transplants. For kidney transplantation, such an index is already even available as a smart-phone app. But in truth, the validity of such indices is questionable and the proportion of variability in transplant outcome that they actually capture may be limited. Effective incorporation of these kinds of tools into allocation policy seems likely to require more accurate and specific tests of organ biological age and status. Even if we had a perfect method of evaluating a given organ, it seems likely that ethical debate around how best it be used would continue. An ethical organ allocation scheme should aim to achieve maximum equality of access for all potential recipients to this precious and limited resource. A system favouring (in terms of quality of organ allocated) those who already have a better health status and disadvantaging those already in a worse state of health cannot be ethically acceptable. The counterpressures towards such a system are represented in part by the compulsorily reported outcomes of individual units and of the national programme as a whole. Units are accountable for their outcomes in terms of function, patient and graft survival. The ethical requirement to be fair to all individual patients pushes very hard in the opposite direction to 'getting the best results'.

Practical incorporation of patient choice in an allocation system

Minimal scientific evidence exists on the views of the key stakeholders in allocation policy – the patients themselves. The only study of note investigated 128 transplant recipients and 104 dialysis patients. Participants selected which of two hypothetical patients should be allocated a deceased donor kidney based on eight scenarios.[23] Patients in this study disagreed with several aspects of current allocation systems. The numerous current transplant allocation algorithms do not factor in individual preferences, and recipients feel that they are given little information on donor characteristics. Whilst some recipients may be happy to receive a marginal allograft and therefore reduce the time spent on the waiting list, other recipients may want to hold out for an organ with more favourable characteristics (e.g. better HLA matching from a younger donor). By empowering patients, the burden of responsibility could be potentially shared in deciding whether a marginal organ may be appropriate for any particular patient. To incorporate patient choice in an allocation system, Su et al.[24] developed a system in which patients will declare which range of kidneys will be *acceptable* for transplantation, called the UNOS/CHOICE. This system would ensure that organs will only be offered to candidates willing to accept them, and it is proposed as an extension to the UNOS policy for allocation of marginal allografts. There are disadvantages with this system, notably a significant increase in the complexity of the kidney allocation process, which may be difficult for some transplantation candidates to comprehend. The integration of *donor advocates* in the living donor process in transplant centres enables a non-biased professional to represent the patient's interests, and should be available when transplant teams discuss transplant options with potential candidates. A similar system could also be considered internationally. The interpretation of equity may vary considerably between patients and healthcare professionals. Involving the choice of the recipient in organ transplantation could potentially improve outcomes relative to current allocation policies.

Gains achieved by incorporating patient choice will outweigh the concerns of more complex algorithms and in time may lead to the development of a more equitable allocation policy.

Ethical presentation of risk: where, when and how?

Patients have the right to receive all necessary information regarding the risks and benefits of a transplant, marginal or standard, and be informed of alternative treatment options. The patient's status and suitability for transplantation require regular assessment as their clinical condition can deteriorate or improve on multiple occasions during what might be a long period on the transplant waiting list. On occasion, the risk of the procedure may, perhaps temporarily, outweigh the benefit of having the transplant and a process exists whereby the patient is 'suspended' or removed from the waiting list.

Historically, counselling for entry to the waiting list assumed an optimal organ but this is clearly no longer appropriate. Transplant recipients have to be counselled about the potential risks of accepting an organ from an ECD or DCD donor, both in general terms at listing and then once again at the exact time of transplantation, with whatever information has become available regarding the exact organ offered. The complexity of this decision and the process of consent has therefore increased enormously from previous decades. Proper, informed consent and respect for a patient's autonomy require time for the person to consider the complexities of the proposed transplant, to understand them, and to judge the possible effects on their life and health in the short, medium and long term.

In practice, situations like this may be helped by acts of paternalism. The reality of such situations would see patients trying to carefully weigh up highly complex risks and benefits – potentially beyond their understanding – shortly after being urgently summoned to the transplant centre in a state of surprise and very reasonable anxiety. This sort of process has the real potential to cause distress to patients. The requirement for such processes is, at least in part, medicolegal in origin. Avoiding the potential harm requires an ongoing resolve to provide patients with information that is accessible, understandable and in a form that they are comfortable with. This too is constantly evolving as the informational preferences of a 70-year-old in 2012 are likely to be different than those of a 25-year-old brought up in the Internet age. Managing the ethical implications of organ quality also requires flexibility. Technology and public policy change the issues around allocation and consent for transplant. In the 1990s it was widely believed that genetically modified pigs might provide a limitless supply of organs for transplantation. To hypothesise an extreme scenario, if limitless, quality-controlled xenografts were available for a patient waiting for a kidney transplant, the nature of information required by a recipient would shift completely and discussions around variability of organ quality and its evaluation would be replaced by new and distinct risks to consider.

Transplant professionals have an ethical responsibility to keep pace with these changes and to provide their patients with the appropriate information and counselling as technology and other external factors 'move the goalposts'!

Living donation

Living donation presents an essentially unique medical situation. One individual undergoes an invasive procedure with the inherent risks of morbidity or even mortality, predominantly for the benefit of another. Since the first successful living-donor kidney transplant, many transplant and medical professions have expressed discomfort with the concept of living donation, yet it has expanded and become a major treatment for kidney and liver failure, with various other organs also able to be transplanted from living donors. The principle of non-maleficence weighs against living donation, yet this becomes a matter of the magnitude and likelihood of any harm actually encountered. Research indicates that committed potential kidney donors may find a level of risk of death of 50% acceptable in living kidney donation.[25] This clearly would not be acceptable to any surgeon and the real-world risk of living kidney donation, and more recently living liver donation, is very well defined and far smaller. Risk of death from living kidney donation, estimated at 1 in 3500, has clearly become ethically acceptable in the view of society as a whole.

However, watching the deterioration of a relative with organ failure may lead to an atmosphere of unintended coercion. Clearly, for an ethical living donation programme there must be safeguards to protect individuals in a situation like this. In the UK, the Human Tissue Authority is currently the responsible body and has a specific approval process for any living donor transplant. This process also regulates the prohibition of financial incentives for living donors, which is discussed below.

Altruistic donation

Spousal and parental living donors clearly have the potential to gain indirect benefit from their donation. A life caring for a dialysis patient is very different from life alongside a healthier, successfully transplanted patient. The benefits may come in the capability for shared physical experiences or in the economics of fitness for employment, but benefits may be real and go beyond the feeling of well-being brought on by an act of altruism.

In the UK, the Human Tissue Act created the legal possibility of true altruistic donation in which an individual could choose – through a pure wish to benefit society and a needy individual – to donate their kidney. This facility has proved both popular and beneficial, but not, of course, without throwing up its own new set of ethical questions. The concept of directed altruistic donation in which a patient may publicise their need for a transplant and another individual, on becoming aware of this, offers to donate their own body part in an act of directed altruism was clearly not foreseen by those drafting the legislation; however, current legal interpretations suggest that such a transplant would not be illegal per se. Whether such a transplant is ethically acceptable is clearly a separate question, since sanctioning of such a process runs the risk of a transplant popularity concept with individuals advertising their worthiness or attractiveness to receive a living donor transplant and vying for the favour of any potential directed altruistic donor. In modern society, social media entities like Facebook and Twitter take this sort of ethical conundrum to a higher level and the ethical questions of the 21st century's second decade are beginning to be played out on the Internet.

Perhaps the most relevant example of this is the concept of facilitated directed organ donation – which conceptually at least may veer towards organ donation 'brokerage'. The Flood Foundation (www.floodsisters.org/index.php) describes itself as 'a not for profit corporation whose mission is to educate the public on kidney disease and inspire many to donate the greatest gift one could give … life'. This organisation charges a registration fee and is dedicated to bringing together altruistic donors and recipients. Its formation followed the successful transplantation of the Flood sisters' father, Daniel, after the placement of an advert on the website, Craigslist. Initially working in the USA, the foundation has recently contacted several UK transplant units regarding facilitation of a live donor kidney transplant for a UK-based patient.

Whilst this foundation may represent the purest of altruistic motives, the potential for unethical transplantation inherent in the process it espouses makes many UK transplant professionals deeply uncomfortable. It remains to be seen if this concept establishes itself in the UK but the Flood Foundation website shows various American patients who have received and benefited substantially from transplants coordinated through the corporation.

Implications of the living donor work-up

There are additional ethical controversies surrounding the work-up of potential living donors. A frequent occurrence sees multiple family members undergoing work-up for donation to another family member. One or more may be secretly unwilling to donate but equally unwilling to openly state his true opinion due to guilt or perceived likely impact on family relationships. In such a situation, the responsible clinician may be faced with the ethical dilemma of whether to lie to other family members and allude to some sort of 'incompatibility' or other contraindication to proceeding with the donation. This situation highlights the interesting differences between deontological and consequentialist approaches: a lie would be a clear breach of duty in deontological terms but the opposite can be concluded from a consequentialist standpoint, given that good comes from preventing the harm of a reluctant donation and avoiding emotional upset within the family. Systems have evolved to try to avoid exposing transplant clinicians to this kind of ethical dilemma.

Perhaps the best example is the phenomenon of misattributed paternity. Living-donor transplantation work-up often entails HLA typing for the evaluation of immunological risk. This has the side-effect of being a relatively crude test of parentage, not sensitive or specific enough to stand against the legally recognised parentage tests incorporating extremely polymorphic short tandem repeat sequences within

telomeres, but effectively confirming or refuting parentage with a small error frequency.

Extensive debate surrounds the ethics and best practice of handling such a situation. In the UK, donation on the basis of emotional relationship alone is well established in the form of spousal or platonic friend donation. On that basis, the HLA typing can be considered to be performed for immunological risk stratification rather than as a confirmation of the assumed genetic relationship. It has been argued, therefore, that to proceed in such situations without necessarily disclosing the non-paternity may be ethical; however, the UK living-donor authorisation now stipulates that the potential donor should record how they would wish such a finding to be handled in terms of disclosure. The price of this clarity for the transplant team in the not infrequent situation of misattributed paternity is clearly some awkward conversations for the majority and on some occasions stress and emotional upset within families where doubt regarding parentage may exist.

However, not withstanding all the ethical controversies around it, living donation has the potential to revolutionise the treatment of organ failure on multiple levels. The number of healthy individuals on earth renders the number of potential recipients negligible. If safety and attendant harm were equally negligible – or at least acceptably small – could it be argued that only a lack of incentive would prevent people coming forward to offer to be live donors for every patient in need?

Human organs as a commodity: incentivisation and payment for organ donation

The concept of incentivisation for living (and indeed deceased) donation is perhaps the greatest modern ethical controversy in transplantation. This is in part because adequate incentivisation represents a theoretical solution for all, but furthermore the broad spectrum of routes by which incentivised living donation might be constructed within any society contains some dark and dangerous side roads.

Globally, and particularly in the developed world, it is abundantly clear that the deficit in the availability of solid organs is increasing rapidly and will continue to do so as the population demographic shifts towards older age groups.[26] It is unlikely that the current organ procuring systems, even with 'expansion' (maximising the use of expanded criteria donors, paired matching, opt-out systems, etc.), will be able to reverse this trend. The numbers of people living with and dying from organ failure will therefore grow and the statistics are indeed sobering (**Fig. 1.1**). Many commentators argue that to combat such a burden of misery, radical solutions are required and justified. One such solution is to encourage people to become organ vendors.

It is fair to assert that the majority of the medical and transplant communities remain against payment for donation. Various groups have come out strongly against (WHO,[27] Nuffield Council of Bioethics,[28] Participants in the International Summit on Transplant Tourism and Organ Trafficking[29]). The practice also remains illegal in the vast majority of countries. There are, however, prominent voices arguing in favour of a controlled market in organs.[30-34] The debate has recently come to the fore again in the UK as a result of an opinion piece in the BMJ.[35]

No one would disagree that, in an ideal world, no individual should have to subject themselves to the risk and pain of living-organ donation. The reality of altruistic living-organ donation has resulted from a utilitarian approach to the problem of causing an individual harm by removing an organ – the consequence of the action has a 'benefit' (suffering in the recipient will be greatly alleviated) at a modest 'cost' to the donor (who may also gain some spiritual, social or psychological benefit). The problem is therefore one of a moral economy – at the *individual and societal level*. Do the positives that result from paid donation transplantation outweigh the negatives? When considering this equation, in terms of an analysis of consequentiality, it is absolutely crucial to consider *all consequences to all those involved*, not just the recipient. This includes organ vendor, healthcare team and society at large. The vendor and recipient may have family and dependants who have an important stake.

Part of the difficulty with the debate is defining exactly what is meant by payment. There is indeed a spectrum of 'reward' for donating an organ that extends from a simple explanation of the potential benefits (physical/psychological/social) of living-donor transplantation all the way to a generous monetary award to the donor/vendor. Already, it is deemed ethically acceptable to reimburse certain costs that a donor may incur (travel, for example). So, where to draw the line? The recent report by the Nuffield Council on Bioethics usefully differentiated these incentives using an 'intervention ladder'. Interventions were broadly classified into those that were altruistic focused and those that were non-altruistic focused. The key ethical threshold was deemed crossed when an intervention was aimed at 'recruiting donors' who would not ordinarily have been disposed to act altruistically as opposed to facilitating the decision to donate by individuals who were disposed to act this way.

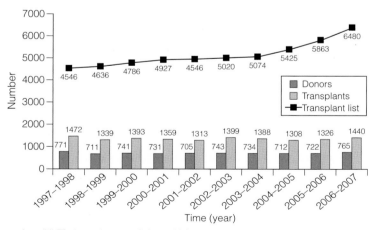

Figure 1.1 • UK Transplant (UKT) data: deceased donor kidney programme in the UK, 1 April 1997–31 March 2007. Number of donors, transplants and patients on the active transplant list at 31 March. Reproduced from Maple NH, Hadjianastassiou V, Jones R et al. Understanding risk in living donor nephrectomy. J Med Ethics 2010; 36:142–7. With permission from BMJ Publishing Group Ltd.

So what are the arguments for and against paying people to donate their organs? A full answer to this question is beyond the scope of this chapter; rather, two *critical* areas of disagreement between those who are for and those who are against paid donation will be discussed in detail. The other arguments are presented in table format.

'Paid organ donation exploits the poor.'

'Preventing people from selling an organ on the grounds that they might they have no choice given their circumstances is paternalistic and ignores the bioethical principle of respect for autonomy.'

For those who argue against paid donation, the potential exploitation of the poor in such a scheme is usually the bedrock of their reasoning. As Matas et al.[36] put it, inevitably a 'power gradient' between vendor and recipient would develop and organs would flow from poor to rich or, as Epstein[37] has written, '[the organ market] creates severe inequities in the distribution of power, benefit and risk'. The notion of exploiting the vulnerable is intimately tied in with the issue of informed consent. Can this really be 'freely given' in the context of a potentially life-changing sum of money? Are the bioethical principles of justice being upheld? An interesting juxtaposition in the context of recent world events concerns the morality of banks issuing loans to those unlikely to be able to repay them. Who is at fault – the creditor or the debtor? Again, to paraphrase Matas et al.: is some state paternalism (seat-belts, crash helmets, financial regulation, etc.) *necessarily* a bad thing?

Proponents of paid-for donation would argue that it is paternalistic to assume that 'we' know what is best for potential vendors. They should be free to make what will usually be 'a hard choice, as opposed to an enforced one'. The principle of respect for autonomy comes first. Is it moral to deprive a person of the 'right to choose' to sell a kidney for money if their circumstances would be significantly improved by that money? Is it more morally acceptable if a vendor's circumstances were *not* dependent on extra cash – i.e. they were relatively wealthy already? Is it better to leave the poor poor rather than to offer them a potential way out? In terms of exploiting the developed world, proposed markets would not be international, they would be national. This would mitigate against a power gradient from developing to developed world.

'The human body is priceless and trading in its irreplaceable parts is an affront to human dignity.'

'Who is to say what an individual can and cannot do with their own body?'

This argument centres on the idea of the integrity of the human body (and the dignity attached to this) and the immorality of violating this integrity for commercial reasons; the body (or its parts), it is contended, is commodified and cheapened. Proponents of paid donation would argue that the weakness of this argument becomes apparent if one considers what it is already considered ethical to 'sell' – hair, ova, sperm and most recently peripherally derived bone marrow stem cells.[38] Is it not ethically inconsistent to be able to, on one hand, accept the sale of these items of human tissue but, on the other, not a kidney? Similarly, does society also not tolerate people being paid to do jobs that are likely to cause a significant violation of bodily integrity (jockeys, deep-sea divers, soldiers, sexual and gestational surrogates, etc.)? Opponents would argue that there is an important distinction to be made between a regenerable body *product* and a unique body *part*. In the vast majority of dangerous jobs, the violation of integrity is a possibility and not a certainty and, critically, the person doing that job at least has some degree of control over events. Jobs (e.g. a professional boxer) that entail a certainty of bodily harm are often felt to reflect poorly on society.

Examples of some other arguments and their counter arguments are summarised in Tables 1.1 and 1.2.

For the moment, paid donation remains a matter for debate and is not an imminent possibility. It is also clear that an organ market could never work without the explicit (in as far as this is possible) assent of the public and the individuals involved in delivering the service. It does, however, appear that what was once taboo is no longer.

Is the current organ donation programme in its multiple forms a 'house of cards' that may be irreparably damaged by unsavoury incidents arising from corruption of an ethical programme of incentivised

Table 1.1 • Arguments for paid donation

Arguments for paid donation	Counter argument
The organ supply would increase and the suffering of thousands would be alleviated. There would also be cost savings associated with this as it is widely accepted that transplantation is more cost-effective than dialysis – even after a generous financial 'incentive'.	Do the ends justify the means? It is not sufficient to consider these facts alone. The potential harm to vendors, vendors' relations and society in general must be weighed against the benefits to recipients. There is a greater moral issue at stake.
Why should donors be the only people involved in transplantation who do not benefit materially?	They usually do benefit materially by a return to a degree of normality within their family/marriage/partnership/friendship. Moral/spiritual gains for donors and society are important. Truly altruistic 'stranger' donations have alternative motives.
Like the debate over the illegal drug trade, a legitimate organ trading market will make redundant the illegal one. Vendor care will improve.	Morally relativistic. This is choosing between the lesser of two evils, a false dichotomy has been created. Vendor care in the official markets may improve, but evidence from tobacco and alcohol suggests that a 'black market' would continue to exist and may be pushed even further underground.
We already have elements of paid donation – meeting of expenses, etc.	Important difference as per the Nuffield council on difference between altruist-centred and non-altruistic-centred approach. Wigmore et al. – important semantic difference between donor and vendor.

Table 1.2 • Arguments against paid donation

Arguments against paid donation	Counter argument
The image of medicine and transplant medicine may be tarnished with a resultant loss of trust – many examples of this in the history of medical research.	No way of knowing this is true. Financial transactions are commonplace throughout the world in medicine and do not necessarily tarnish the doctor–patient relationship at the individual level or societal level. A system that used a monopsonistic buyer (single purchaser – to avoid the ugly 'wrongful gain' of private transactions) would mitigate here.
Paid donation and organ trafficking are inalienably linked.	This is perhaps the case until now. It does not follow that a future tightly regulated organ market in a mature and functional healthcare system would necessarily be tarnished by previous scandal in other jurisdictions.
Paid donation would cause a reduction in the quality of donors – people would lie about their medical history in order to become organ vendors. Outcomes would be worse for recipient and donor – there is evidence for this.	Stringent checks and regulations within the framework of a functional regulatory body should minimise the risks. The evidence for poor vendor outcome relates to the experience in India, Pakistan, the Philippines, etc. where the markets were created in suboptimal conditions.
Look at the examples of India, Pakistan, the Philippines, China and to a certain extent Iran.	These are not examples of what is being proposed. Regulatory authorities were insufficiently equipped to police systems properly. Problems of poverty are particularly acute in these countries. A poor human rights record exists in some of these countries.
Altruistic donation is morally superior and has positive social consequences.	Paid donation would not devalue altruistic donation. Paid donation would still be a 'good act' in terms of its final consequences for the recipient and financial status of the recipient. There are positive social consequences from having more organs available.

(Continued)

Table 1.2 • *(cont.)* Arguments against paid donation

Arguments against paid donation	Counter argument
Paid for donation would reduce altruistic donation.	Maybe. Evidence from Iran suggests that this is the case. But this may reduce coercive living-related transplantation. People could be doubly altruistic and donate their fee too if they so desired. There will still be a major need for other organs where paid donation is not possible – this should drive the continuing need for a cadaveric programme. Perhaps fewer expanded criteria donors will be needed, thereby improving results. People may still prefer an altruistic donor – they may want to know their donor, or a particular donor may want to know their recipient.
Vendors' long-term health needs are uncertain and they may suffer in the long term.	These concerns apply to altruistic donation. Mechanisms to assure follow-up, provide lifelong health insurance and to ensure priority in transplant waiting lists could be implemented.
This is a slippery slope. Once a market was established, it would be very difficult to reverse.	A pilot would be planned and desirable, with a subsequent temporary moratorium until results for recipients and vendors were assessed.

living donation? Is a step in the direction of testing the effects of paid donation irreversible? These questions are central to the ethical debate that seems likely to continue as future generations of transplant professionals enter and mature within the ethically richest of medical fields.

References

1. President's Council on Bioethics. Controversies in the determination of death: a white paper by the President's Council on Bioethics. 2008; The Presidential Commission for the Study of Bioethical Issues, Washington, DC.

2. Dhanani S, Hornby L, Ward R, et al. Variability in the determination of death after cardiac arrest: a review of guidelines and statements. J Intensive Care Med 2012;27(4):238–52.

3. Lamb D. Brain death and brainstem death. Soc Soc Hist Med Bull (Lond) 1985;37:90–2.

4. Hornby K, Hornby L, Shemie SD. A systematic review of autoresuscitation after cardiac arrest. Crit Care Med 2010;38(5):1246–53.

5. Sundin-Huard D, Fahy K. The problems with the validity of the diagnosis of brain death. Nurs Crit Care 2004;9(2):64–71.

6. Academy of Medical Royal Colleges. A code of practice for the diagnosis and confirmation of death. 2011.

7. Riad H. Elective ventilation for organ donation. Br J Hosp Med 1993;50(8):438, 441–2.

8. Rithalia A, McDaid C, Suekarran S, et al. A systematic review of presumed consent systems for deceased organ donation. Health Technol Assess 2009;13(26):iii, ix–xi, 1–95.

9. Cotter H. Increasing consent for organ donation: mandated choice, individual autonomy, and informed consent. Health Matrix Clevel 2011;21(2):599–626.

10. Human Tissue Act 2004. London: HMSO; 2011.

11. Human Tissue (Scotland) Act 2006. Edinburgh: Scottish Government; 2011.

12. Rosenblum AM, Horvat LD, Siminoff LA, et al. The authority of next-of-kin in explicit and presumed consent systems for deceased organ donation: an analysis of 54 nations. Nephrol Dial Transplant 2012;27(6):2533–46.

13. Douglass GE, Daly M. Donor families' experience of organ donation. Anaesth Intensive Care 1995;23(1):96–8.

14. Dominguez-Gil B, Haase-Kromwijk B, Van LH, et al. Current situation of donation after circulatory death in European countries. Transpl Int 2011;24(7):676–86.

15. Reznik O, Bagnenko S, Scvortsov A, et al. The use of in-situ normothermic extracorporeal perfusion and leukocyte depletion for resuscitation of human donor kidneys. Perfusion 2010;25(5):343–8.

16. Sheth KN, Nutter T, Stein DM, et al. Autoresuscitation after asystole in patients being considered for organ donation. Crit Care Med 2012;40(1):158–61.

17. Caplan A. The use of prisoners as sources of organs – an ethically dubious practice. Am J Bioeth 2011;11(10):1–5.

18. Ysebaert D, Van BG, De GK, et al. Organ procurement after euthanasia: Belgian experience. Transplant Proc 2009;41(2):585–6.

19. Hoffenberg R, Lock M, Tilney N, et al. Should organs from patients in permanent vegetative state be used for transplantation? International Forum for Transplant Ethics. Lancet 1997;350(9087):1320–1.

20. www.uktransplant.org.uk/ukt/statistics/transplant_activity_report/current_activity_reports/ukt/activity_report_2010_11.pdf; [accessed 16.08.12].

21. Weber M, Dindo D, Demartines N, et al. Kidney transplantation from donors without a heartbeat. N Engl J Med 2002;347(4):248–55.

22. Veatch RM. Transplanting hearts after death measured by cardiac criteria: the challenge to the dead donor rule. J Med Philos 2010;35(3):313–29.

23. Geddes CC, Rodger RS, Smith C, et al. Allocation of deceased donor kidneys for transplantation: opinions of patients with CKD. Am J Kidney Dis 2005;46(5):949–56.

24. Su X, Zenios SA, Chertow GM. Incorporating recipient choice in kidney transplantation. J Am Soc Nephrol 2004;15(6):1656–63.

25. Maple NH, Hadjianastassiou V, Jones R, et al. Understanding risk in living donor nephrectomy. J Med Ethics 2010;36:142–7.

26. Galliford J, Game DS. Modern renal transplantation: present challenges and future prospects. Postgrad Med J 2009;85(1000):91–101.

27. WHO. WHO Guiding Principles on Human Cell, Tissue and Organ Transplantation. WHA63.22, 2010. Available at: http://www.who.int/transplantation/publications/en/index.html.

28. Nuffield Council on Bioethics. Human bodies: donation for medicine and research. Nuffield Council on Bioethics Report; 2011.

29. Steering Committee of the Istanbul Summit. Organ trafficking and transplant tourism and commercialism. Declaration of Istanbul. Istanbul Summit 2012.

30. Matas AJ. The case for living kidney sales: rationale, objections and concerns. Am J Transplant 2004;4(12):2007–17.

31. Hippen BE, Taylor JS. In defense of transplantation: a reply to Nancy Scheper-Hughes. Am J Transplant 2007;7(7):1695–7.

32. Radcliffe-Richards J, Daar AS, Guttmann RD, et al. The case for allowing kidney sales. International Forum for Transplant Ethics. Lancet 1998;351(9120):1950–2.

33. de Castro LD. Commodification and exploitation: arguments in favour of compensated organ donation. J Med Ethics 2003;29:142–6.

34. Erin CA, Harris J. An ethical market in human organs. J Med Ethics 2003;29(3):137–8.

35. Roff SR. We should consider paying kidney donors. Br Med J 2011;343:d4867.

36. Matas AJ, Adair A, Wigmore SJ. Paid organ donation. Ann R Coll Surg Engl 2011;93(3):188–92.

37. Epstein M. Sociological and ethical issues in transplant commercialism. Curr Opin Organ Transplant 2009;14(2):134–9.

38. Cohen IG. Selling bone marrow – Flynn v. Holder. N Engl J Med 2012;366(4):296–7.

2

Organ donation in the UK: recent progress and future challenges

Christopher J. Rudge

Introduction

In the previous edition of this book the acute shortage of deceased donors in the UK was described, together with the 14 recommendations of the Organ Donation Taskforce.[1] These recommendations were based on an analysis of the entire donation pathway: donor identification, referral, consent and management, and organ retrieval. Taken together, the recommendations were designed to build a UK model for donation that was expected to provide a robust infrastructure that could support improvements at all the key stages. The chapter concluded that 'Successful implementation of the recommendations will undoubtedly be a challenge but they offer the most realistic opportunity for many years to make the step-change in UK donation and transplant rates that is so clearly needed.' Overall implementation of the recommendations was overseen by the Programme Delivery Board (PDB) established by the Department of Health that brought together all the relevant stakeholders, including professional bodies and societies, NHS Blood and Transplant (NHSBT), the four UK health administrations, and others. The PDB sat from June 2008 until January 2011, and was further supported by designated groups in Scotland, Wales and Northern Ireland.

The Taskforce Report has been central to all efforts to improve organ donation in the UK, and this chapter will review the extent to which the recommendations have been implemented 3 years later, together with the impact on deceased donor numbers that

has been seen. It will also describe the current understanding of areas of clinical practice where the new infrastructure provides opportunities to increase further the number of deceased donors, and the number of available organs that are suitable for transplantation. This occurs at a time of great change to the NHS in England that results from the reforms currently being introduced – changes that introduce new challenges but also potential new opportunities. It is also essential to manage expectations as to what is realistically achievable, in terms both of the number of deceased donors and the 'quality' of donated organs. Whilst transplant surgeons (and their patients) may yearn for more organs from younger donors who have died following cerebral trauma, international comparisons suggest that much of the possible increase in donation will come from greater use of older donors – for example, for donors over the age of 70, the Spanish rate is 8.2 per million population (pmp) compared with 1.3 pmp in the UK.[2,3]

Recent progress

The Department of Health has recently reported on progress made in the first 3 years of implementation of the 14 recommendations from the Organ Donation Taskforce.[4] What follows is largely based on this report.

Recommendations 1 and 2:
A UK-wide Organ Donation Organisation should be established. The establishment of the Organ

Donation Organisation should be the responsibility of NHS Blood and Transplant.

This has been fully implemented. NHSBT management arrangements have been developed to reflect its role as the Organ Donation Organisation. This is delivered through the Organ Donation and Transplantation Directorate (ODT), which builds on and expands the previous role of UK Transplant. ODT continues to have the specific responsibilities previously held by UK Transplant in terms of organ allocation, data collection and analysis, monitoring transplant outcomes and the NHS Organ Donor Register.

Recommendation 3:

Urgent attention is required to resolve outstanding legal, ethical and professional issues in order to ensure that all clinicians are supported and are able to work within a clear and unambiguous framework of good practice. Additionally, an independent UK-wide Donation Ethics Group should be established.

Legal issues

Many clinicians caring for patients who are dying but not yet dead, whilst supportive of donation, expressed genuine anxieties about the legality of steps to facilitate donation under the Mental Capacity Act 2006 and the Adults with Incapacity Act 2001. These concerns related principally to potential donors after circulatory death (DCD; previously known as non-heartbeating donors). The Taskforce recognised the strength and importance of these concerns and in response the health administrations have published important guidance. The Department of Health and the Welsh Assembly Government published jointly *Legal Issues Relevant to Non-Heartbeating Donation* in November 2009,[5] and Scottish Guidance was circulated under cover of a Chief Medical Officer letter,[6] which should be used in conjunction with Operational Guidelines for controlled non-heartbeating organ donation that were circulated to intensive care clinicians across Scotland in November 2009.

Northern Ireland is not covered by the Mental Capacity Act, but guidance on legal issues relevant to donation after circulatory death was published by the Department of Health, Social Services and Public Safety Northern Ireland in March 2011.[7]

Ethics

The UK Donation Ethics Committee has been established and is hosted by the Academy of Medical Royal Colleges to assure its independence. The Committee met for the first time in February 2010 and issued its first major consultation document in January 2011. The two main areas of interest to date have been donation after circulatory death and the possibility of cardiac retrieval from such donors. In December 2011 the Committee published 'An Ethical Framework for Donation after Circulatory Death'.[8] Additionally, the Scottish Transplant Group's Ethics Subgroup continues to meet quarterly to consider legal and ethical issues relevant to organ donation in Scotland.

Recommendation 4:

All parts of the NHS must embrace organ donation as a usual, not an unusual, event. Local policies, constructed around national guidelines, should be put in place. Discussions about donation should be part of all end-of-life care when appropriate. Each Trust should have an identified clinical donation champion and a Trust donation committee to help achieve this.

The Taskforce envisaged that the main vehicles for change at local level would be clinical leaders (now called clinical leads for organ donation – CLODs) supported by a local donation committee. Progress has been remarkable. By 31 March 2011:

- 96% of acute trusts/health boards had established a Trust donation committee and appointed donation committee chairs.
- 98% of clinical leads for organ donation (referred to as clinical donation champions in the original recommendation) had been appointed.
- New UK standards for critically ill children state that all paediatric intensive care units should each have a lead consultant for organ donation.

The support and maintenance for the clinical leads and donation committees has become part of 'business as usual' for NHSBT. In order to provide systematic support for donation committees NHSBT has established a network of regional organ donation collaboratives, and re-structured the Donation Advisory Group as a national donation committee with representation from regional committees. In many ways this mirrors the Spanish model of local, regional and national action. Donation committees are now being asked to work with their specialist nurses for organ donation (SN-OD, previously called donor transplant coordinator) to develop an annual plan for organ donation within their organisation, and draft templates have been developed.

Similar arrangements are also in place in Scotland, Wales and Northern Ireland, reflecting the varying organisational structures in these countries.

Work is under way across all government health departments and relevant parts of the NHS to ensure that organ donation and end-of-life care policies are aligned and linked where appropriate. For example, in Wales organ donation prompts have been included in the All Wales End of Life Care Pathway and reference is made in the draft quality requirements for end-of-life care.

Recommendation 5:

Minimum notification criteria for potential organ donors should be introduced on a UK-wide basis. These criteria should be reviewed after 12 months in the light of evidence of their effect, and the comparative impact of more detailed criteria should also be assessed.

The original Taskforce Report included two proposals for models that would guarantee comprehensive potential donor identification in UK intensive care units. These models, which were endorsed by the Intensive Care Society, were:

1. When no further treatment options are available or appropriate, and there is a plan to confirm death by neurological criteria, the SN-OD should be notified as soon as sedation/analgesia is discontinued, or immediately if the patient has never received sedation/analgesia. This notification should take place even if the attending clinical staff believe that donation (after death has been confirmed by neurological criteria) might be contraindicated or inappropriate.

2. In the context of a catastrophic neurological injury, when no further treatment options are available or appropriate and there is no intention to confirm death by neurological criteria, the SN-OD should be notified when a decision is made by a consultant to withdraw active treatment and this has been recorded in a dated, timed and signed entry in the case notes. This notification should take place even if the attending clinical staff believe that death cannot be diagnosed by neurological criteria, or that donation after cardiac death might be contraindicated or inappropriate.

This work is being taken forward by clinical leads at local level.

Recommendation 6: Donation activity in all trusts should be monitored. Rates of potential donor identification, referral, approach to the family and consent to donation should be reported. The Trust donation committee should report to the Trust board through the clinical governance process and the medical director, and the reports should be part of the assessment of trusts through the relevant healthcare regulator. Benchmark data from other Trusts should be made available for comparison.

Disseminating donation activity data

An assessment of local donation activity is issued to individual hospitals by NHSBT every 6 months, using data from the Potential Donor Audit (PDA). The activity reports are passed through CLODs and donation committees to Trust boards and SHA medical directors or board chief executives in Scotland. The data provide information about how their own hospital is performing in comparison to other hospitals and indications for where improvements could be made. This process has received high-level support from relevant groups in all four health administrations. It is important, though, to recognise both the strengths and the weaknesses of the PDA data, and clinical leads are encouraged to collaborate with specialist nurses in the compilation of the PDA returns. It is also necessary to ensure that effective reporting links are in place within each organisation's governance and executive structure, and that the data are used to develop both an annual report on organ donation and a plan for the next year.

Work is under way within NHSBT to improve the accuracy and reliability of the PDA data and this will be vital for continued clinician confidence in the statistics that are regularly circulated.

Healthcare regulator assessments

The changing structure of healthcare regulation in England has presented a challenge to successful implementation of this part of Recommendation 6.

The Healthcare Commission has been replaced by the Care Quality Commission since the Taskforce Report was published, and further changes are likely as the NHS reforms develop. However, the National Institute for Health and Clinical Excellence (NICE) has recently published clinical guidelines on donor identification and consent,[9] and this will help to ensure that organ donation is included in the healthcare regulator assessments, as trusts are inspected against adherence to NICE guidance. NICE has also been asked to develop quality indicators for organ donation. Again, trusts are inspected against adherence to quality indicators, so should these be introduced they will also become part of the regulator's assessment process. A recent initiative has been the development of a series of donation-related metrics that have been introduced by the West Midlands Strategic Health Authority as a CQUIN (Commissioning for Quality and Innovation) with anticipated values (dependent on hospital activity) in the region of £120 000–£317 000 per annum.[10] Once again, similar steps have been taken to incorporate donation activity within the regulatory framework in the devolved administrations of the UK.

Recommendation 7:

Brain stem death testing should be carried out in all patients where brain stem death is a likely diagnosis, even if organ donation is an unlikely outcome.

The PDA demonstrates that, in 2010/11, brain stem death tests were not conducted in 467 patients out of a total of 1672 where the criteria for testing appeared to be met (28%).[11] Whilst in some circumstances this may have been entirely appropriate, and it cannot be assumed that these patients had the same donation potential as those who were tested, this remains an area where significant improvements appear to be possible.

The Professional Development Programme for CLODs and donation committees, run by NHSBT during 2010/11, gave considerable emphasis to this. Donation committees have been supported to develop and implement local mechanisms to ensure that brain stem death tests are performed whenever is appropriate. Clinical leads are encouraged to be involved in the investigation of all local cases of patients who are not tested when brain stem death appears to be a likely diagnosis. A face-to-face Masterclass on the Diagnosis of Death was delivered

as a module of the Programme, and this material is now available to clinical leads to use in their own environment. Clinical pathways describing the diagnosis of brain stem death have been developed and are available through the Map of Medicine.

Recommendation 8:

Financial disincentives to Trusts facilitating donation should be removed through the development and introduction of appropriate reimbursement.

NHSBT undertook an analysis of costs involved in the management of potential organ donors, and Trusts are now entitled to claim approximately £2000 to cover the cost of managing a potential organ donor, even if the donation does not actually proceed (for example, for clinical reasons). This reimbursement occurs on a quarterly basis, and the costs of managing potential organ donors are kept under review.

Further details of the reimbursement scheme are available at www.organdonation.nhs.uk/ukt/ members/pdfs/letter_290708.pdf.

Donation committees are being supported to use the reimbursement monies to further the cause of donation in their organisations.

In Scotland, the reimbursement of donation hospitals had never been removed.

Recommendation 9:

The current network of donor transplant coordinators (DTCs) should be expanded and strengthened through central employment by a UK-wide Organ Donation Organisation. Additional coordinators, embedded within critical care areas, should be employed to ensure a comprehensive, highly skilled, specialised and robust service. There should be a close and defined collaboration between DTCs, clinical staff and Trust donation champions. Electronic online donor registration and organ offering systems should be developed.

This, together with the following recommendation, were undoubtedly two of the most radical and far-reaching changes that came from the Taskforce and it is to the great credit of all the organisations and individuals concerned that such rapid and successful progress has been made. Two major changes were required to the coordinator network: firstly, that all staff working as donor coordinators should focus exclusively on organ donation rather than also performing a role within a transplant centre as a recipient coordinator; and, secondly, that all donor coordinators should be employed and managed by NHSBT.

As part of these changes, the term 'donor transplant coordinator' has been amended to 'specialist nurse for organ donation' (SN-OD). This new term is more closely aligned with wider NHS terminology. The transfer of employment to NHSBT was completed across the UK by 2011, and recruitment of additional SN-ODs has been highly successful: overall the total SN-OD workforce and support staff has more than doubled. Increasingly, the SN-ODs are being embedded within critical care teams and the network has been reconfigured into 12 regional teams. In addition to involvement with potential and actual deceased donors, SN-ODs also play a key role in training and raising awareness with key stakeholder organisations and the general public.

Reorganisation on this scale inevitably produces difficulties as well as advantages during the transitional phase, and perhaps the most inevitable of these has been the incorporation of a large number of excellent but relatively inexperienced new SN-ODs into the system over a relatively short period. However, the structure is now in place and most of the difficulties are being resolved.

NHSBT has developed and deployed a new Electronic Offering System (EOS). This system is available to all SN-ODs and transplant teams and is becoming more widely used. It requires adaptation to make best use of new technology such as tablet computers and smart phones, with the possibility of simultaneous offering to all transplant centres an achievable goal.

Recommendation 10:
A UK-wide network of dedicated organ retrieval teams should be established to ensure timely, high-quality organ removal from all heartbeating and non-heartbeating donors. The Organ Donation Organisation should be responsible for commissioning the retrieval teams and for audit and performance management.

Building on early work by the British Transplantation Society, NHSBT developed and commissioned the National Organ Retrieval Service (NORS), which came into effect on 1 April 2010. There are seven dedicated abdominal retrieval teams and six dedicated cardiothoracic retrieval teams. Whilst these are all based on existing transplant centres, innovative arrangements mean that some teams are provided jointly by two centres. Teams may now have to travel outside their local area to attend a donor if the local team is already retrieving, thus reducing the waiting time for families and donor hospitals – for example, the Scottish retrieval zone now covers some areas within Northern Ireland and provides back-up to teams in England as and when necessary. An as yet unresolved issue is the provision of anaesthetic and donor management support to the retrieval teams and donor hospitals. The physiological and haemodynamic management of a brain-dead potential organ donor is a very important aspect of organ donation that has perhaps received less attention than it deserves, and NHSBT now has a lead clinician to help resolve these difficulties.

Recommendation 11:
All clinical staff likely to be involved in the treatment of potential organ donors should receive mandatory training in the principles of donation. There should also be regular update training.

The response to this recommendation has perhaps been less integrated and coordinated than originally hoped, but nonetheless significant progress has been made.

In the short term, the Professional Development Programme (PDP) for CLODs and donation committee chairs, led by NHSBT, covered both clinical issues relevant to deceased organ donation and the professional and leadership skills required to effectively lead change within hospitals. The material was designed and delivered by senior clinicians and the content was approved by an Expert Reference Group that included representatives from relevant professional bodies such as the Intensive Care Society, the Royal College of Anaesthetists, the College of Emergency Medicine, and the Royal College of Paediatrics and Child Health. This 12-month programme involved face-to-face workshops, self-study and regional events aimed at building leadership and changing management skills, and to advance clinical expertise and capability.

Other outputs of the PDP include a toolkit for organ donation that includes education material based upon the various modules of the PDP, and a description of clinical pathways for organ donation that are available online on the Map of Medicine platform. In Scotland, NHS Education for Scotland has developed an online educational resource with the primary aim of helping clinicians involved in organ donation, and clinical leads established a series of training initiatives for professional staff across trusts in Northern Ireland.

In the longer term, the relevant professional bodies now incorporate training in organ donation in their postgraduate specialist curricula, and perhaps the two most relevant bodies are the recently established Faculty of Intensive Care Medicine (FICM) and the College of Emergency Medicine. For example, the FICM includes all aspects of organ donation in the syllabus and core competencies for the Certificate of Completion of Training in Intensive Care Medicine. The Paediatric Intensive Care Society has also made training in organ donation a mandatory competence.

It would clearly be beneficial if awareness of, and knowledge about, organ donation were to be included at an earlier stage, in the medical (and probably nursing) undergraduate curricula. Although this is not yet universal it is gradually becoming more widespread.

Recommendation 12:
Appropriate ways should be identified of personally and publicly recognising individual organ donors, where desired. These approaches may include national memorials, local initiatives and personal follow-up to donor families.

There are many ways in which donors and their families are personally and publicly recognised, ranging from local events and non-denominational services of remembrance and thanks, to national memorials. In the UK there is a Gift of Life memorial stone in Cardiff, a love seat in Glasgow and a 'New Life Garden' in Northern Ireland. The garden is a symbol of remembrance, thanks and hope.

However, there are many more ways in which society's recognition of the gift of donation could be recognised and three recent developments are:

- An online book of remembrance developed by the Donor Family Network.
- The Royal College of Physicians (RCP) has published a very moving book of recipient letters, thanking their anonymous donors for the gift of life. The book, *Thank You – For Life*, was published in November 2010 and will be given to future donor families.
- In a pilot scheme, six donation committees were asked to provide a public commemorative plaque in a prominent position in their hospitals, recognising the gift of life made by donors and using the phrase 'In their final moments they gave a lifetime'.

Recommendation 13:
There is an urgent requirement to identify and implement the most effective methods through which organ donation and the 'gift of life' can be promoted to the general public, and specifically to the BME population. Research should be commissioned through Department of Health research and development funding.

Promotion of organ donation remains one of the key functions of NHSBT and a high-profile, multimedia campaign to promote organ donation was launched in November 2009. Recent financial restraints have limited the use of such major media campaigns, although the Scottish government have run multimedia organ donation media and advertising campaigns in 2009/10 and in 2010/11, and the Wales and Northern Ireland groups have also been active in a wide range of projects.

In early 2009 an updated Organ Donation Teaching Resource Pack for schools in Scotland was launched. The aim of the Pack is to educate young people about the complex moral and ethical issues associated with organ donation and transplantation.

It has been recognised for a number of years that the wide range of faiths and cultures in the UK leads to an equally wide range of understanding of, and attitudes towards, organ donation. The second Taskforce Report[12] included a detailed assessment of this subject and provided a valuable basis for future work. This has been continued through a wide range of activities involving engagement with leaders of the 17 major faiths within the UK, to raise their awareness of the issues surrounding organ donation and encourage discussion from a faith perspective, public engagement events at various religious centres and festivals in Scotland, and a 'peer educator' project, where local high-profile community leaders were educated about the issues surrounding organ donation and encouraged to continue the debate and raise awareness with their local communities.

The implementation programme was also able to ensure funding for three major academic research projects to explore factors that influence the bereaved family's decision about donation, medical professionals' attitudes to organ donation and to further investigate attitudes within black and minority ethnic communities to organ donation.

Recommendation 14:

The Department of Health and the Ministry of Justice should develop formal guidelines for coroners concerning organ donation.

The Department of Health worked with the Ministry of Justice, other UK Health Departments, the Coroners' Society and other stakeholders to develop guidance for coroners regarding organ donation. The guidance is available at www. dh.gov.uk/en/Publicationsandstatistics/Publications/ PublicationsPolicyAndGuidance/DH_114804.

In Scotland, close working relationships are in place with the Crown Office of the Procurator Fiscal (COPFS) and it was not felt necessary to issue guidance. An existing agreement between the Scottish Transplant Group (STG) and the COPFS regarding organ and tissue donation is currently being revised by the STG ethics subgroup.

It is not only implementation of these 14 specific recommendations that has led to significant developments over the past 3 years. Perhaps one of the most important changes is the ever-increasing awareness, by clinicians caring for patients who are likely to die, that organ donation can and should be seen as an integral part of the end-of-life care for such a patient whenever it is appropriate.[13] For many years the promotion of donation has been based very strongly on the needs of those on transplant waiting lists and the benefits that they receive from a transplant. Increasingly, however, it is now being argued that donation is appropriate in its own right. If it is known that an individual wanted to donate their organs after death, whether by active registration on the NHS Organ Donor Register or through discussion about their wishes and preferences with their family, then donation is the right thing and should happen whenever it is appropriate, lawful and ethical. This may seem a somewhat artificial distinction but it is not – it is putting the wishes of the individual at the centre of decision-making about that individual. The individual's motives are of course very likely to be to save the lives of others, but donation is being facilitated in order to meet the person's wishes rather than solely for the benefit of others. Many of the perceived ethical and practical difficulties associated with donation take on a very different perspective when things are seen in this light. This distinction is at the heart of the legal guidance published by the Department of Health, where the 'best interests' of a patient are

seen to reflect a much wider range of issues than simply the 'best medical management'. The same thread runs through two consensus documents produced by professional societies in association with NHSBT and the Department of Health – A Consensus Document Regarding Donation after Circulatory Death by the British Transplant Society and the Intensive Care Society in December 2010,[14] and the Role of Emergency Departments in Organ Donation produced by the British Transplantation Society and the College of Emergency Medicine in November 2011.[15]

Progress

The Taskforce Report was published in January 2008 and the donor numbers for 2007/8 serve as the baseline year against which progress should be measured. **Figure 2.1** shows the number of deceased donors in the UK from 2000/01 to 2010/11, and demonstrates the steady increase that has followed implementation of the recommendations. The total number of donors has risen from 809 to 1088 – a 34% increase in 4 years – after many years of falling or static activity. However, an unforeseen aspect of this has been that virtually the entire increase has come from DCD donors (**Fig. 2.2**). In 2011/12 there were 652 DBD donors (down from a peak of 716 in 2002/3) compared with 609 in 2007/8 (an increase of 7.1%) – the corresponding numbers for DCD donors are 436 and 200 (an increase of 118%).

So whilst the overall increase is to be welcomed it is clear that this has had little impact on the number of suitable heart donors. Moreover, whilst results of kidney transplantation from DCD donors

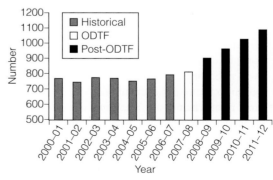

Figure 2.1 • Deceased donors in the UK.

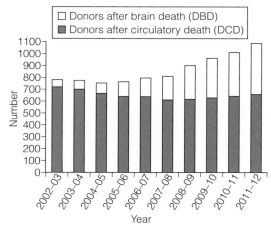

Figure 2.2 • Number of DBD and DCD donors.

appear to be broadly equivalent to those using donation after brain death (DBD) donors (at least in the short term), this is not the case for liver recipients. There is considerable speculation – but little good evidence – as to whether DCD donors represent a pool of 'new' donors, who hitherto would not have donated organs, or whether they are patients who could or would in the past have progressed to become DBD donors. The answer is probably a combination of these two possibilities, but more detailed information than is currently available is needed before conclusions can be drawn.

Future challenges

Whilst much has been achieved, and deceased donor numbers have risen significantly for the first time in many years, the underlying problem of the shortage of organs for transplantation remains. This is particularly true for organs from DBD donors, where the decline of recent years has been halted but little increase has been seen. The Taskforce Report identified and recognised the barriers to organ donation through an analysis of the donor 'pathway' but made recommendations – consciously or unconsciously – primarily about the necessary organisational changes that were required to enable progress to be made rather than addressing the specific details of each stage of the pathway. For example, the important issue of consent was identified and the recommendation was that there should be more donor transplant coordinators, better trained and

managed. The Report outlined the possible benefits of having more coordinators but did not recommend specific changes to the consent process that could be introduced through the new coordinator network. During implementation of the recommendations, and specifically during the Professional Development Programme for clinical leads and others, six aspects of clinical practice have emerged as being key to further progress, and have become known as the 'six big wins'.[13] These, together with many other aspects of the diagnosis of death and organ donation, were reviewed in a superb supplement of the *British Journal of Anaesthesia* in December 2011.[16] The six key areas are shown in Box 2.1.

These are the areas where the challenges now lie – how to use the new infrastructure in practice to make improvements at each stage of the pathway. Recent changes to the PDA have started to provide much more information, and making improvements requires not only the development of clear and agreed practical, detailed proposals, but also the ability to translate those changes into daily clinical practice. It is at the bedside that decisions are made about individual patients that either preserve the possibility of subsequent organ donation or rule it out. The new structures provide an excellent mechanism for developing the necessary detailed proposals, mainly through the regional collaboratives of clinical leads and SN-ODs and the National Donation Committee that has replaced the Donation Advisory Group at NHSBT. The same structure also allows for implementation of change.

Very importantly, the PDP provided a focus for improved clinical leadership and change management skills for clinical leads and donation committee chairs to enable them to overcome barriers to change (human, political, organisational, economic and geographical). This should facilitate not only

Box 2.1 • The 'six big wins'

1. Increased consent/authorisation rates
2. Increased diagnosis of brain stem death
3. Increased donation after circulatory death
4. Greater involvement of emergency departments
5. Increased referral according to minimum notification criteria
6. Better donor management

local improvements in 'traditional' donation (i.e. DBD donors), but also the introduction of new donation programmes such as DCD donation or donation from the emergency department. Changing the way individuals or organisations work is far more complex than simply coming up with a new plan (however good it may be) and announcing to the world that this is how things are to happen from now on, and it requires skills that can be taught and learnt. Fundamental to this is a sympathetic understanding, on the part of those who work to increase donation, of the perspective of those who care for dying patients. Organ donation remains a rare event in all but the very largest critical care centres, knowledge and experience of donation may inevitably be limited, and the ethical dilemma that may be posed by donation should not be underestimated.[17,18] What seems straightforward and uncontroversial to the enthusiast may be deeply troubling to clinicians who experience donation as a small part of a much wider picture of critical care. NICE, for example, recognises this in saying 'Although donation occurs after death, there are steps that healthcare professionals may need to take before the death of the patient if donation is to take place. This guidance covers such steps, and in the case of clinical triggers for referral, refers to actions that might take place even beforethe inevitability of death has been recognised. These actions may result in challenges and tensions for the healthcare teams but they can and indeed should be incorporated into local hospital policies in order to better promote donation as part of end-of-life care.'

Very few clinicians are opposed to donation in principle – and it is therefore essential to listen to their concerns, almost invariably carefully considered, and to find mutually acceptable solutions. It is here that the wishes of the individual patient about donation – either known directly or established from others – can be seen as common ground and a sound basis for agreeing what is appropriate action to meet those wishes.

Increased consent/authorisation rates

Figure 2.3 shows the consent rates for potential DBD and DCD donors over the past 2 years. It is clear that for DBD donors in the UK as a whole there has been no sustained improvement over this

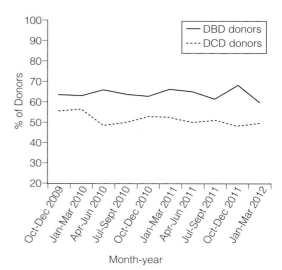

Figure 2.3 • Consent rates for potential donors.

time period, although an analysis of consent rates in individual hospitals shows a number with a rate in excess of 80% (unadjusted data). The consent rate for DCD donors is a cause for concern – it is lower than for DBD donors, and the rate appears to have fallen over this time period. In several European countries consent rates exceed 75%, reaching approximately 85% in Spain.[19] There is much debate about how best to try to improve the situation in the UK, including some data which appear to show a higher rate when a SN-OD is involved,[20] although this is at odds with the ACRE Study.[21] This is perhaps the aspect of donation where the greatest gains could be made if a coherent strategy is developed and introduced. Vincent and Logan[20] have suggested a series of practical steps based on current evidence and experience:

• an approach pre-planned by the coordinator/specialist nurse and healthcare team to consider specific individual circumstances – the 'team huddle';
• requesting by individuals known to the family;
• requesting by team members with the required training and expertise to provide the right information in a sensitive and empathic manner – in the UK, this should be the SN-OD and a senior doctor;
• requesting at a time separate to that when the family are informed of the death or its inevitability, in an unhurried manner in an appropriate setting;

- use of unapologetic and positive language, emphasising the benefits of donation;
- ensuring the family are given specific information, and that (where appropriate) the concept of brain death has been fully explained.

NICE clinical guidelines aim to assist teams in implementing such a model. This guidance[9] states that a multidisciplinary team (MDT) should be responsible for planning the approach and discussing organ donation with those close to the patient. The MDT should include the medical and nursing staff involved in the care of the patient, led throughout the process by an identifiable consultant, the specialist nurse for organ donation and local faith representative(s) where relevant. Cultural and religious issues that may have an impact on consent should be identified,[22] and the approach to those close to the patient should be made in a setting suitable for private and compassionate discussions.

Discussions about organ donation with those close to the patient should only take place when it has been clearly established that they understand that death is inevitable or has occurred, and they must be given sufficient time to consider the information. At all times assurance must be given that the primary focus is on the care and dignity of the patient (whether the donation occurs or not), with explicit confirmation and reassurance that the standard of care received will be the same whether they consider giving consent for organ donation or not.

Increased diagnosis of brain stem death

In a major review, Smith[23] points out that although it is more than 40 years since the concept of brain death was first introduced into clinical practice, many of the controversies that surround it have not been settled. These include the relationship between brain death and death of the whole person, the international differences in the nomenclature and criteria for the determination of brain death, and the inextricable links between brain death and organ donation.[24] Smith goes on to say 'Although guidelines are available in many countries to standardise national processes for the diagnosis of brain death, the current variation and inconsistency in practice make it imperative that an international consensus is developed. As a minimum,

this should clarify the criteria for the determination of brain death and provide specific instructions about the clinical examination necessary and the conduct of the apnoea test. It should also stipulate the role and type of confirmatory investigations, identify the training and experience of those able to determine death by neurological criteria, and detail the required level of documentation. This is likely to require the UK to reconsider its reliance on the brain stem formulation of brain death, but this should not prevent us from enthusiastically embracing the debate. An international consensus on the determination of brain death is desirable, essential and long overdue.'

These anxieties may, in part, explain why not all patients in the UK in whom neurological death appears to be a likely diagnosis (i.e. those who meet four criteria: apnoea, coma from known aetiology, ventilated and with unresponsive fixed pupils) are in fact tested formally (**Fig. 2.4**).[11] There are a range of reasons for this, some of which are entirely appropriate or which could be resolved through better guidance on, for example, the use of ancillary tests when the clinical tests are not possible. However, the impression remains that at least a proportion of these patients could and probably should have been tested, and as such (if the tests confirmed neurological death) could have progressed to DBD donation. A small number become DCD donors which, as has been noted, are less satisfactory from the recipients' perspective. The hospital donation committees are

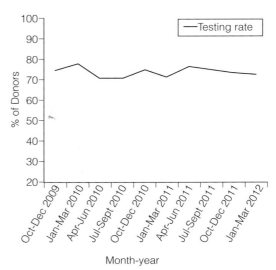

Figure 2.4 • BSD testing rate for potential DBD donors.

being asked to review every suitable patient who was not tested, and to introduce measures to support testing in difficult clinical situations.

Increased donation after circulatory death

DCD differs in many aspects from donation after brain death and poses specific challenges. However, where DCD is practised widely, organ donation is often considered a routine part of end-of-life care.[25] The timing of treatment withdrawal may be controversial, and there is significant variation in how treatment withdrawal is managed in adult critical care units, particularly with regard to airway management and the use of pharmacological comfort cares. The Intensive Care Society and the British Transplantation Society produced a joint Consensus Statement on DCD donation in 2010 which, whilst not resolving every issue, lays out a national framework for the care of such patients and calls on local groups to develop consistent approaches to the identified areas of uncertainty.[14] As with all other DCD guidelines, it is recommended that the decision to withdraw cardiorespiratory support should always be independent, and made before any consideration of organ donation. The PDA is likely to be least accurate in data relating to DCD donors as a result of a degree of subjectivity in the definitions used, but nonetheless suggests that only 50–60% of patients who may become such donors are referred to the SN-OD network for assessment and an approach to the next of kin. It would appear, therefore, that there is the possibility to almost double the number of potential DCD donors through widespread adoption of the Consensus Statement. There is also a clearly identified need for transplant programmes to adopt the consistent approaches recommended in the Statement, and for NHSBT to resolve the delays and frustration that result from a protracted 'offering' sequence for the organs. There appears to be great potential to increase the number of lung transplants from DCD donors, possibly utilising ex-vivo lung perfusion, and there is also growing interest in the possibility of heart donation and the associated ethical issues. NICE guidance stresses that it is essential for those close to the patient to understand the rationale behind the decision to withdraw or withhold life-sustaining treatment, how the timing

will be coordinated to support organ donation, and the process of organ donation and retrieval. They must also be fully informed about the interventions that may be required between consent and organ retrieval, where and when organ retrieval is likely to occur and the reasons why organ donation may not take place, even if consent is granted.

Greater involvement of emergency departments

Whilst the Taskforce Report recognised that 'Intensive care should not be the only focus for organ donation; all areas where end-of-life care is provided should be included', the specific recommendations did not place particular emphasis on the role of the emergency department (ED). This omission has become increasingly apparent, not least because of the rapid increase in the availability of high-quality brain scans and the facility for remote radiological and neurological assessment of treatment options. A number of centres have promoted a greater role for EDs and in 2011 the PDA was extended to include all EDs in the UK. In November 2011 the College of Emergency Medicine and the British Transplantation Society published a joint report on the Role of Emergency Departments,[15] and the challenge now is to introduce the findings of this report as widely as possible. There are, in general terms, two ways in which EDs can contribute:

- Firstly, through the robust identification of the donation potential of those patients whose catastrophic brain injuries (medical or traumatic) are clearly not survivable. In these circumstances, rather than have life-sustaining treatment withdrawn, the legal wishes of the patient – either recorded on the Organ Donor Register or with their closest relatives orally or in written form – should guide the ED to early referral of the patient to the specialist nurses for organ donation. It is in the best interests of the patient that they be cared for in a critical care environment to allow a full assessment of their donation potential.
- Secondly, and less commonly, if admission to the ICU is not appropriate or possible, for the entire donation pathway prior to transfer to theatre for organ retrieval to be managed from within the ED.

Even in large departments, donation is likely to be a relatively infrequent event. The most important specific recommendations are that:

- All EDs should consider the identification of a lead clinician with an interest in donation.
- All EDs should be represented on the local donation committee, and thus engage the support of the Trust/health board.
- Trusts/health boards should review data from the Potential Donor Audit (PDA) on the potential for organ donation from the ED every 6 months, and the potential for donation should be reviewed as part of the standard discussion that follows every death within the ED.
- Local policies and guidelines should be developed based on a national template, but reflecting local factors such as the likely frequency of potential donors and the resources that are available or will be needed.
- Neurosurgery/neurosciences should be part of these developments both nationally and locally.
- These policies should include the care of a ventilated patient, the transfer of patients to intensive care for further assessment, and the withdrawal of life-sustaining treatment within EDs.

Increased referral according to minimum notification criteria

Whilst the definitions used in the PDA are to some extent subjective, particularly with respect to potential DCD donors, there remain patients who may be potential donors who are not referred to the SN-OD network (**Fig. 2.5**). NICE guidance[9] states that it is important to identify all patients who are potentially suitable donors as early as possible, through a systematic approach. While recognising that clinical situations vary, identification should be based on either of the following criteria:

1. Defined clinical trigger factors in patients who have had a catastrophic brain injury, namely:
   - the absence of one or more cranial nerve reflexes; and
   - a Glasgow Coma Scale (GCS) score of 4 or less that is not explained by sedation;
   unless there is a clear reason why the above clinical triggers are not met or a decision has been made to perform brain stem death tests.

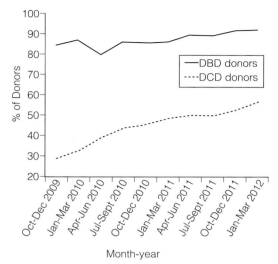

Figure 2.5 • Referral rates for potential donors.

2. The intention to withdraw life-sustaining treatment in patients with a life-threatening or life-limiting condition that will, or is expected to, result in circulatory death.

NICE recognises that a proportion of the patients who are identified by these clinical triggers will survive, and this guidance therefore goes significantly further than the minimal notification criteria detailed in the Taskforce Report. Many clinicians involved in the care of patients with major brain injuries have in the past expressed concerns about such early identification and/or referral, as it could be seen to represent the conflict of interests between treating the patient actively in the hope or expectation of survival and considering the patient primarily as a potential donor that they, and the public, so fear. Whilst in practice this conflict is extremely unlikely to affect the delivery of active treatment, the perception of it can be very real. It will be for local teams to develop local policies that should incorporate the minimal notification criteria as a starting point, and move towards the criteria suggested by NICE as and when they can satisfy themselves and the patient's family that there is no reduction in their commitment to active treatment until it is no longer felt to be appropriate and in the patient's best interests.

Better donor management

McKeown et al.[26] have recently reviewed all aspects of the management of the haemodynamic and physiological changes that occur in association with brain stem death. They conclude that appropriate support before and after brain death can improve the number and quality of donor organs. Such support is intensive and time-consuming and should be introduced as soon as possible after the diagnosis of death – not simply during the retrieval operation itself. The organisational aspects of donor management, and in particular the division of responsibility between clinicians at the donor hospital and the retrieval teams, are important but have not all been resolved and implemented fully. Despite the publication of such guidelines and the efforts of many SN-ODs there still seems to be a degree of inertia in optimising all donors that is limiting, in particular, the number of hearts that are deemed suitable for transplantation. All organ retrieval teams – both abdominal and cardiothoracic – are now commissioned by NHSBT and it is to be hoped that this will provide the necessary momentum for change. Legal guidance[5] has clarified some aspects of the management of potential DCD donors but there remain unresolved issues such as the administration of pre-mortem heparin or other agents that will require further guidance from the Departments of Health.

Other issues

Whilst implementation of the Taskforce recommendations has been the main focus over recent years, a number of other relevant changes have occurred:

1. The European Directive on standards of quality and safety of human organs intended for transplantation.[27] In force since August 2012, this requires all member states to develop a framework for quality and safety, licence procurement organisations and transplant centres, ensure appropriate organ and donor characterisation, meet certain requirements for the transport of organs, and to have in place rigorous traceability and reporting systems for serious adverse events. The Human Tissue Authority is the designated competent authority in the UK. The Directive acknowledges the organ shortage and the overall benefits of transplantation, and the need for clinicians to make a risk–benefit assessment in judging whether an organ is suitable for transplantation, and its stated aim is to reduce the risks and maximise the benefits. It has,

however, added a layer of bureaucracy that many feel is of less benefit to the UK than to some of the emerging members of the European Union.

2. The NHS reforms. Following the establishment of the coalition government in 2010 major, and controversial, reforms of the NHS in England were introduced. At the time of writing the details of the new NHS, and particularly of the NHS Commissioning Board, remain unclear. However, the general principle of greater local autonomy in both commissioning and service provision may present a challenge to the maintenance of a national focus on organ donation that has been so important over recent years. It will be important to identify and use the various levers within the new system, such as the Outcomes Framework and Quality Standards, which will influence the Commissioning Board and acute hospitals. The operating framework's five domains include the need to reduce avoidable and premature deaths, improve the care of patients with long-term conditions and improve care for acute illnesses – organ transplantation belongs clearly in all three of these domains, and it is to be hoped that this will ensure the necessary focus on increasing organ donation.

3. Opting out. For several years the Welsh government has been exploring the possible introduction of some form of opting-out legislation in Wales, and in late 2011 it published a White Paper for consultation, with a clear intent to introduce legislation in due course.[28] The proposals suggest a 'soft' opt-out scheme, which will apply to people aged 18 or over who live and die in Wales. Adults will have the opportunity to make an objection to donation of their organs and tissues, there will be an effective and secure system for individuals to make an objection should they wish to, and after death families will be involved in the decision-making process around donation. There remain a number of significant practical and organisational challenges to the introduction of the scheme but its impact will of course be followed very closely in the other countries of the UK.

Managing expectations

The last 10 years have seen changes to the potential donor pool and to donor characteristics in the UK over and above the rapid rise in the number of DCD donors.

The potential donor pool

The PDA provides an estimate of the number of patients who meet criteria that suggest testing for neurological death would be appropriate. There is limited information as to why patients are not tested, and there is no doubt that it cannot be assumed that those not tested have the same donation potential as those who were tested, but nonetheless it is noteworthy that there appears to have been a reduction of nearly 30% in the number of such patients between 2004/5 and 2009/10.[13] A more definitive figure is the 26% reduction in the number of patients whose death was confirmed on neurological criteria, and who were therefore possible DBD donors.[13] This reduction may be explained – at least in part – by developments in neuroradiology and neurosurgery that have significantly changed the management of patients with subarachnoid haemorrhage and raised intracranial pressure. Similar experience has been reported from the USA,[29] with similar observations that changes in clinical practice, especially in management of patients with severe brain injury, may account for the increased proportion of DCD donors and the falling number of possible DBD donors. Unpublished data[30] suggest that the number of patients in the New England Organ Bank area whose death has been confirmed on neurological criteria has fallen by approximately 25% in recent years. These are welcome developments, but they have resulted in a fall in the number of possible DBD donors. It is noteworthy that during this time of change the percentage of patients whose death was confirmed on neurological criteria that subsequently became actual solid-organ donors has risen from 46% in the earlier time period to 54% in 2010/11. This is sometimes called the conversion rate and it is now identical to the overall figure of 54% in Spain for the period 1998–2009, although more recently the Spanish rate has approached 60%.[31]

Donor characteristics

Unsurprisingly, solid-organ donors in the UK are becoming older and more obese. In the last 10 years the proportion of donors over the age of 60 has risen from 16% to 30% and of donors with a body mass index (BMI) of 30 or more from 12% to 20%.[3] Once again, there are marked differences between the UK and Spain. For donors under the age of 45 the rates in the two countries are broadly similar. For ages 45–60 the rates are 10.4 and 6.2 pmp in Spain and the UK, respectively. The corresponding rates for donors aged 61–70 are 6.7 and 3.3 pmp, and for donors over the age of 70 they are 8.2 and 1.3 pmp.[32]

Summary/conclusions

For well over a decade Spain's donor rate of 30–35 pmp has been the highest in the world, and more recently the rate in Portugal has reached a similar level. The Taskforce learnt in detail about the Spanish model, much of which has now been incorporated into the UK. However, the clear implication of the data presented above is that Spain has a higher donor rate because there are more patients who are certified dead by neurological criteria, and this in turn may be a consequence of the greater number of critical care beds – 87.5 per million population compared with 27 per million population in the UK (excluding coronary care, neonatal and burns units).[23] There are also likely to be different admission criteria for ITU[33] (with fewer beds in the UK, those with a poor prognosis, who are therefore more likely to be potential donors, are less likely to be admitted to ITU) and different end-of-life practices (in the UK it is considered good practice to withdraw life-sustaining treatment before brain stem tests are carried out if treatment is no longer benefiting the patient, whereas this is very much less common in Spain). This situation could change with recent Spanish legislation on withdrawal of life support, which could make patient and family requests to withdraw ventilation more common.[34] To summarise these data, they show that if *every* patient in the UK who appeared to meet the criteria for neurological testing were to be tested and death confirmed, and *every* patient subsequently became an organ donor, the UK DBD donation rate would be approximately 22 per million population (pmp) compared with the current *actual* Spanish DBD rate of 29.3 pmp and the rate in Portugal of 30.2 pmp. It would seem that there are major differences in the broader healthcare systems between the UK and Spain that lead to the very apparent differences in donation activity, and that notwithstanding the obvious success of the Spanish donation model it is not realistic to expect to achieve comparable DBD donor rates in the two countries.

The conversion rate for potential DCD donors is based on data that remain more subjective despite recent changes to improve the accuracy of the PDA. Nevertheless, the published figure of 12% for 2010/11[9] suggests that there is considerable scope to increase further the number of DCD donors. It is interesting to speculate what could be achieved if the referral rate and approach rate (to the family) for possible DCD donors matched those currently seen for possible DBD donors. Overall donor numbers in the UK could reach approximately 2000 (32 pmp), of which two-thirds would be DCD donors. Realistically this would appear to be the likely limit, unless in addition significant improvements could be made to the consent rate. For example, a consent rate of 75% for both DBD and DCD donors would lead to a higher theoretical UK donor rate of 45 pmp – but nearly 75% of donors would be DCD donors.

Whilst this is – at present – a less satisfactory form of donation for liver transplantation and does nothing to meet the need to increase heart donation, it is to be hoped that developments such as ex-vivo (probably normothermic) perfusion will lead to improved outcomes for all organs transplanted from DCD donors.[35]

So the three challenges for the coming years are to convert more potential DBD donors into actual donors (limited scope for increases), convert more potential DCD donors into actual donors (considerable scope for increases), and to improve consent rates to those seen in countries such as Spain, Poland and the Republic of Ireland.[19] These are major challenges, but if they can be met there is no doubt that the deceased donation rate in the UK can continue to increase, that more people who wish to donate their organs after death can in fact do so, and that more patients can receive a transplant and fewer die in vain whilst waiting and hoping.

Key points

- Implementation of the Organ Donor Taskforce recommendations is largely complete.
- Deceased organ donor numbers have increased by 34% in 4 years.
- The increase in DCD donors (118%) has been much greater than the increase in DBD donors (7.1%). This may in part be the result of a falling number of patients meeting the criteria for the diagnosis of death on neurological criteria.
- There is a considerable evidence base on which to develop strategies to increase further donor numbers: increasing the consent rate for donation is the single step that would have the greatest impact.
- More systemic differences in healthcare suggest that at present the DBD donor rate in the UK is unlikely to reach that currently seen in Spain and Portugal.

Acknowledgements

The developments described in this chapter would not have been possible without the active support and commitment of many stakeholder organisations and individuals too numerous to mention, but the author would like to recognise the particular roles played by the Intensive Care Society, the Royal College of Anaesthetists, the College of Emergency Medicine, the Faculty of Intensive Care Medicine and the British Transplantation Society.

References

1. Organs for transplants: a report from the Organ Donation Taskforce, http://www.dh.gov.uk/en/Publicationsandstatistics/Publications/PublicationsPolicyAndGuidance/DH_082122; [accessed 8.09.12].

2. http://www.ont.es/infesp/Memorias/Memoria_Donantes_2010.pdf; [accessed 8.09.12] (in Spanish)].

3. Transplant activity in the UK, http://www.uktransplant.org.uk/ukt/statistics/transplant_activity_report/current_activity_reports/ukt/activity_report_2010_11.pdf; [accessed 8.09.12].

4. Organ donation: working together to save lives, https://www.wp.dh.gov.uk/health/2011/12/organ-donation-taskforce-report/; [accessed 8.09.12].

5. Legal issues relevant to non-heartbeating organ donation, www.dh.gov.uk/en/Publicationsandstatistics/Publications/PublicationsPolicyAndGuidance/DH_108825; [accessed 8.09.12].

6. Guidance on legal issues relevant to donation following cardiac death, http://www.sehd.scot.nhs.uk/cmo/CMO(2010) 11.pdf; [accessed 8.09.12].

7. Legal issues relevant to donation after circulatory death (non-heart-beating organ donation) in Northern Ireland, http://www.dhsspsni.gov.uk/donation-after-circulatory-death-legal-guidance-march-2011.pdf; [accessed 8.09.12].

8. An ethical framework for donation after circulatory death, http://www.aomrc.org.uk/publications/reports-a-guidance/doc_details/9425-an-ethical-framework-for-controlled-donation-after-circulatory-death.html

9. Organ donation for transplantation: improving donor identification and consent rates for deceased organ donation. Issued: December 2011. NICE Clinical Guideline 135; www.nice.org.uk/cg135; [accessed 8.09.12].

10. CQUIN templates. Available from http://www.westmidlands.nhs.uk/CQUINTemplates.aspx, uk/CQUINTemplates.aspx.

11. http://www.organdonation.nhs.uk/ukt/statistics/potential_donor_audit/pdf/pda_report_1011.pdf

12. The potential impact of an opt out system for organ donation in the UK: an independent report from the Organ Donation Taskforce, http://www.dh.gov.uk/en/Publicationsandstatistics/Publications/PublicationsPolicyAndGuidance/DH_090312; [accessed 8.09.12].

13. Murphy PG, Smith M. Towards a framework for organ donation in the UK. Br J Anaesth 2012;108(Suppl. 1):i56–67.

14. Donation after circulatory death, http://www.bts.org.uk/transplantation/standards-and-guidelines/; [accessed 8.09.12].

15. The Role of Emergency Medicine in Organ Donation, http://www.bts.org.uk/transplantation/publications/; [accessed 8.09.12].

16. Diagnosis of death and organ donation. Br J Anaesth 2012;108(Suppl. 1).

17. Simpson PJ. What are the issues in organ donation in 2012? Br J Anaesth 2012;108(Suppl. 1):i3–6.

18. Farsides B. Respecting wishes and avoiding conflict: understanding the ethical basis for organ donation and retrieval. Br J Anaesth 2012;108(Suppl. 1):i73–9.

19. Council of Europe. International Figures on Donation and Transplantation – 2010. Newsletter Transplant 2011;16(1).

20. Vincent A, Logan L. Consent for organ donation. Br J Anaesth 2012;108(Suppl. 1):i80–7.

21. ACRE Trial Collaborators. Effect of 'collaborative requesting' on consent rate for organ donation: randomised controlled trial (ACRE trial). Br Med J 2009;339:b3911.

22. Randhawa G. Death and organ donation: meeting the needs of multiethnic and multifaith populations. Br J Anaesth 2012;108(Suppl. 1):i88–91.

23. Smith M. Brain death: time for an international consensus. Br J Anaesth 2012;108(Suppl. 1):i6–9.

24. Gardiner D, Shemie S, Manara A, et al. International perspective on the diagnosis of death. Br J Anaesth 2012;108(Suppl. 1):i14–28.

25. Manara AR, Murphy PG, O'Callaghan G. Donation after circulatory death. Br J Anaesth 2012;108(Suppl. 1):i108–21.

26. McKeown DW, Bonser RS, Kellum JA. Management of the heartbeating brain-dead organ donor. Br J Anaesth 2012;108(Suppl. 1):i96–107.

27. Directive 2010/53 of the European Parliament and of the Council of 7 July 2010 on standards of quality and safety of human organs intended for transplantation, http://ec.europa.eu/health/blood_tissues_organs/organs/index_en.htm

28. Proposals for legislation on organ and tissue donation. A Welsh Government White Paper; http://wales.gov.uk/consultations/healthsocialcare/organ; [accessed 8.09.12].

29. Saidi RF, Bradley J, Greer D, et al. Changing pattern of organ donation at a single center: are potential brain dead donors being lost to donation after cardiac death? Am J Transplant 2010;10(11): 2536–40.

30. Personal communication, Dr Frank Delmonico.

31. http://www.ont.es/infesp/DocumentosCalidad/Memoria%20PGC_2011.pdf

32. Derived from unpublished data supplied by NHSBT and see Ref. 3.

33. Bion JF, Nightingale P, Taylor BL. Will the UK ever reach international levels of organ donation? Br J Anaesth 2012;108(Suppl. 1):i10–3.

34. Rodríguez-Arias D, Wright L, Paredes D. Success factors and ethical challenges of the Spanish model of organ donation. Lancet 2010;376:1109–12.

35. Watson CJE, Dark JH. Organ transplantation: historical perspective and current practice. Br J Anaesth 2012;108(Suppl. 1):i29–42.

3

Immunology of graft rejection

George Tse
Lorna Marson

Introduction

The study of transplantation has played a pivotal role in defining fundamental immunological phenomena, which in turn have provided a rationale for the development of clinical transplantation and immunosuppression. The first concepts of histocompatibility date back to the observations of Gaspero Tagliacozzi in the 16th century, who described 'force and power of individuality' after being able to successfully perform skin autografts, but not allografts.

The reality of transplantation progressed with the introduction of immunosuppressive agents alongside a more comprehensive appreciation that rejection of donor tissue was a consequence of actively acquired immunity against differences in genetically encoded histocompatibility antigens.

In this chapter, we will discuss the molecular and cellular events that lead to graft rejection, including the alloimmune and effector responses and injury occurring around the time of transplantation. We will go on to describe clinical rejection and look at potential therapeutic targets.

Basic concepts and nomenclature of immunology

In order to understand the alloimmune response, it is necessary to understand how the host recognises and responds to danger. In the context of transplantation, this relates to the recipient's ability to distinguish between self and non-self.

Recognition of danger

In Matzinger's model of immune activation, 'danger' to the host (danger-associated molecular patterns, DAMP) is sensed through pattern recognition receptors (PRRs) on antigen-presenting cells (APCs).[1,2] APCs are made up of a variety of innate cells, including tissue resident macrophages and dendritic cells (DCs). APCs engulf, process and present peptide antigen on their cell surface in the context of major histocompatibility complex (MHC) antigens. They then migrate to lymphoid tissue and present the antigen to T cells. The resulting adaptive response is determined by the balance between co-stimulatory and co-inhibitory signals received alongside this specific antigenic stimulus; this will be discussed in more depth later.

Histocompatibility

Histocompatibility antigens were first defined on the basis of their preventing transplantation between outbred members of the same species. In pioneering work, Snell and Higgins identified that the genes responsible for rejection were found on chromosome 17 at just one locus (H2); this complex of murine genes was termed the major histocompatibility complex (MHC).[3] The characterisation of MHC in humans was later identified at the same locus and the nomenclature of human leucocyte antigens (HLAs) was adopted after the first Histocompatibility meeting in 1964.

Differences between donor and recipient MHC antigens significantly contribute to rejection, despite significant progress in immunosuppressive therapy.[4] Furthermore, numerous minor histocompatibility systems also exist and can result in allograft rejection; this is particularly problematic in bone marrow transplantation (see Chapter 4).

Major histocompatibility complexes

There are two main types of MHC molecules, MHC class I and II (see **Fig. 3.1**). In humans, the genetic sequences for these glycoproteins are found on the short arm of chromosome 6, with the exception of the light chain β_2-microglobulin, which is encoded on chromosome 15. There are six main loci in the human MHC: HLA-A, HLA-B and HLA-C belong to HLA class I, while HLA-DP, HLA-DQ and HLA-DR belong to HLA class II.

The MHC system has a high degree of polymorphism, which is defined as the presence of more than one allele at the same locus. There are hundreds of variants of MHC proteins, and all of them are relatively common in the population. This is useful in the context of combating pathogenic microorganisms, but constitutes a significant challenge to preventing rejection in transplantation.

MHC class I proteins are cell-surface glycoproteins expressed on all nucleated cells and present peptides derived from intracellular proteins. They are formed by a highly polymorphic heavy chain (45 kDa) and a less variable light chain, β_2-microglobulin, which is bound non-covalently to the heavy chain. Endogenous antigens are digested into peptides by proteosomes, and loaded on to class I MHC, as shown in **Fig. 3.2a**. MHC class I proteins present antigen to CD8-positive (cyotoxic) T cells, which have important roles in the defence against viral infection and malignancy.

MHC class II proteins are found constitutively on the surface of APCs and B cells, but can also be induced by the process of inflammation on endothelial cells. Exogenous antigen is engulfed, degraded within endosomes and presented on the cell surface in the context of MHC class II (see **Fig. 3.2b**). Antigen processed in this way is recognised by CD4-positive (helper) T cells; these cells are important in the defence against extracellular infection and have been linked to the development of autoimmunity.

Assembly of the MHC–peptide complex

The specific structure of the binding groove of MHC class I or II determines which peptide can be bound to it. In evolutionary terms, the extreme polymorphism in MHC proteins probably reflects the need to bind a vast array of rapidly mutating pathogens. The assembly of the MHC–peptide complex, as shown in Fig. 3.2, involves a sophisticated mechanism of antigen uptake, processing and transport.

Other histocompatibility genes in rejection

MHC class I chain-related A (MICA) antigens are surface glycoproteins with functions related to innate immunity.[5] The genes are located within the class I region of the chromosome and are highly polymorphic. The contribution of MICA antigens to rejection is controversial, with some studies showing no effect on rejection,[6] while other large studies have demonstrated that the presence of MICA antibodies was associated with rejection.[7,8]

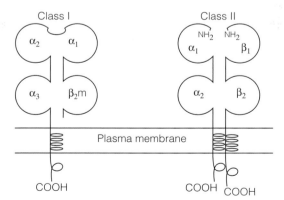

Figure 3.1 • Structure of MHC class I and II molecules. α_1, α_2, α_3 of MHC class I are membrane integral and form a non-covalent bond with β_2-microglobulin 9 (β_{2-M}), which is not membrane bound. MHC class II is formed from α and β chains, each with two domains and each membrane integral.

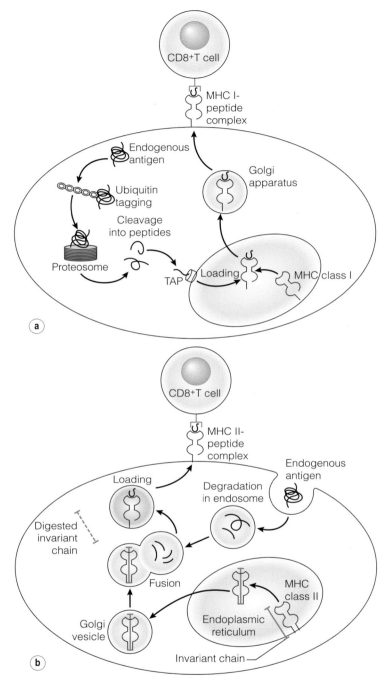

Figure 3.2 • Antigen processing and presentation in the MHC class I and II pathways. **(a)** Processing of endogenous antigens occurs primarily via the class I pathway. Peptides are produced and loaded into MHC class I proteins as shown. **(b)** Processing of exogenous antigens occurs primarily via the class II pathway. Antigens are taken up into intracellular vesicles. MHC class II proteins are synthesised in the endoplasmic reticulum, and fuse with vesicles containing peptide. MHC, major histocompatibility complex; TAP, transporters associated with antigen processing.

Minor histocompatibility antigens (miH) are distinct from MHCs; they are less polymorphic and typically induce a weaker response than disparities in the MHC. The male-specific H-Y antigen is the most well-defined miH antigen and has been shown to play a role in the rejection of bone marrow and in rodent models of transplantation. The role in solid organ transplantation is not yet fully understood, with some studies suggesting that it may only have an effect on short- but not long-term outcomes following renal transplantation.[9]

T cells

T cells play a major role in cell-mediated immunity and are pivotal in defence against a wide range of pathologies, including infection and malignancy. They display high specificity in their T-cell receptor (TCR) repertoire, which has been honed by both positive and negative selection to avoid the recognition of self; defects in this process lead to autoimmunity. T cells recognise peptide antigen bound to MHC displayed on the surface of APCs, and upon receiving the appropriate co-stimulatory signals are capable of either direct cytotoxic activity or coordinating the innate immune response; the importance of these co-stimulatory signals will be explored in more depth later.

CD8-positive T cells

CD8-positive (CD8+) or cytotoxic T cells respond to antigenic peptide derived from intracellular protein bound to MHC class I. Their function is to lyse cells that display peptide recognised as foreign; this may occur in cells infected with viruses (their main purpose) or following organ transplantation.

CD4-positive T cells

CD4-positive (CD4+) or helper T cells engage antigenic peptide derived from extracellular protein and bound to MHC class II. These cells have an array of functions, including coordinating the efficacy and vigour of the innate immune response, promoting the activation and proliferation of CD8+ T cells, and in antibody class switching in B cells.

CD4+ T-cell activation by DCs and their subsequent effector responses are central to many forms of allogeneic rejection. In some rodent models, the absence of CD4+ T cells can abolish rejection, despite the presence of CD8+ T cells and fully allogeneic MHC class I mismatches.

Early inflammatory response

Inflammation lies at the centre of rejection and begins even prior to organ transplantation, with the haemodynamic and neuroendocrine responses associated with brain stem death, the process of multiorgan retrieval and subsequent cold preservation (see **Fig. 3.3**). During the transplantation procedure itself, there is a further period of warm ischaemia and reperfusion. This compound injury results in the release of DAMPs and stimulates an inflammatory response, which promotes and shapes alloantigen-specific immunity and has an effect on long-term graft survival.[10]

The importance of these events in transplantation is illustrated by the superior outcome of live donor transplants even in the face of significant MHC mismatch, the impact of cold ischaemia time on graft outcome[11] and the higher rates of rejection observed in individuals with delayed graft function.[12] Indeed, in experimental syngeneic transplantation, graft histology very similar to that seen in chronic allograft damage may be reproduced by prolonged ischaemia.

Ischaemia–reperfusion injury

Ischaemia–reperfusion injury (IRI) is an inevitable consequence of organ retrieval as the organ is temporarily deprived of its blood supply before being reperfused and reoxygenated following transplantation. IRI is responsible for a spectrum of early organ dysfunction after transplantation and the mechanisms involved are summarised in **Fig. 3.4**.

Ischaemic injury

Cessation of arterial supply results in oxygen deprivation and a switch to anaerobic metabolic pathways. There is also a build-up of toxic metabolic byproducts, including lactate, H+ and inorganic phosphate. High-energy phosphates, such as adenosine triphosphate (ATP), are vital for most cellular functions. Their depletion inhibits the Na+/K+ pump, thereby impairing the ability of the cell to maintain its membrane potential and subsequently the integrity of the cell membrane.[13] Acidosis occurs

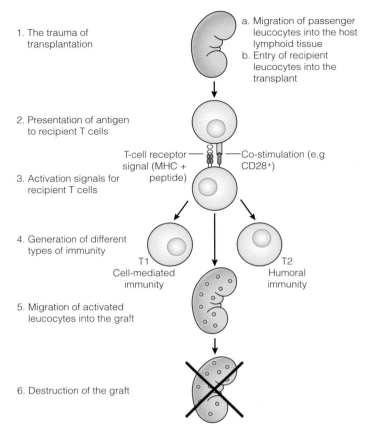

1. The trauma of transplantation

   a. Migration of passenger leucocytes into the host lymphoid tissue
   b. Entry of recipient leucocytes into the transplant

2. Presentation of antigen to recipient T cells

   T-cell receptor signal (MHC + peptide) —— Co-stimulation (e.g CD28+)

3. Activation signals for recipient T cells

4. Generation of different types of immunity

   T1 Cell-mediated immunity

   T2 Humoral immunity

5. Migration of activated leucocytes into the graft

6. Destruction of the graft

Figure 3.3 • The evolution of the immune response following kidney transplantation.

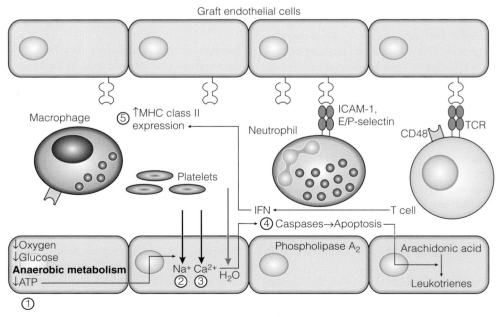

Graft endothelial cells

Macrophage

⑤ ↑MHC class II expression

Platelets

Neutrophil

ICAM-1, E/P-selectin

CD48   TCR

IFN ←—— T cell

④ Caspases→Apoptosis

↓Oxygen
↓Glucose
Anaerobic metabolism
↓ATP

Na+ Ca2+ H_2O
② ③

Phospholipase A_2

Arachidonic acid

Leukotrienes

①

Figure 3.4 • Mechanisms of ischaemia reperfusion injury. (1) Anaerobic metabolism. (2) Breakdown of Na+/K+ pump, with resultant cellular oedema. (3) Acidosis leads to Ca^{2+} influx, and mitochondrial injury. (4) Activation of phospholipase A2 and caspases. (5) Increased MHC class II expression, which intensifies the immune response.

as an immediate result of anaerobic glycolysis and has been shown to correlate well with tissue injury.[14] This is one of a number of mechanisms that causes an influx of calcium into the cell, leading to mitochondrial injury as well as activation of proteases and phospholipases, including caspases and phospholipase A2. The generation of free radicals also contributes directly to tissue injury.

Reperfusion injury

Ischaemia induces an acute inflammatory response, leading to endothelial activation with increased permeability and adhesion molecule expression. On reperfusion, circulating inflammatory cells become adherent to the activated epithelium, with a resulting increase in release and expression of proinflammatory mediators (cytokines, chemokines and adhesion molecules), leading to further recruitment and activation of leucocytes.[15,16]

During the hours or days following the ischaemic insult, repair and regeneration occur alongside apoptosis (characterised by nuclear fragmentation, plasma membrane blebbing and cell shrinkage), autophagy cell-associated death (with loss of organelles and accumulation of vacuoles) and necrosis (with plasma membrane rupture and leakage of proteases extracellularly). The fate of the organ will depend on whether regeneration or cell death prevails.[17]

Sterile inflammation

IRI is a form of sterile inflammation, in which endogenous DAMPs are released into the extracellular compartment as a result of tissue injury.[18] These DAMPs signal through various pattern-recognition receptors, such as Toll-like receptors (TLRs), and result in the activation of effector pathways, including the production of proinflammatory cytokines and chemokines.[19]

This early phase of sterile inflammation is characterised by the rapid infiltration of innate inflammatory cells, including neutrophils, macrophages and monocytes. The functional contributions of these cells may depend upon the sequence of events surrounding their priming, but in this early phase will include propagation of the immune response, phagocytosis of damaged cells and antigen presentation.

As a result of natural antibodies, innate recognition proteins can react to self in a process known as innate autoimmunity; this leads to the activation of complement. The complement system is an immune surveillance system set up to detect cellular debris, apoptotic cells and non-self, and plays an important role in the amplification of the immune response seen in sterile inflammation, and as such is an attractive target for therapy.[20,21]

Adaptive immune response to IRI

There is evidence for the role of CD4+ T cells in the pathogenesis of IRI. This has been shown in a number of models of IRI, including renal,[22] hepatic,[23] cardiac[24] and cerebral.[25] In contrast, regulatory T cells may have a protective effect in IRI, with evidence emerging in models of ischaemic stroke[26] and renal IRI.[27]

Through this wide range of mechanisms, IRI leads to increased expression of HLA antigens by the graft, as well as the release of proinflammatory chemokines, cytokines and adhesion molecules within the graft; this leads to increased recruitment of effector immune cells into the graft and is likely to increase the risk of rejection.[10]

The alloimmune response

Recognition of alloantigen by T cells

Alloimmunity refers to the initiation of an immune response against antigen from the same species. The most common form of alloimmune injury is initiated when donor alloantigens are presented to recipient T cells by APCs. T cells engage MHC with their receptors either directly on donor-derived APCs, or indirectly as processed peptide in the context of self-MHC. A third 'semi-direct' pathway has more recently been elucidated, and all three are illustrated in **Fig. 3.5**.

Direct allorecognition

Donor-derived APCs (typically dendritic cells), known as passenger leucocytes, carry donor antigens from the transplanted organ to the recipient's draining lymph nodes. These donor-derived APCs express high levels of MHC class I and II laden with antigen and are capable of activating both CD4+ and CD8+ T cells. This pathway of allorecognition is characterised by a high frequency of responder T cells (100-fold greater than for a response to

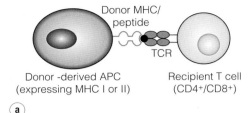

Direct antigen presentation

Donor MHC/
peptide

TCR

Donor -derived APC
(expressing MHC I or II)

Recipient T cell
(CD4+/CD8+)

(a)

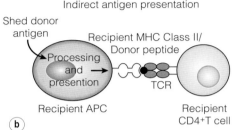

Indirect antigen presentation

Shed donor
antigen

Recipient MHC Class II/
Donor peptide

Processing
and
presentation

TCR

Recipient APC

Recipient
CD4+T cell

(b)

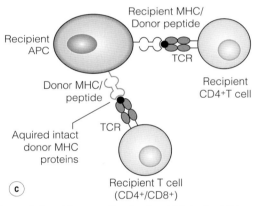

Semi-direct antigen presentation

Recipient MHC/
Donor peptide

Recipient
APC

TCR

Donor MHC/
peptide

Recipient
CD4+T cell

Aquired intact
donor MHC
proteins

TCR

Recipient T cell
(CD4+/CD8+)

(c)

Figure 3.5 • Allorecognition by direct **(a)**, indirect **(b)** and semi-direct **(c)** pathways.

conventional antigens) and is critical in the initiation of the alloresponse. CD4[+] T cells with exclusively direct allospecificity can effect transplant rejection, in the absence of the indirect pathway, and CD8[+] cytotoxic T cells,[28] and indeed may contribute to the development of chronic rejection.[29]

Indirect allorecognition

The indirect pathway refers to recognition of processed peptides of allogeneic histocompatibility antigens presented by self-MHC in a restricted manner.[30] Thus, donor protein is processed and presented in the context of MHC class II by recipient APCs, such

as dendritic cells and macrophages, to CD4[+] T cells. There is evidence to demonstrate the involvement of the indirect pathway in both acute[31,32] and chronic[33] graft rejection.

Semi-direct allorecognition

These two seemingly distinct pathways of allorecognition suggest that there is no crosstalk between T cells activated by direct or indirect means. However, CD4[+] T cells with indirect anti-donor specificity can amplify or reduce direct pathway CD8[+] T-cell responses.[34] This observation points to interactions between direct and indirectly activated T cells during graft rejection. Thus, a third semi-direct pathway has been proposed, in which recipient APCs can acquire functional MHC molecules from donor cells and this acquired MHC is capable of stimulating antigen-specific T-cell responses.[35] This allows a single APC to stimulate both direct CD8[+] T cells and indirect pathway CD4[+] T cells.[36] Recent work supports this hypothesis, demonstrating the presence of cells expressing both donor MHC class I and II molecules, allowing indirectly activated CD4[+] T cells to regulate directly activated CD8[+] T cells.[37]

Co-stimulation

T cells require two signals to stimulate T-cell activation: signal 1 is the antigen-specific binding of the MHC–peptide complex to the T-cell receptor (TCR) and signal 2 is the engagement of the co-stimulatory molecule. Signalling through the TCR alone is insufficient in itself to lead to T-cell activation and in the absence of co-stimulation (signal 2) may lead to anergy[38,39] (a state of immune unresponsiveness). Targeting co-stimulatory pathways is clearly attractive for anti-rejection therapy and has been the focus of considerable interest both experimentally and in clinical trials (see Chapter 5).

CD28 is the best characterised co-stimulatory molecule and is critical for T-cell proliferation and survival. CD28 is expressed on the surface of T cells and has two main ligands: CD80 (B7-1), which is constitutively expressed, and CD86 (B7-2), which is rapidly up-regulated on activated APCs.[40] CD28 co-signals can stabilise messenger RNA of cytokines and amplify the activation of nuclear factor of activated T cells (NFAT) and nuclear factor κB (NFκB).[41]

Co-inhibitory molecules

More recently, another T-cell surface receptor that binds the same ligands as CD28 has been identified, known as cytotoxic T-lymphocyte antigen-4 (CTLA-4).[42] This is up-regulated on T-cell activation and binds to B7-1 and B7-2 with much higher avidity than CD28. In contrast to CD28, CTLA-4 dampens T-cell responses by several mechanisms: it reverses the 'stop signal' needed for firm contact between T cells and APC, thus limiting their contact,[43] and blocks the formation of microclusters of kinases that is required for effective transmission of signals from the TCR complex.[44] In addition, there is evidence to suggest that CTLA-4 is required for optimal function of regulatory T cells (Tregs).[45]

Other co-inhibitory pathways exist and another potential therapeutic target is a second member of the CD28–CTLA-4 family, programme death-1 receptor (PD-1). Signalling through PD-1 leads to negative regulation of T- and B-cell activity, with decreased proliferation and cytokine production.[46,47] In a murine model of hepatic IRI, blockade of signalling through PD-1 led to a worse injury.[48]

Such co-inhibitory pathways are attractive targets for therapy. The first strategy adopted was to develop a soluble recombinant fusion protein–CTLA–4Ig (abatacept), which was potent at inhibiting B7-1- but not B7-2-mediated T-cell responses.[49] A modified version of CTLA–4Ig, belatacept, was subsequently developed through mutagenesis.[50] In the seminal non-human primate study, Larsen and colleagues tested belatacept as monotherapy and in combination with either basiliximab or MMF and steroids. Belatacept was superior to CTLA-4Ig monotherapy in maintaining renal allograft survival. However, renal function declined during ongoing belatacept treatment, highlighting the need for adjunctive therapies. When used in combination with basiliximab induction, MMF and steroids, belatacept was shown to be safe and efficacious.[50] Recent phase II and III clinical trials have yielded promising results, and this strategy holds promise to improve the care of transplant patients.[51]

T-cell synapse

T-cell receptor engagement through MHC–peptide complex binding (signal 1) and co-stimulation (signal 2) results in the clustering and recruitment by the plasma membrane of many signalling molecules. This molecular arrangement is known as the immunological synapse, and this dynamic protein array modulates T-cell activation, depending on cytoskeletal–cell membrane interactions, and is orchestrated by the coordinated movements of proteins congregated within lipid rafts. This results in an orderly congregation of molecules known as a supramolecular activation complex (SMAC). Although the signal 1/signal 2 model of co-stimulation proved useful, it is increasingly apparent that distinction between adhesion molecules and co-stimulatory molecules is not absolute. The kinetics of TCR binding, non-antigen-specific interactions between T cells and APCs, the presence of cytokines and the state of T-cell maturation all contribute to determining cell fate on TCR engagement.

TCR signalling

Following the formation of the immunological synapse, diverse signalling pathways are activated that ultimately lead to transcriptional activation and de novo expression of a range of genes, including those encoding cytokines and new cell-surface proteins. Relevant pathways include the following:

- phospholipase C-γ1 activates NFAT;
- protein kinase C-θ, which acts through NFκB and activator protein 1 (AP1);
- renin–angiotensin system (RAS)–guanosine-releasing protein (GRP) and the growth factor receptor bound protein 2 complex, which act through RAS.

These signalling pathways coordinate to drive proliferation and differentiation of the T lymphocytes, and can be influenced by different co-stimulatory molecules.

T-cell differentiation: the role of cytokines

The interaction of T cells with APCs is central to the development of the alloimmune response against the graft, and this is mediated through various effector pathways. A productive immune response generally results in the proliferation and differentiation of CD4$^+$ T (helper) cells, that drive and direct antigen-specific immune responses. The type of effector response is defined and shaped by the particular patterns of cytokines delivered to cells of the innate immune system. These effector mechanisms evolved to deliver effective host defence, but at the same time are designed to maintain self-tolerance.

In alloimmune responses, naive helper T cells are polarised towards various cell lineages, including Th1, Th2, Th17 and regulatory T cells (see below), defined according to the cytokine profile they produce (**Fig. 3.6**); this is referred to as signal 3. The antigen load, state of maturation of APCs, as well as the polarisation of T cells to a particular effector or regulatory lineage, ultimately determine the type of effector response and its effect on the transplanted organ.

T-cell responses

T helper 1 (Th1) response

The Th1 respone is characterised by interferon-gamma (IFN-γ) production and is key to driving the cellular immune response, with characteristic features of dense lymphocytic infiltration, tubulitis (in the kidney) and tissue destruction.

T helper 2 (Th2) response

Th2 cells drive the humoral response, with B-cell activation resulting in plasma cell production, antibody release and antibody-dependent cellular cytotoxicity. It is characterised by the production of interleukin-4 (IL-4), IL-5 and IL-13.

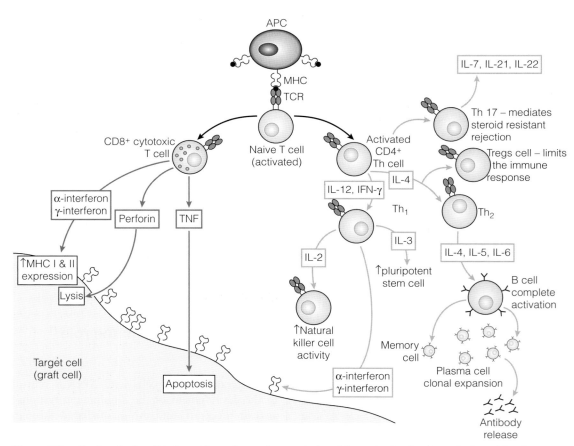

Figure 3.6 • T-cell activation: T helper cells, acting as the conductor of the orchestra, lead to activation of T cells along different pathways, depending on the cytokine milieu, and resulting in cell-mediated rejection, antibody-mediated rejection, or regulation.

T helper 17 (Th17) response

Th17 immunity is characterised by the production of IL-17, IL-21 and IL-22, with subsequent release of a host of proinflammatory cytokines (IL-6, IL-8, tumour necrosis factor (TNF)-α) and chemokines (such as CXCL1, CXCL2, CCL2 and CCL20).[52] IL-17 is a potent stimulator and recruiter of innate immune cells, including neutrophils and monocytes. IL-17-producing cells have been detected in renal allografts undergoing rejection.[53] There is evidence to suggest that they may play a role in acute rejection, particularly when other immune responses are suppressed by conventional immunosuppression.[54]

T regulatory (Treg) response

There is increasing recognition that Tregs are important in self-tolerance and may play a role in transplant tolerance. The manipulation of the Th17–Treg axis is an attractive therapeutic option that has been exploited both experimentally and more recently in early clinical trials.[55]

There are two main subsets of regulatory T cells (Tregs), thymus-derived natural Tregs (nTregs) and induced T regs (iTregs) generated in the periphery from conventional T cells as a consequence of peripheral exposure to antigens in a tolerogenic environment. They are functionally and phenotypically heterogeneous, with varying expression profiles throughout their lifetime. They can be induced to differentiate into pathogenic effector cells, depending on the cytokine milieu; this is termed plasticity.

In order to prove their in vivo capacity, humanised mouse models have been developed, with the reconstitution of immunodeficient mice with human immune cells. Results from these studies have shown promise, with significant reduction in vasculopathy in an incorporated human aortic graft when mice were reconstituted with peripheral blood mononuclear cells (PBMCs) with co-transfer of expanded Tregs compared with PBMCs alone.[56] Recently similar strategies have been introduced into haemopoietic stem cell transplantation, in which ex vivo expanded Tregs were administered following bone marrow transplantation, with evidence to suggest a reduction in the incidence of graft versus host disease.[57] A European trial has recently begun to evaluate the safety of various immunomodulatory cell products in living donor kidney transplantation, and this includes administration of nTregs (the ONE study). The major risk of all cell therapies is the potential for plasticity, in which a protective regulatory cell differentiates into a pathogenic effector in vivo.

The effector arm of the immune response

Migration of activated leucocytes

In order to enter a site of inflammation, activated leucocytes must migrate across the vascular endothelium. This is mediated through a variety of adhesion molecules and chemokines, and by cell-to-cell interactions between the leucocyte and the endothelium. Activated cells and memory cells express a range of chemokine receptors and adhesion molecules that promote migration into peripheral tissues.

Cell-to-cell interactions

The adhesion of leucocytes to the endothelium is a multistep process, involving a series of interactions between the leucocyte and the endothelial cell.[58] Cell adhesion molecules involved are selectins, integrins and immunoglobulin superfamily members, such as intercellular adhesion molecules (ICAMs) and vascular cell adhesion molecules (VCAMs).

The initial step is attachment and rolling; the cell may then detach or be activated, adhere and transmigrate. Rolling of leucocytes along the endothelium allows them to sample the endothelial environment, whilst still being able to detach and travel elsewhere. Attachment is largely mediated by selectin binding, and the passage of leucocytes through the endothelium is mediated by integrins, ICAMs and VCAMs. IRI results in the up-regulation of selectins, ICAM-1 and VCAM-1, and thus the allograft is primed for the subsequent alloimmune response.

Chemokines

Chemotactic cytokines – hence chemokines – are a family of small soluble proteins, which have the ability to induce directed migration of responsive cells (chemotaxis); this may be homeostatic trafficking in the normal immune system, or directed towards sites of inflammation. These can be divided into four groups based on specific sequence motifs:

- *CC chemokines* are important in mononuclear cell recruitment (e.g. MCP-1, RANTES).
- *CXC chemokines* are involved in neutrophil recruitment (e.g. CXCL-9, CXCL-10).

- *C chemokines.* Two chemokines have been defined in this group, XCL1 (lymphotactin-X) and XCL2 (lymphotactin-β). These attract immature T cells to the thymus.
- CX_3C *chemokines* (e.g. *fractalkine* – a potent chemoattractant of monocytes and T cells).

In transplantation, a variety of chemokines are involved in graft infiltration during the alloimmune response.[59] Modest reduction in rejection rates has been observed in mouse models through blockade of specific chemokines, but this has not been borne out in larger animal models, probably due to the involvement of an array of chemokines.

Cellular mechanisms of injury

Antigen-specific cytotoxic CD8-positive T cells

In cell culture, MHC-mismatched lymphocytes proliferate and produce cytokines in response to one another in the mixed lymphocyte reaction (MLR). The resulting cytokine production allows the differentiation of precursor cytotoxic T cells into effector cells (CD8+ T cells) that lyse target cells bearing mismatched antigens. Evidence for the contribution of CD8+ T cells to the effector response includes: delayed onset of graft rejection in the absence of CD8+ cells in some animal models;[60] these cells can be recovered from allografts undergoing rejection;[61] and cloned populations of CD8+ T cells can cause tissue damage similar to that associated with rejection. Graft destruction can, however, occur in their absence, and their presence does not inevitably lead to rejection. CD8+ T cells kill their targets in a variety of ways, including through the action of perforins and granzymes that attack membrane integrity, through Fas-mediated apoptosis and the secretion of TNF-α.

Natural killer (NK) cells

NK cells are recognised to provide an important early innate immune response to viral and bacterial pathogens, and for the surveillance of stressed and transformed autologous cells. The primary paradigm of NK cell killing was the notion of 'missing self', especially regarding deficient autologous MHC I expression. NK cells are known to be mediators of MHC-disparate haematopoietic stem cell rejection, but in the context of solid-organ transplantation, NK cells are neither necessary nor sufficient to mediate allograft rejection independent of an intact adaptive immune system. Nevertheless, they have the potential to enhance adaptive immune responses, through contributing to the maturation of APCs, augmenting the helper T-cell response, and enhancing IRI and endothelial cell injury. Despite a correlation between NK cell reactivity and allograft rejection, NK cells also have important regulatory properties, and can facilitate allograft tolerance induction. This may be mediated by the effect of NK cells on DCs; NK cells can drive DC maturation, but in the right environment NK–DC interaction may also result in the killing of immature DCs. The relative role of NK cells and Tregs in the induction of tolerance has been examined, with a possible role for NK cells in the early post-transplant period, and a requirement for Tregs for long-term allograft survival.[62]

Macrophages

Macrophages are key elements of the innate immune response, and can be classified as M1, or classically activated macrophages, or M2, alternatively activated macrophages. M1 macrophages arise in response to T-cell-produced IFN-γ and TNF-α produced by APCs and are thought of as proinflammatory. M2 macrophages develop in response to IL-4 produced by T cells or granulocytes, and may be involved in tissue repair.

There is increasing evidence of accumulation of macrophages in both acute and chronic allograft injury, but their role is complex, and varies with time and stage of injury.[63] In rodent models of IRI, there is an early accumulation of proinflammatory M1 macrophages, which are F4/80-low and Ly6C-high, and produce IL-6, IL-1 and TNF-α; experimental macrophage depletion at an early stage confers protection, but if performed later may contribute to a delay in repair. This is further supported by evidence of a temporal relationship between M1 and M2 phenotypes in the course of renal IRI.[64] The relative contribution of these cells in organ transplantation is not known, although there are experimental data to suggest that early depletion of monocyte/macrophages may have a beneficial impact.[65]

B cells

B cells are positive regulators of humoral immune responses through their ability to differentiate into antibody-secreting plasma cells. They also appear to have other significant roles in the alloimmune response, such as in antigen presentation, T-cell activation, memory formation and cytokine production. While B-cell depletion is an intuitive objective in desensitisation protocols, the evidence for its effect on outcome following transplantation is controversial, with some work demonstrating a negative impact of B-cell depletion on acute rejection rates,[66] and its role in treating chronic antibody-mediated rejection is unclear.[67] This may be explained by the discovery of IL-10-producing regulatory B cells, which appear to provide protection in models of autoimmunity, including experimental autoimmune encephalomyelitis,[68] collagen-induced arthritis[69] and type 1 diabetes.[70] The role of such 'regulatory' B cells in transplantation remains to be defined.

Different populations of B cells have been described within allografts. Non-cluster-forming, scattered B cells (CD20 negative) observed within the tubular interstitium of kidney transplants are associated with antibody production and are likely to represent the classic antibody-producing plasma cells. Nodular B-cell-rich infiltrates have been identified in chronically rejected renal allografts and in biopsies of acute transplant rejection; these are CD20 positive.[67,71] Such B-cell-rich infiltrates have been associated with the development of tertiary lymphoid tissue (TLT). TLT is histologically similar to secondary lymphoid tissue found in normal lymph nodes and spleen, and contains macrophages, dendritic cells, lymphatics, T lymphocytes and high endothelial venules (HEVs). The function and significance of TLT is unknown, but may have a protective role in the allograft.[72]

Endothelial cells

Endothelial cells of donor origin are uniquely located at the interface between donor and recipient circulations, and have been implicated in graft rejection.[73] Endothelial cells may promote allorecognition by a crosstalk mechanism, which involves recruitment and transformation of recipient monocytes into efficient APCs, which then mature and present antigen via the indirect pathway. Endothelial cells express MHC class I and II molecules, and have been shown to be capable of directly stimulating CD8+ T cells, thereby triggering acute rejection.[74] However, there is evidence to suggest that activated endothelial cells

may be able to tolerise T cells activated via the direct pathway of allorecognition.[75]

Rejection of the allograft

Classical experiments first demonstrated the specificity of tissue rejection. By fusing the embryos from mice of two different genetic origins the tissues of the resulting mosaic offspring were made up of patches of cells from each parental type. Skin from the heterozygous offspring was then grafted to mice of either parental origin, resulting in the cells of the other-parent type being rejected, leaving cells of recipient type intact. From these initial experiments we have come to understand and investigate the non-specific (innate) and specific (adaptive) mechanisms of rejection.

Cell-mediated rejection

Acute allograft rejection is most commonly cell mediated and initiated when donor antigens are presented to the T cells of the recipient by APCs, as described earlier in the chapter. Interstitial mononuclear cells, including CD4+ and CD8+ T cells, and inflammatory cytokines and chemokines accumulate in sites of acute cellular rejection. Activated macrophages secrete proinflammatory cytokines such as IL-1, IL-12, IL-18, TNF-α and IFN-γ, which impair the function of the graft and intensify T-cell-mediated rejection.[76] T cells mediate cytotoxicity directly through contact with allograft epithelial cells and the effects of locally released cytokines indirectly activate inflammatory and vascular endothelial cells. CD8+ T cells release perforin, which directly perforates target-cell membranes, allowing secreted granzymes-A and -B to enter cells and induce caspase-mediated apoptosis. The Fas ligand on CD8+ cells activates Fas receptor on cells of the allograft, also inducing caspase-mediated apoptosis. CD4+ T cells can attack cells expressing minor MHC antigens and can also secrete TNF-α and TNF-β, which bind to TNF receptors on endothelial or epithelial cells, causing them to undergo apoptosis. The resulting T-cell-mediated rejection is characterised by interstitial infiltration, intimal arteritis and, in the kidney, tubulitis (see **Fig. 3.7**). Chronic T-cell-mediated rejection results in arterial intimal fibrosis with mononuclear cell infiltration and formation of a neointima.

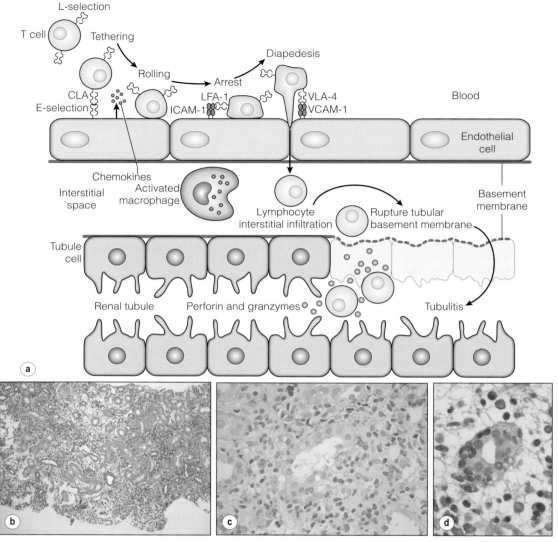

Figure 3.7 • Cell-mediated rejection (plus histology). **(a)** Mechanism of cell-mediated rejection. **(b)** Low power picture of acute rejection, showing dense lymphocytic infiltrate. **(c)** Tubulitis. **(d)** Arteritis.

Antibody-mediated rejection (AMR)

Hyperacute AMR results from preformed antibodies resulting from prior sensitisation, such as foetal–maternal reactivity, previous allografts or blood transfusions. Immediately following perfusion of the allograft with recipient blood, deposition of antibodies against HLA antigens expressed on the endothelium of the microvasculature occurs.

Similarly, acute AMR requires the synthesis of 'recall' antibodies to HLA antigens by memory B cells and generation of plasma cells; this may occur days or months following transplantation. The damaged endothelial cells release and display cell-surface DAMPs, including von Willebrand factor and P-selectin, which promote platelet aggregation, secretion of cytokines and chemokines, and the chemoattractants of complement C3a and C5a. C4d is a marker of classic complement activation and is frequently found in organ capillary

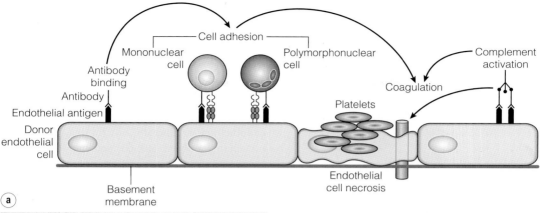

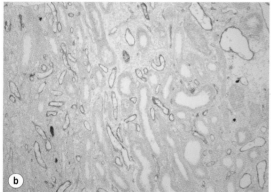

Figure 3.8 • Antibody-mediated rejection (plus histology). **(a)** Mechanism of antibody-mediated rejection. **(b)** C4d-positive staining, suggestive of antibody mediated rejection.

beds, specifically peritubular capillaries in the kidney (see **Fig. 3.8**). C5b triggers the assembly of the membrane-attack complex, which causes localised endothelial necrosis and apoptosis, and detachment of endothelial cells from the basement membrane. With continuing injury to the vasculature, microthrombi form resulting in haemorrhage, arterial-wall necrosis and infarction.[77] Increasingly it has been recognised that antibody-mediated changes may coincide in parallel with the classically defined process of cellular rejection. Furthermore, it is increasingly speculated that chronic AMR is responsible for insidious subclinical allograft injury.[78]

Studies in human renal transplantation have been important in providing evidence for a role of circulating antibodies in this process, including a large prospective study in which de novo production of donor HLA-specific antibodies was found in 51% of 112 renal transplant recipients with graft failure compared to 2% of 123 stable controls. Furthermore, the presence of alloantibodies predicted the subsequent development of chronic allograft rejection and graft loss.[79]

Classification of rejection

Various classifications of rejection have existed over the years, based on timing following transplantation (hyperacute, acute and chronic), on pathophysioloical changes (interstitial, vascular), or on severity/response to treatment. With the diversity of these methods there has been a move to standardise classification. The process of rejection in the renal allograft is the most well studied as it is the most frequently transplanted solid organ. The Banff classification was first proposed in 1993 to standardise pathological diagnoses of rejection and this has since been widely adopted.[80] Other solid-organ transplants, which include liver, pancreas, heart and lung, have tended to follow the structure of the renal classification, reflecting the similar underlying immune–pathological processes, as shown in Box 3.1.[81]

Future developments

Tolerance

Tolerance, defined as the ability of the allograft to survive in the long term in the absence of immunosuppression, has been termed the 'holy grail' of allo-transplantation. Virtually all patients receive maintenance immunosuppression in an attempt to maximise the function and survival of the allograft. However, the long-term use of immunosuppressive agents is associated with undesirable side-effects that have the potential to limit the survival of the patient and transplanted organ, as well as to compromise quality of life. Tolerance remains a rarity in clinical transplantation and we currrently lack both a therapeutic regimen to induce tolerance or a validated biomarker pattern that is predictive of tolerance.[82] Strategies that have shown tolerogenic effects in animal models and are ready for clinical trial include the combination of co-stimulatory blockade reagents and T-cell depletion. Early clinical trials are under way to try and capitalise on the anti-inflammatory and tolerogenic properties of Tregs;[83] it is hoped that they may promote graft survival through the induction of tolerance.

There is also growing evidence that several immune pathways previously regarded purely as graft destructive can also participate in tolerance induction. Although the presence of proinflammatory and cytolytic activity usually correlates with allograft injury, there is increasing evidence that there is also a regulatory role for many of these effector cells, such as T cells,[84] B cells,[85] macrophages[86] and NK cells.[87]

Accommodation

In blood group incompatible renal transplantation perioperative removal of antibodies from the recipient can result in successful transplantation. Subsequently, anti-blood group antibodies can rise to pretreatment levels, adhere to the microvasculature and activate complement, but interestingly the endothelium is generally not injured.[88] This phenomenon has been termed 'accommodation', but the mechanisms responsible are not entirely understood. Possible explanations include a change in the effector properties of antibodies directed against the donor, a change in the properties or expression of antigen targeted by anti-graft antibodies, modification of the complement cascade such that its effector functions cause little or no injury to graft endothelium or an acquired resistance of an organ or tissue to injury by complement or other noxious factors.[89]

Privileged sites are those in which tissue allografts appear to elicit a weak immune response and consequently there may be prolonged allograft survival. These sites include the anterior chamber of the eye, the cornea, the brain and the testis. They are typified by absent or limited lymphatic drainage. The degree of 'privilege' seems to vary depending on the nature of the transplanted tissue as well as the site of transplantation. The liver is an unusual vascularised graft in that, despite its extensive blood supply and high immune cell content, it often fails to elicit rejection and may protect co-transplanted organs from rejection despite their usual immunogenicity. Outbred pigs often fail to reject orthotopic liver allografts and simultaneous renal allografts from the same donor show prolonged survival despite the fact that they would otherwise have been rejected. In rat strain combinations, in which an orthotopic liver allograft is not rejected, the graft may even overcome a previously existing state of sensitisation of the host against donor histocompatibility antigen.[90] Similarly, although crossmatching has been demonstrated to be of some relevance in liver transplantation outcome, implanted grafts survive well despite a positive CDC crossmatch.

Xenotransplantation

All animals apart from Old World primates and man possess a cell-surface antigen containing the epitope 'alpha-Gal' to which humans produce complement-fixing antibodies. These antibodies cause immediate rejection of animal cells when transplanted into humans, and have been a significant obstacle to the development of xenotransplantation. The immune rejection of cellular xenotransplants is usually stronger and more immediate than with allotransplants. Advances in the genetic engineering of pigs have resulted in pigs that do not present the alpha-Gal epitope and they have been the subjects of recent studies. The reactivity of human T cells for pig MHC antigen in these animals is still being investigated, with evidence to suggest that the response is similar in strength and specificity to a T-cell or HLA-specific antibody allogeneic response.[91]

Xenografting has been used in clinical practice for many years, with the use of frame-mounted porcine and bovine heart valves. Here animal tissue undergoes fixation with glutaraldehye, which was originally thought to reduce immunogenicity through the cross-linking of antigens. It may be that evading the immune system, rather than inducing tolerance or immunosuppression, would be a more desirable strategy in xenotransplantation.

This strategy of immune evasion may be more amenable to cellular transplants compared to solid organs. Porcine islet transplants in humans have been reported: intrahepatic transplantation of foetal pig islets using systemic immunosuppression has been performed with no discernible clinical effect.[92] In two different studies, co-transplantation of porcine islets and Sertoli cells either in a subcutaneous pre-vascularised device or protected by microencapsulation have been tried in type 1 diabetic humans with some clinical benefit derived; hypoglycaemic unawareness in particular seemed amenable to the microencapsulation approach.[93,94]

Porcine corneal transplantation has gathered interest owing to the perceived low immunogenicity and implantation into an immune-privileged site reflected by low rejection rate in human allografts. To date, neither corneal nor solid organs have undergone experimental human xenotransplantation.

Tissue engineering

In recent years, there has been considerable progress in the translation of engineered tissues into clinical application. Using autologous urothelial and muscle cells grown in culture and seeded on to a biodegradable bladder-shaped scaffold made of collagen, bladder augmentation has been performed.[95] Donor tissue has also been used (following decellularisation, using a human donor trachea colonised by autologous cultured epithelial cells and mesenchymal stem-cell-derived chondrocytes) to replace a segment of trachea.[96] Experimentally decellularised organs have been successfully used as scaffolds for heart and liver stem cells or precursors to populate,[97] but these have not yet undergone in vivo studies. The ultimate goal is to reduce or ameliorate immunogenicity by removing MHC antigens from donor tissue or constructing a patient's own tissue de novo.

Improvements in IRI

Reduction in IRI aims to reduce acute injury and delayed graft function, which consequently may reduce cellular and humoral responses aginst the graft.

Ischaemic pre-conditioning (IPC) is a surgical manoeuvre in which an organ is paradoxically protected by a brief period of ischaemia and reperfusion immediately prior to a longer index ischaemic event, which by itself would normally lead to injury.[11,12] Several small randomised controlled trials have looked at the effectiveness of IPC in both liver transplantation and resection; subsequent Cochrane reviews conclude that further trials are still required to evaluate its role in hepatic and transplant surgery.[13,14] Human cardiac clinical studies so far have been unable to reproduce the profound tissue-protective effects observed in animal studies.[98,99]

Soluble agents perfused into the donor organ or given systemically are also currently undergoing clinical investigation, including heme arginate, which was shown to be protective in an animal model of renal IRI.[100] Therapeutic gases including hydrogen, nitric oxide, hydrogen sulphide and carbon monoxide have been tested experimentally and shown to reduce oxidative stress. In a small trial, inhaled nitric oxide reduced IRI with restoration of liver function and lowered hepatocyte apoptosis following liver transplantation.[101]

Recent interest has turned to micro RNAs (miRNAs), which are post-transcriptional regulators that bind to complementary sequences on target messenger RNA transcripts and usually result in translational repression or target degradation and gene silencing. Expression of specific miRNAs may alter IRI, and in a mouse model of myocardial ischaemia injury was reduced with exogenous miRNA administration.[102]

Ex vivo perfusion techniques of solid organs are gaining interest. A randomised controlled trial of cold perfusion of kidneys has shown reduced delayed graft function compared to standard cold storage, presumably due to some reduction in IRI.[103] Specific benefit has been shown in the field of lung transplantation with ex vivo lung perfusion (EVLP) for donors of marginal quality (Maastricht category II); results from randomised trials are required before this strategy can be recommended.[104]

Acknowledgements

We would like to thank David McMorran and Lucinda Bell for preparing the figures.

Key points

- The fundamental principle of transplant immunology is based on the body's ability to recognise 'non-self' as foreign.
- The role of MHC antigens is to present foreign peptide to T cells, and they exist in two classes: MHC class I (HLA-A, -B and -C) and MHC class II (HLA-DP, -DQ and -DR).
- Ischaemia–reperfusion injury, occurring as an inevitable consequence of events around the time of transplantation, causes endothelial cell damage within the graft, up-regulation of HLA molecules, and sets the scene for the alloimmune response.
- Antigen is presented in the context of MHC class I to CD8$^+$ T cells, and MHC class II to CD4$^+$ T cells, through the direct, indirect or semi-direct pathways of allorecognition.
- Following antigen presentation to the T-cell receptor (signal 1), a second co-stimulatory signal is required in order for T cells to undergo activation. Co-stimulatory and co-inhibitory pathways are being targeted in the development of new therapies.
- Following T-cell activation, naive T cells are induced to various cell lineages, which have important roles in the shaping of the immune response to the graft.
- Cell-mediated rejection is characterised by the infiltration of CD4$^+$ and CD8$^+$ T cells into the allograft, giving rise to inflammatory cytokine production and apoptosis.
- Antibody-mediated rejection involves the production of antibodies, which often target donor-specific HLA antigens; this results in endothelial damage, the activation of complement and microthrombi formation.
- Important future developments in transplantation include tolerance induction, tissue engineering and development of strategies to combat IRI.

References

1. Matzinger P. Friendly and dangerous signals: is the tissue in control? Nat Immunol 2007;8:11–3.

2. Matzinger P. Tolerance, danger, and the extended family. Annu Rev Immunol 1994;12:991–1045.

3. Snell GD, Higgins GF. Alleles at the histocompatibility-2 locus in the mouse as determined by tumor transplantation. Genetics 1951;36:306–10.

4. Opelz G, Dohler B. Effect of human leukocyte antigen compatibility on kidney graft survival: comparative analysis of two decades. Transplantation 2007;84:137–43.
   The study of UNOS data showed a significant improvement in graft survival over recent years, with HLA matching remaining a major contributor irrespective of the interval investigated.

5. Bahram S, Bresnahan M, Geraghty DE, et al. A second lineage of mammalian major histocompatibility complex class I genes. Proc Natl Acad Sci USA 1994;91:6259–63.

6. Lemy A, Andrien M, Lionet A, et al. Posttransplant major histocompatibility complex class I chain-related gene A antibodies and long-term graft outcomes in a multicenter cohort of 779 kidney transplant recipients. Transplantation 2012;Mar 29. Epub ahead of print.

7. Zou Y, Stastny P, Susal C, et al. Antibodies against MICA antigens and kidney-transplant rejection. N Engl J Med 2007;357:1293–300.

8. Cox ST, Stephens HA, Fernando R, et al. Major histocompatibility complex class I-related chain A allele mismatching, antibodies, and rejection in renal transplantation. Hum Immunol 2011;72:827–34.

9. Kim SJ, Gill JS. H-Y incompatibility predicts short-term outcomes for kidney transplant recipients. J Am Soc Nephrol 2009;20:2025–33.

10. Tilney NL, Guttmann RD. Effects of initial ischemia/reperfusion injury on the transplanted kidney. Transplantation 1997;64:945–7.

11. Quiroga I, McShane P, Koo DD, et al. Major effects of delayed graft function and cold ischaemia

time on renal allograft survival. Nephrol Dial Transplant 2006;21:1689–96.

12. Yarlagadda SG, Coca SG, Formica Jr RN, et al. Association between delayed graft function and allograft and patient survival: a systematic review and meta-analysis. Nephrol Dial Transplant 2009;24:1039–47.

13. Mangino MJ, Tian T, Ametani M, et al. Cytoskeletal involvement in hypothermic renal preservation injury. Transplantation 2008;85:427–36.

14. Kon ZN, Brown EN, Grant MC, et al. Warm ischemia provokes inflammation and regional hypercoagulability within the heart during off-pump coronary artery bypass: a possible target for serine protease inhibition. Eur J Cardiothorac Surg 2008;33:215–21.

15. Carden DL, Granger DN. Pathophysiology of ischaemia–reperfusion injury. J Pathol 2000;190:255–66.

16. Linfert D, Chowdhry T, Rabb H. Lymphocytes and ischemia–reperfusion injury. Transplant Rev 2009;23:1–10.

17. Kosieradzki M, Rowinski W. Ischemia/reperfusion injury in kidney transplantation: mechanisms and prevention. Transplant Proc 2008;40:3279–88.

18. Lu CY, Winterberg PD, Chen J, et al. Acute kidney injury: a conspiracy of toll-like receptor 4 on endothelia, leukocytes, and tubules. Pediatr Nephrol 2012;27(10):1847–54.

19. Chen GY, Nunez G. Sterile inflammation: sensing and reacting to damage. Nat Rev Immunol 2010;10:826–37.

20. Huang Y, Qiao F, Atkinson C, et al. A novel targeted inhibitor of the alternative pathway of complement and its therapeutic application in ischemia/reperfusion injury. J Immunol 2008;181:8068–76.

21. Patel H, Smith RA, Sacks SH, et al. Therapeutic strategy with a membrane-localizing complement regulator to increase the number of usable donor organs after prolonged cold storage. J Am Soc Nephrol 2006;17:1102–11.

22. Day YJ, Huang L, Ye H, et al. Renal ischemia–reperfusion injury and adenosine 2A receptor-mediated tissue protection: the role of CD4+ T cells and IFN-gamma. J Immunol 2006;176:3108–14.

23. Caldwell CC, Okaya T, Martignoni A, et al. Divergent functions of CD4+ T lymphocytes in acute liver inflammation and injury after ischemia–reperfusion. Am J Physiol Gastrointest Liver Physiol 2005;289:G969–76.

24. Yang Z, Day YJ, Toufektsian MC, et al. Infarct-sparing effect of A2A-adenosine receptor activation is due primarily to its action on lymphocytes. Circulation 2005;111:2190–7.

25. Yilmaz G, Arumugam TV, Stokes KY, et al. Role of T lymphocytes and interferon-gamma in ischemic stroke. Circulation 2006;113:2105–12.

26. Liesz A, Suri-Payer E, Veltkamp C, et al. Regulatory T cells are key cerebroprotective immunomodulators in acute experimental stroke. Nat Med 2009;15:192–9.

27. Gandolfo MT, Jang HR, Bagnasco SM, et al. Foxp3+ regulatory T cells participate in repair of ischemic acute kidney injury. Kidney Int 2009;76:717–29.

28. Pietra BA, Wiseman A, Bolwerk A, et al. CD4 T cell-mediated cardiac allograft rejection requires donor but not host MHC class II. J Clin Invest 2000;106:1003–10.

29. Nadazdin O, Boskovic S, Wee SL, et al. Contributions of direct and indirect alloresponses to chronic rejection of kidney allografts in nonhuman primates. J Immunol 2011;187:4589–97.

30. Liu Z, Braunstein NS, Suciu-Foca N. T cell recognition of allopeptides in context of syngeneic MHC. J Immunol 1992;148:35–40.

31. Tugulea S, Ciubotariu R, Colovai AI, et al. New strategies for early diagnosis of heart allograft rejection. Transplantation 1997;64:842–7.

32. Fangmann J, Dalchau R, Fabre JW. Rejection of skin allografts by indirect allorecognition of donor class I major histocompatibility complex peptides. J Exp Med 1992;175:1521–9.

33. Vella JP, Spadafora-Ferreira M, Murphy B, et al. Indirect allorecognition of major histocompatibility complex allopeptides in human renal transplant recipients with chronic graft dysfunction. Transplantation 1997;64:795–800.

34. Lee RS, Grusby MJ, Glimcher LH, et al. Indirect recognition by helper cells can induce donor-specific cytotoxic T lymphocytes in vivo. J Exp Med 1994;179:865–72.

35. Smyth LA, Herrera OB, Golshayan D, et al. A novel pathway of antigen presentation by dendritic and endothelial cells: implications for allorecognition and infectious diseases. Transplantation 2006;82:S15–8.

36. Herrera OB, Golshayan D, Tibbott R, et al. A novel pathway of alloantigen presentation by dendritic cells. J Immunol 2004;173:4828–37. Crosstalk between T cells with direct and indirect allospecificity suggests that a third pathway of allorecognition exists. This paper provides evidence of a third semi-direct pathway in which recipient dendritic cells acquire intact donor MHC molecules as well as presenting processed peptide in the context of host MHC.

37. Brown K, Sacks SH, Wong W. Coexpression of donor peptide/recipient MHC complex and intact donor MHC: evidence for a link between the direct and indirect pathways. Am J Transplant 2011;11:826–31.

38. Baxter AG, Hodgkin PD. Activation rules: the two-signal theories of immune activation. Nat Rev Immunol 2002;2:439–46.

39. Jenkins MK, Schwartz RH. Antigen presentation by chemically modified splenocytes induces antigen-specific T cell unresponsiveness in vitro and in vivo. J Exp Med 1987;165:302–19.

40. Lenschow DJ, Walunas TL, Bluestone JA. CD28/B7 system of T cell costimulation. Annu Rev Immunol 1996;14:233–58.

41. Rudd CE, Taylor A, Schneider H. CD28 and CTLA-4 coreceptor expression and signal transduction. Immunol Rev 2009;229:12–26.

42. Linsley PS, Brady W, Urnes M, et al. CTLA-4 is a second receptor for the B cell activation antigen B7. J Exp Med 1991;174:561–9.

43. Schneider H, Downey J, Smith A, et al. Reversal of the TCR stop signal by CTLA-4. Science 2006;313:1972–5.

44. Schneider H, Smith X, Liu H, et al. CTLA-4 disrupts ZAP70 microcluster formation with reduced T cell/APC dwell times and calcium mobilization. Eur J Immunol 2008;38:40–7.

45. Wing K, Onishi Y, Prieto-Martin P, et al. CTLA-4 control over Foxp3+ regulatory T cell function. Science 2008;322:271–5.

46. Agata Y, Kawasaki A, Nishimura H, et al. Expression of the PD-1 antigen on the surface of stimulated mouse T and B lymphocytes. Int Immunol 1996;8:765–72.

47. Fisicaro P, Valdatta C, Massari M, et al. Antiviral intrahepatic T-cell responses can be restored by blocking programmed death-1 pathway in chronic hepatitis B. Gastroenterology 2010;138:682–93.93 e1–4

48. Ji H, Shen X, Gao F, et al. Programmed death-1/B7-H1 negative costimulation protects mouse liver against ischemia and reperfusion injury. Hepatology 2010;52:1380–9.

49. Linsley PS, Greene JL, Brady W, et al. Human B7-1 (CD80) and B7-2 (CD86) bind with similar avidities but distinct kinetics to CD28 and CTLA-4 receptors. Immunity 1994;1:793–801.

50. Larsen CP, Pearson TC, Adams AB, et al. Rational development of LEA29Y (belatacept), a high-affinity variant of CTLA4-Ig with potent immunosuppressive properties. Am J Transplant 2005;5:443–53.
This important paper describes the evolution to belatacept and provides in vitro and in vivo evidence for this efficacy in renal transplantation.

51. Wekerle T, Grinyo JM. Belatacept: from rational design to clinical application. Transpl Int 2012;25:139–50.

52. Peters A, Lee Y, Kuchroo VK. The many faces of Th17 cells. Curr Opin Immunol 2011;23:702–6.

53. Loverre A, Tataranni T, Castellano G, et al. IL-17 expression by tubular epithelial cells in renal transplant recipients with acute antibody-mediated rejection. Am J Transplant 2011;11:1248–59.

54. Abadja F, Sarraj B, Ansari MJ. Significance of T helper 17 immunity in transplantation. Curr Opin Organ Transplant 2012;17:8–14.

55. Mitchell P, Afzali B, Lombardi G, et al. The T helper 17–regulatory T cell axis in transplant rejection and tolerance. Curr Opin Organ Transplant 2009;14:326–31.

56. Issa F, Hester J, Goto R, et al. Ex vivo-expanded human regulatory T cells prevent the rejection of skin allografts in a humanized mouse model. Transplantation 2010;90:1321–7.
This animal study first described the potential for regulatory T cells to prevent rejection.

57. Trzonkowski P, Bieniaszewska M, Juscinska J, et al. First-in-man clinical results of the treatment of patients with graft versus host disease with human ex vivo expanded CD4+ CD25+ CD127− T regulatory cells. Clin Immunol 2009;133:22–6.

58. Butcher EC, Picker LJ. Lymphocyte homing and homeostasis. Science 1996;272:60–6.

59. Inston NG, Cockwell P. The evolving role of chemokines and their receptors in acute allograft rejection. Nephrol Dial Transplant 2002;17:1374–9.

60. Madsen JC, Peugh WN, Wood KJ, et al. The effect of anti-L3T4 monoclonal antibody treatment on first-set rejection of murine cardiac allografts. Transplantation 1987;44:849–52.

61. Bradley JA, Mason DW, Morris PJ. Evidence that rat renal allografts are rejected by cytotoxic T cells and not by nonspecific effectors. Transplantation 1985;39:169–75.

62. Beilke JN, Gill RG. Frontiers in nephrology: the varied faces of natural killer cells in transplantation – contributions to both allograft immunity and tolerance. J Am Soc Nephrol 2007;18:2262–7.

63. Famulski KS, Kayser D, Einecke G, et al. Alternative macrophage activation-associated transcripts in T-cell-mediated rejection of mouse kidney allografts. Am J Transplant 2010;10:490–7.

64. Lee S, Huen S, Nishio H, et al. Distinct macrophage phenotypes contribute to kidney injury and repair. J Am Soc Nephrol 2011;22:317–26.

65. Qi F, Adair A, Ferenbach D, et al. Depletion of cells of monocyte lineage prevents loss of renal microvasculature in murine kidney transplantation. Transplantation 2008;86:1267–74.

66. Clatworthy MR, Watson CJ, Plotnek G, et al. B-cell-depleting induction therapy and acute cellular rejection. N Engl J Med 2009;360:2683–5.

67. Thaunat O, Patey N, Gautreau C, et al. B cell survival in intragraft tertiary lymphoid organs after rituximab therapy. Transplantation 2008;85:1648–53.

68. Matsushita T, Yanaba K, Bouaziz JD, et al. Regulatory B cells inhibit EAE initiation in mice while other B cells promote disease progression. J Clin Invest 2008;118:3420–30.

69. Gray M, Miles K, Salter D, et al. Apoptotic cells protect mice from autoimmune inflammation by the induction of regulatory B cells. Proc Natl Acad Sci U S A 2007;104:14080–5.

70. Hussain S, Delovitch TL. Intravenous transfusion of BCR-activated B cells protects NOD mice from type 1 diabetes in an IL-10-dependent manner. J Immunol 2007;179:7225–32.

71. Zarkhin V, Kambham N, Li L, et al. Characterization of intra-graft B cells during renal allograft rejection. Kidney Int 2008;74:664–73.

72. Brown K, Sacks SH, Wong W. Tertiary lymphoid organs in renal allografts can be associated with donor-specific tolerance rather than rejection. Eur J Immunol 2010;41:89–96.

73. Briscoe DM, Alexander SI, Lichtman AH. Interactions between T lymphocytes and endothelial cells in allograft rejection. Curr Opin Immunol 1998;10:525–31.

74. Kreisel D, Krupnick AS, Gelman AE, et al. Non-hematopoietic allograft cells directly activate CD8+ T cells and trigger acute rejection: an alternative mechanism of allorecognition. Nat Med 2002;8:233–9.

75. Marelli-Berg FM, Scott D, Bartok I, et al. Activated murine endothelial cells have reduced immunogenicity for CD8+ T cells: a mechanism of immunoregulation? J Immunol 2000;165:4182–9.

76. Paul LC, Saito K, Davidoff A, et al. Growth factor transcripts in rat renal transplants. Am J Kidney Dis 1996;28:441–50.

77. Nankivell BJ, Alexander SI. Rejection of the kidney allograft. N Engl J Med 2010;363:1451–62.

78. Colvin RB, Smith RN. Antibody-mediated organ-allograft rejection. Nat Rev Immunol 2005;5:807–17.

79. Worthington JE, Martin S, Al-Husseini DM, et al. Posttransplantation production of donor HLA-specific antibodies as a predictor of renal transplant outcome. Transplantation 2003;75:1034–40. **This original article outlines the importance of post-transplant monitoring of donor-specific antibodies and the effect they have on graft outcome.**

80. Sis B, Mengel M, Haas M, et al. Banff'09 meeting report: antibody mediated graft deterioration and implementation of Banff working groups. Am J Transplant 2010;10:464–71.

81. Solez K. History of the Banff classification of allograft pathology as it approaches its 20th year. Curr Opin Organ Transplant 2010;15:49–51.

82. Newell KA, Phippard D, Turka LA. Regulatory cells and cell signatures in clinical transplantation tolerance. Curr Opin Immunol 2011;23:655–9.

83. Knechtle SJ. Immunoregulation and tolerance. Transplant Proc 2010;42:S13–5.

84. Wood KJ, Bushell A, Jones ND. Immunologic unresponsiveness to alloantigen in vivo: a role for regulatory T cells. Immunol Rev 2011;241:119–32.

85. Newell KA, Chong AS. Making a B-line for transplantation tolerance. Am J Transplant 2011;11:420–1.

86. Hutchinson JA, Riquelme P, Sawitzki B, et al. Cutting edge: immunological consequences and trafficking of human regulatory macrophages administered to renal transplant recipients. J Immunol 2011;187:2072–8.

87. Kroemer A, Edtinger K, Li XC. The innate natural killer cells in transplant rejection and tolerance induction. Curr Opin Organ Transplant 2008;13:339–43.

88. Delikouras A, Dorling A. Transplant accommodation. Am J Transplant 2003;3:917–8.

89. Lynch RJ, Platt JL. Accommodation in organ transplantation. Curr Opin Organ Transplant 2008;13:165–70.

90. Kamada N, Davies HS, Roser B. Reversal of transplantation immunity by liver grafting. Nature 1981;292:840–2.

91. Mulder A, Kardol MJ, Arn JS, et al. Human monoclonal HLA antibodies reveal interspecies crossreactive swine MHC class I epitopes relevant for xenotransplantation. Mol Immunol 2010;47:809–15.

92. Ryan EA, Lakey JR, Rajotte RV, et al. Clinical outcomes and insulin secretion after islet transplantation with the Edmonton protocol. Diabetes 2001;50:710–9.

93. Wang DZ, Skinner S, Elliot R, et al. Xenotransplantation of neonatal porcine islets and Sertoli cells into nonimmunosuppressed streptozotocin-induced diabetic rats. Transplant Proc 2005;37:470–1.

94. Valdes-Gonzalez RA, White DJ, Dorantes LM, et al. Three-year follow-up of a type 1 diabetes mellitus patient with an islet xenotransplant. Clin Transplant 2007;21:352–7.

95. Atala A, Bauer SB, Soker S, et al. Tissue-engineered autologous bladders for patients needing cystoplasty. Lancet 2006;367:1241–6.

96. Macchiarini P, Jungebluth P, Go T, et al. Clinical transplantation of a tissue-engineered airway. Lancet 2008;372:2023–30.

97. Ott HC, Matthiesen TS, Goh SK, et al. Perfusion-decellularized matrix: using nature's platform to engineer a bioartificial heart. Nat Med 2008;14:213–21.

98. Botker HE, Kharbanda R, Schmidt MR, et al. Remote ischaemic conditioning before hospital admission, as a complement to angioplasty, and effect on myocardial salvage in patients with acute myocardial infarction: a randomised trial. Lancet 2010;375:727–34.

99. Grenz A, Eckle T, Zhang H, et al. Use of a hanging-weight system for isolated renal artery occlusion during ischemic preconditioning in mice. Am J Physiol Renal Physiol 2007;292:F475–85.

100. Ferenbach DA, Nkejabega NC, McKay J, et al. The induction of macrophage hemeoxygenase-1 is protective during acute kidney injury in aging mice. Kidney Int 2011;79(9):966–76.

101. Lang Jr. JD, Teng X, Chumley P, et al. Inhaled NO accelerates restoration of liver function in adults following orthotopic liver transplantation. J Clin Invest 2007;117:2583–91.

102. Wang JX, Jiao JQ, Li Q, et al. miR-499 regulates mitochondrial dynamics by targeting calcineurin and dynamin-related protein-1. Nat Med 2011;17:71–8.

103. Moers C, Smits JM, Maathuis MH, et al. Machine perfusion or cold storage in deceased-donor kidney transplantation. N Engl J Med 2009;360:7–19.

104. Cypel M, Yeung JC, Liu M, et al. Normothermic ex vivo lung perfusion in clinical lung transplantation. N Engl J Med 2011;364:1431–40.

4

Testing for histocompatibility

Phil Dyer
Ann-Margaret Little
David Turner

Introduction

Immunity

The immune system exists to protect an individual from morbidity and mortality following pathogen infection and from emergent malignancy; this conflicts with the need for viviparity and the artificial state of successful allogeneic cell, tissue and organ transplantation.

Histocompatibility

ABO-A and -B blood group substances function as histocompatibility antigens as they are expressed as structurally variable carbohydrates, linked to glycoproteins or to glycolipids. The ABO blood group system is unique in that alloantibodies develop naturally in neonates, reaching adult levels within a few years of life, in response to carbohydrates present in the diet. Consequently, ABO-O individuals usually develop antibodies to both ABO-A and -B antigens, ABO-A to -B, ABO-B to -A, but ABO-AB individuals have no ABO blood group antibodies. In the early days of transplantation, pioneers who were aware of the danger of ABO incompatible blood transfusions assumed ABO compatibility should be adopted for organ transplantation. Therefore, the 'rules' governing blood transfusion were applied to organ transplantation. It is now known that ABO blood group substances are expressed on endothelium. There has never been a randomised controlled trial of ABO blood group compatible versus incompatible organ transplantation because the risks are perceived to be too high. Of interest is the successful transplantation of ABO blood group incompatible hearts into neonates and the successful transplantation of ABO incompatible kidneys in adults found to have unexpectedly low titre ($\leq 1:4$) naturally occurring ABO blood group antibodies. Both of these experiences indirectly support the role of ABO blood group substances as histocompatibility antigens in transplantation. In recent years, pre-transplant antibody removal protocols to circumvent the antibody-mediated response to ABO blood group incompatibility in kidney transplantation have been successful.[1]

To counter the myriad of pathogens that an individual may encounter, the immune system has responded to environmental pressures by selective, adaptive evolutionary processes resulting in the immunogenetic system, which is central to the initial recognition and response to an alloantigen. Human leucocyte antigen (HLA) genes encode highly polymorphic glycoproteins that are expressed on the surface of all nucleated cells, to varying degrees depending on cell function and state of activation. In the natural situation, HLA proteins bind and present self or non-self peptides to T cells, resulting in a respective anergic or vigorous immune response to the antigen presenting cell. Because of their high degree of polymorphism, HLA proteins are also the primary trigger for an alloimmune response (see Chapter 3) and that is why development of clinical transplantation has driven our understanding of HLA gene and allele structure and protein function. Consequently, HLA protein disparity between donor and recipient cells is a barrier to successful allotransplantation, which is only overcome by interventional modulation of the immune response (see Chapter 5).

Sensitisation

Individuals are at risk of developing IgM and IgG alloantibodies reactive with non-self HLA protein allotypes when exposed to:

- leucocytes and platelets in blood transfusion(s);
- paternal HLA proteins in pregnancy;
- HLA protein incompatible transplantation.

Subsequently, these antibodies can disappear from the circulation, making the identification of prior sensitisation impossible. Infection, which elicits a heightened immune response, can reveal pre-existing HLA reactive alloantibodies because of antigenic epitopes shared between HLA and viral proteins. Furthermore, T cells will be primed to HLA alloantigens. The presence of donor specific HLA reactive IgG antibodies at the time of kidney transplantation conveys a high risk of immediate antibody-mediated hyper-acute rejection (HAR), making the detection and definition of HLA reactive sensitisation an essential component of histocompatibility laboratory services. A crossmatch assay, involving incubation of patient serum with donor target cells, to detect the presence of donor-specific sensitisation is also a prerequisite for successful kidney transplantation in the absence of a virtual crossmatching programme.

While there are claims of roles for other alloantigenic systems in clinical transplantation, none are routinely addressed in most transplant centres, since they have significantly less impact than the ABO blood group and HLA systems. They are sometimes implicated when humoral rejection in the post-transplant period cannot be ascribed to development of HLA reactive antibodies.

This chapter aims to explain how HLA phenotyping, HLA reactive alloantibody detection and definition

and donor–recipient crossmatching, along with well-established organ allocation policies, are used to support effective cell, tissue and organ transplantation.

HLA: history of clinical application and technical development

Working independently in the mid-20th century, Rose Payne in California, Jon van Rood in Leiden and Jean Dausset in Paris detected antibodies reactive with non-self leucocytes in serum from multigravid women and from multitransfused patients. Linking of these findings to the understanding of the function of the immune system stimulated a rapid expansion of effort to define the immunogenetic basis of allosensitisation. In parallel, clinical transplant teams were attempting to overcome the immune response to allogeneic organ transplantation since they had established effective surgical techniques for organ implantation. The successful transplantation of a kidney between monozygotic twins, by Murray and colleagues in 1954 in Boston, USA, indicated that the alloimmune response is genetically encoded. The aspiration was to identify the gene(s) responsible for alloimmunity and subsequently to avoid their mismatching and so establish clinical tolerance of allogeneic tissues. Full tolerance has still to be achieved due to the plasticity of the immune response.

> ✓ Immunogeneticists persisted with their endeavours through a series of collaborative International Histocompatibility Workshops, which continue to support the World Health Organisation HLA Nomenclature Committee that maintains the universally applied HLA language.[2]

The culmination of six decades of HLA research is a complete resolution of the major histocompatibility complex of approximately 3.5 megabases of DNA containing at least 25 HLA gene loci coding for in excess of 7000 HLA allele sequences. This is the most polymorphic system in the human genome and exists because of the persistent infections that humans encounter throughout life (**Fig. 4.1**).

The elucidation of HLA polymorphisms was pursued to support matching, or minimising mismatching, for clinically relevant transplantation since this reduces T-cell activation and minimises the risk of acute cellular rejection. The detection and definition

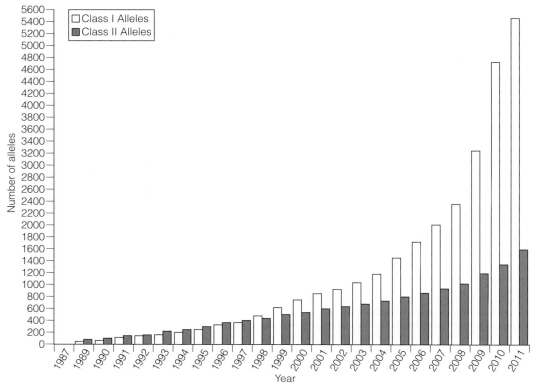

Figure 4.1 • Polymorphism of the HLA system. Adapted from Robinson J, Mistry K, McWilliam H et al. The IMGT/HLA Database. Nucleic Acids Res 2011; 39(Suppl 1):D1171–6;[40] Robinson J, Malik A, Parham P et al. IMGT/HLA – a sequence database for the human major histocompatibility complex. Tissue Antigens 2000; 55:280–7.[41]

of antibodies to HLA protein allotypes in patients' serum was soon shown to be an important component of histocompatibility.

To identify circumstances when HAR is likely to occur, Patel and Terasaki developed the complement-mediated lymphocytotoxicity assay (CDC).[3] In outline, this assay comprises a two-stage incubation of donor lymphocytes, as a source of donor HLA proteins, with the potential recipient's serum and addition of heterologous (rabbit) complement. The CDC assay detects lysis of the target donor lymphocytes through binding of HLA reactive antibody, present in recipient serum, with donor cell surface HLA proteins, mediated by complement-dependent cytotoxicity. When a CDC assay detected recipient serum lysis of donor lymphocytes (a 'positive' test), then HAR was shown to be highly likely to occur.[4]

The CDC assay was subsequently used to define the specificity of the HLA protein allotypes present on recipient and donor lymphocytes to establish the HLA phenotype – a process known at the time as 'tissue typing', a term that is no longer useful. This approach was dependent on the availability of sera containing well-defined reactivity to one, or more, HLA protein allotypes, as typing reagents. Again, the worldwide histocompatibility community collaborated by exchanging such sera, sourced from HLA alloimmunised individuals, most often gravid women. Despite significant challenges, HLA typing serology technology allowed identification of most "broad" HLA protein allotypes. Serological typing still has a role, primarily because it is a rapid assay and monospecific monoclonal antibodies are now available as commercial reagents, and it is used in some centres to support identification of organ donor HLA phenotypes alongside more comprehensive molecular biological testing.

In the early 1990s, the development of the polymerase chain reaction (PCR), which generates millions of identical copies of genomic DNA, revolutionised the identification of HLA alleles. A series of techniques was developed, with two remaining commonly used. Sequence-specific primers (SSPs) are short, artificially designed DNA sequence reagents that are used in a PCR reaction to generate copies of DNA with exclusivity for a unique (HLA) gene sequence. A battery of SSPs is designed and a corresponding number of PCR reactions are set up utilising DNA extracted from cells from the individual for whom an HLA phenotype is to be identified. Identification of positive PCR amplifications is visualised by gel electrophesis and indicates presence of a specific polymorphic HLA gene sequence. Subsequently, HLA alleles can be allocated to the DNA tested and an HLA type to the individual. PCR-SSP is used to type for all HLA loci but the resolution achieved is sometimes limited.

The second current molecular HLA typing technique employs xMAP® technology, commercially available as the Luminex platform.[5] In essence, commercially available kits of Luminex microbeads (5.6 μm), with inherent unique fluorochromasia, are coated with oligonucleotide probes that will hybridise exclusively to the DNA hypervariable region encoding specific HLA alleles. Multiple bead populations, each bearing known HLA-specific oligonucleotide probes, are identified in a multiplex assay by an internal and specific fluorochrome dye and visualised in a flow cytometer with laser light stimulation. Hybridisation to target HLA DNA sequences is revealed by a fluorochrome-tagged streptavidin conjugate that binds to biotin incorporated in the primers used to amplify the HLA locus of interest.

Conventional gene sequencing technologies can also be used to detect HLA gene polymorphisms, especially in the context of haemopoietic progenitor stem cell transplantation when complete identity between the stem cell donor and the patient HLA is preferable to limit rejection and graft versus host disease.

For the detection and definition of HLA reactive allosensitisation, histocompatibility testing laboratories have developed specific and sensitive assays, with the current technology of choice again employing the xMAP® technology. In essence, commercially available microbeads with multiple or single HLA proteins attached to their surface are incubated with patient serum and any HLA reactive antibody bound is detected by addition of a fluorochrome-labelled secondary antibody. The Luminex platform is used to identify individual microbeads by their inherent fluorochromasia and positive binding of antibody to HLA proteins on the beads by flow cytometry.

HLA genes and proteins: structure and genetics relevant to transplantation

✔ The human major histocompatibility complex (MHC), located on the short arm of chromosome six (6p21.3), is an extremely gene-dense region of the human genome, being home to over 250 expressed genes.[6]

There are two types of HLA genes within the human MHC: HLA class I and HLA class II. HLA class I genes encode a single-polypeptide heavy chain that associates with β-2-microglobulin to form an HLA class I protein. HLA class II genes encode both an α (DRA) and a β chain (DRB1, 3, 4, 5), which associate non-covalently to form an HLA class II protein. Both HLA class I and class II proteins are expressed at the cell surface and are bound to a short processed peptide within a peptide-binding site formed by the membrane distal domains of the HLA protein (**Fig. 4.2**).

HLA class I proteins are expressed on all nucleated cells and are also present on some non-nucleated cells such as platelets. HLA class II proteins have a restricted cell expression found on the surface of cells involved in antigen presentation, such as dendritic cells and macrophages. However, HLA class II protein expression can be up-regulated on other cell types, including endothelial cells, in response to stimulation by immune mediators such as γ-interferon at the time of immune activation.[7]

Three types of HLA class I proteins (HLA-A, HLA-B and HLA-C) and three types of HLA class II proteins (HLA-DR, HLA-DQ and HLA-DP) have a role in the generation of immune reactions that influence transplant outcome.

The HLA genes are the most polymorphic expressed genes within our genome. Polymorphism within HLA genes is not random and the variation found within DNA sequences is predominantly non-synonymous. Most of the protein variation observed impacts on the function of the HLA protein either by influencing the structure of peptides bound and/or influencing interactions with T-cell and natural killer cell receptors.

The well-defined WHO nomenclature system is key to the description of HLA allele and protein variation. For description, HLA allele names are broken down into numerical fields that are separated by colons (**Fig. 4.3**).

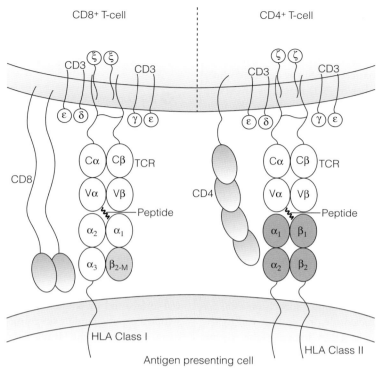

Figure 4.2 • Diagrammatic representation of HLA class I and class II proteins presenting peptide to CD8-positive and CD4-positive T cells. HLA class I and II molecules interact with the T-cell receptor (TCR) complex. The TCR complex consists of the TCR α and β chains; the CD3 γ, δ, and ε chains and 2 ζ chains. Cα and Cβ = Constant region of the α and β TCR chains respectively and Vα and Vβ = Variable region of α and β TCR chains respectively. β2M = β2-microglobulin. Figure prepared and donated by Catherine Wilson.

✔ Depending on the testing methodology, the HLA type may be obtained at different levels of resolution:

• low;
• high;
• allelic resolution.[8]

Intermediate resolution is often used to describe anything between low and high resolution.

✔ Some HLA alleles are high frequency; HLA-A*02:01 is the most common HLA-A allele found in about 50% of European Caucasoids, while other HLA alleles may only have been identified in a single individual.[9,10]

For organ transplantation, it is usually sufficient for donor and recipient typing to be at low resolution for HLA-A, -B, -C, -DRB1 and -DQB1. In the UK there is a requirement for histocompatibility laboratories to report deceased organ donor HLA types at this level to facilitate a consistent national process of organ allocation.

Not all defined HLA alleles occur at the same frequency.

The WHO system for assigning names to HLA alleles does not consider allele frequency and therefore efforts have been made to establish databases that contain information on the frequency of HLA alleles in different populations. Within a given population there will be a number of common HLA alleles and a number of rare HLA alleles. The organ allocation system within the UK defaults rare HLA types to their most common structurally related HLA type to reduce the bias in organs being provided to the patients with the most common HLA types. For example, DR9, which has a frequency of 2.6% in kidney patients, is structurally

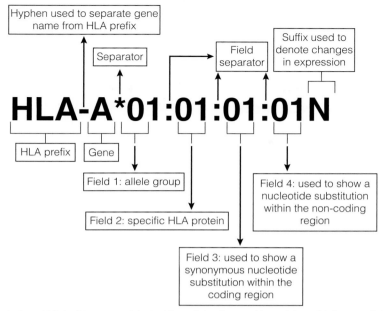

Figure 4.3 • Description of HLA allele name. Adapted from: http://www.ebi.ac.uk/imgt/hla/nomenclature/index.html; Robinson J, Mistry K, McWilliam H et al. The IMGT/HLA Database. Nucleic Acids Res 2011; 39(Suppl 1):D1171–6;[40] Robinson J, Malik A, Parham P et al. IMGT/HLA – a sequence database for the human major histocompatibility complex. Tissue Antigens 2000; 55:280–7.[41]

related and defaulted to DR4, which has a phenotype frequency of 29.8%, so that DR9-positive patients have access to the kidney donor pool more frequently.

HLA genes are inherited following Mendelian genetics and as they are co-located within the MHC, they are inherited 'en bloc' as a haplotype. It follows that any two siblings have a 1 in 4 chance of inheriting both the same or different HLA haplotypes from their parents.

Some combinations of HLA alleles are found on haplotypes at a higher frequency than would be predicted from random association of alleles.[11] This observation is called linkage disequilibrium and may result from one or more events, such as:

• selective pressures biasing particular combinations of alleles;
• non-random mating;
• suppression of recombination events.

A well-known example of linkage disequilibrium within the European Caucasoid population is the haplotype HLA-A*01-C*07-B*08-DRB1*03-DQB1*02, which is highly conserved and occurs in approximately 10% of individuals.

As explained later, understanding of HLA reactive antibodies at the epitope levels can precipitate the need for histocompatibility laboratories to define HLA alleles at high resolution and to include the alleles encoded by DQA1, DPA1 and DPB1.

HLA reactive antibodies, causes of sensitisation and antibody epitopes

Antibodies and rejection

HLA reactive antibody definition is an important element of histocompatibility laboratory testing to support transplantation, and testing has evolved in both sensitivity and specificity. Whilst the presence of high-titre HLA reactive antibodies at the time of transplantation can lead to HAR, lower level donor HLA reactive antibodies can cause acute antibody-mediated rejection (AMR). Therefore, defining the specificity of HLA reactive antibodies in patients reduces the risk of both HAR and AMR. Before transplantation, defined HLA reactive antibodies are recorded as 'unacceptable antigens', which are donor HLA proteins to be avoided for that patient. HLA reactive antibodies produced *de novo* following transplant are also associated with graft loss.

Alloimmunisation to HLA proteins

HLA reactive antibody production as a result of the different modes of sensitisation is variable. Clinical emphasis has been placed on IgG antibodies but IgM antibodies can be produced and there is evidence that the relevance of IgM antibodies may have been underestimated.

Passenger leucocytes in transfused blood can stimulate HLA class I and II reactive antibody production. HLA class I expression on platelets can also act as a source of antigen, although the presence of leucocytes seems to be required for antibody production.[12] Leucoreduction is associated with a reduction in the frequency of HLA reactive antibody formation but does not prevent antibody production after red blood cell (RBC) transfusion.[13] When tested using CDC assays, 9.6% of cardiac surgery patients negative for HLA reactive antibodies prior to surgery became positive after leucodepleted RBC transfusion. In patients who had not experienced any previous allogeneic exposure, the rate of sensitisation was reduced to 5.3%.[14] There is evidence that HLA reactive antibodies produced as a result of transfusion alone are less able to fix complement,[15] in contrast to transplant-induced sensitisation.

HLA proteins expressed on foetal cells can induce HLA class I and II reactive antibodies in mothers following transfer to the maternal circulation. This is a common cause of HLA sensitisation. Using Luminex testing it has been shown that HLA reactive antibody sensitisation increases with the number of pregnancies from under 10% in nulliparous women to over 40% in women with three or more pregnancies.[16]

HLA mismatched transplantation is an important route of HLA sensitisation. In kidney transplantation 10–15% of recipients who are negative for HLA reactive antibodies prior to transplant develop *de novo* donor HLA-specific antibody (DSA).[17,18] The timing of post-transplant HLA-DSA production in patients who were DSA negative pre-transplant has also been described; in one study class I

reactive antibodies appeared at 3.3±2.7 years and class II at 2.3±2.1 years. Furthermore, HLA class II DSA rather than class I dominates after kidney transplantation. In patients who have rejected a kidney transplant, DSA levels are higher post-nephrectomy than pre-nephrectomy.[19] In contrast, in a liver transplant study 4.2% of recipients developed DSA post-transplant[20] and there are reports of HLA-DSA occurring post-transplant in recipients of islet and pancreas transplants.

HLA proteins are essentially a collection of antigenic epitopes and HLA reactive antibodies are produced against non-self epitopes present on intact non-self HLA proteins. Some HLA proteins are structurally closely related because they share epitopes, a result of the mechanisms underlying the production of new HLA alleles during DNA replication. The sharing of epitopes between HLA proteins is the cause of HLA cross-reactivity when antibodies raised as a result of exposure to one HLA protein can react with other HLA proteins that share the common immunogenic epitope. In recent years attempts have been made to elucidate immunogenic HLA epitopes using monoclonal antibodies for analysis.[21]

> ✔ Theoretical computer models of HLA epitopes, particularly the Matchmaker programme developed by Duquesnoy, have also been used.[22]

Studies using Matchmaker software have shown that the ability of a patient to mount an antibody response against mismatched HLA proteins is dependent upon the number of theoretical 'eplets' that are mismatched between donor and recipient. Cases where there is an apparent high degree of antigen mismatching can paradoxically be at low risk of antibody production because of HLA epitope sharing between the mismatched proteins.

Establishing antibody reactivity

The selection of donor cells from a local population, reflecting the local deceased organ donor pool, facilitates an estimate of a patient's reactivity against potential donors. This percentage reactivity was termed the 'panel reactive antibody (PRA)' status of the patient. The 'PRA' was used for many years as an indicator of the likelihood of a patient being crossmatch positive with a donor. Now that a patient's HLA reactive antibody status can be determined with precision, using Luminex technology, it is possible to identify the percentage of the deceased organ donor pool to which a patient has antibodies. In the UK this calculation results in the 'calculated reaction frequency (cRF)', which is a more accurate representation of a patient's chance of receiving an offer of a transplant.

Solid-phase technologies have mostly replaced CDC assays and the result is increased sensitivity and specificity of HLA reactive antibody detection and definition. Some histocompatibility laboratories continue to use CDC-based screening to delineate clinically relevant complement (C') fixing, high-titre antibodies from other antibodies that are potentially less clinically significant.

Microbeads with single antigen specificities allow a rapid, semiquantitative and specific analysis of patient sera but there are some problems associated with their use. There is evidence that the attachment of recombinant antigen to beads can alter antigen structure and expose non-clinically relevant epitopes, leading to false-positive reactions.[23] High-titre C' fixing antibodies can also give false-negative results, potentially as a result of C' fixation affecting binding of secondary detection reagents.[24] The clinical value of Luminex microbead antibody detection and definition has been questioned as over-sensitive in the clinical situation and there is debate of the relevance of low-level DSAs detected solely by this method.[25] Despite these genuine concerns, the benefits of X-map Luminex technology, which include rapidity, high throughput, semiquantitation and better reproducibility, make it the preferred assay employed for HLA reactive antibody definition. Newer versions of antibody definition kits allow the differentiation of C'-fixing from non-C'-fixing antibodies and there is evidence that these may exclusively identify clinically relevant HLA reactive antibodies.[26]

Crossmatching

In the CDC-XM, T- and B-cell populations are separated prior to incubation with recipient sera, allowing assessment of reactivity against HLA class I (expressed on T and B cells) and HLA class II (expressed on B cells). The CDC-XM can identify the presence of relatively high-titre HLA reactive antibodies that are C' fixing. These represent the most deleterious antibodies in the immediate post-transplant period and therefore the CDC-XM can be used to identify those patients at risk of HAR. However, when used alone to decide whether a transplant should proceed, the CDC-XM may not identify patients with lower level HLA reactive antibodies that are still relevant to early AMR risk. Despite the CDC-XM remaining the 'gold standard' for pre-transplant testing it has a number of drawbacks:

- low-level clinically relevant antibodies are not identified;
- non-HLA and auto-reactive antibodies can give false-positive results;
- non-C'-fixing antibodies are not detected.

Most histocompatibility laboratories still undertake CDC-XM as part of their strategy to assess risk prior to transplant.

The flow cytometry crossmatch (FC-XM) was introduced in the UK in the 1990s;[27] in essence, donor lymphocytes, from peripheral blood or spleen or lymph nodes, are incubated with patient sera. Three-colour FC-XM methods allow the distinction of T and B cells using anti-CD3 and -CD19 fluorochrome-labelled antibodies and the measurement of patient antibody bound to donor cells. The key difference from the CDC-XM is the increased sensitivity. This means that the FC-XM can identify antibodies that may not be apparent using CDC-XM and therefore it helps in risk stratification.

Clinical relevance of HLA reactive antibodies

Antibodies before kidney transplantation

Pre-formed, IgG donor-specific HLA reactive antibodies are relevant at the time of kidney transplantation, causing either HAR or early AMR.

> ✔✔ In the UK, a consensus exists as to the likely immunological risk for a transplant and a useful reference table is available.[28]

Luminex technology can identify low-level DSAs not revealed in a CDC or FC-XM and the impact of these antibodies on initiating AMR is now recognised.[29]

De novo donor-specific antibodies after kidney transplantation

> ✔✔ Kidney transplant failure is usually preceded by the appearance of HLA reactive antibodies.[30]

There is some debate over the clinical utility of regular HLA reactive antibody screening after transplantation. The essential question is whether the development of HLA-DSA post-transplant can be used to predict those patients who may need enhanced immunosuppression or other forms of intervention to prevent antibody-mediated rejection and graft loss. In a study of HLA reactive antibody production up to 1 year post-transplant in 70 patients who were antibody negative pre-transplant, 11% produced DSA at a median of 30 days. Although associated with a shorter time to rejection the antibody production was seen concomitantly with clinical signs of dysfunction and was therefore not useful as a predictor of early rejection.[17] However, development of HLA reactive antibodies in the first year after kidney transplantation is probably a marker of long-term chronic rejection and graft loss.[31] Patients who develop HLA reactive antibodies within the first post-transplant year are seven times more likely to lose their grafts.

> ✔✔ Appearance of HLA reactive antibody at later time points, usually to HLA class II, has also been associated with reduced graft survival.[32]

There is some evidence that reducing de novo HLA reactive antibody levels in patients with acute rejection can improve long-term survival,[33] but no data exist on the effect of reducing HLA reactive antibody levels in patients with stable graft function on long-term survival. Therefore, many centres use HLA reactive antibody testing to confirm suspicion of clinically identified rejection rather than testing prospectively.

HLA reactive antibodies in transplantation of other organs

A number of studies address the role of HLA reactive antibodies after transplantation of heart, lung, liver or pancreas. Similarly, there are cases of sensitisation to HLA protein allotypes after pancreatic islet transplants that indicate that the developing field of cell and tissue transplantation should include well-planned studies to monitor the clinical relevance of reactivity to HLA allogeneic proteins.

Antibody removal to facilitate transplantation

There are now established clinical protocols that aim to reduce or remove antibodies to both ABO and HLA antigens (Chapter 5). There is no consensus as to which protocol is the most effective as patient-specific factors dictate the most suitable intervention. Monitoring of antibody levels is an important component of these protocols, giving the histocompatibility expert a key role in achieving a successful outcome. Reduction or removal of antibodies pre-transplant to permit antibody incompatible transplantation to proceed and post-transplant to rescue an organ undergoing AMR is possible.

Other antibodies and their clinical relevance

Antibodies directed against a number of polymorphic systems have been implicated in rejection and graft loss. The targets include the products of the MHC class I chain-related (MIC) genes, the angiotensin type II receptor and endothelial cell antigens.[34]

> ✔✔ Recent work suggests that a significant cause of antibody-mediated chronic damage after kidney transplantation is the exposure to donor chemokines and intracellular matrix proteins.[35]

Despite a number of studies indicating that some cases of rejection and graft loss appear to be caused by these antibodies, few histocompatibility laboratories routinely test for them pre-transplant. A commercial test has been developed that uses endothelial cell precursors from donor peripheral blood as a target to measure patient reactivity against endothelial cells (ECs).[36] This assay has not been utilised widely for a number of reasons:

- it requires a large amount of donor peripheral blood;
- the presence of HLA reactive antibodies can interfere with the assay;
- described associations with rejection are not convincingly applicable in the clinic.

Organ allocation and histocompatibility

Organs are usually allocated by compliance with the rules of blood transfusion for ABO blood groups. In practice it is preferable, for allocation of organs from deceased donors, to achieve ABO blood group *identity* so that ABO-O patients do not accumulate on the transplant eligibility list, as would happen if ABO-O organs were allocated to ABO-A, -B or -AB patients, who would be ABO biologically compatible. In living organ donation of a kidney or lobe of liver, ABO compatibility is perfectly possible. In specific instances, patients may be preconditioned for an ABO incompatible organ transplant by removal of ABO reactive antibody using a protocol of plasmapheresis preceded by ablation of B cells with an anti-CD20 therapeutic antibody such as rituximab. In rare cases emergency ABO incompatible liver transplantation, without conditioning, has been used with moderate success.

The next level of allocation, which also meets the essential requirement of biological/immunological compatibility, is the need for an immediate pre-transplant negative crossmatch. This test establishes the *absence* of IgG antibody in pre-transplant serum reactive with mismatched donor HLA antigens, so the risk of HAR is avoided. Again, this situation can be achieved with a conditioning regime with the aim of removing harmful antibodies from the circulation. This is an increasingly frequent option in HLA incompatible living donation kidney transplantation but has been used in the challenging circumstances of deceased donation.

> ✔✔ For patients who have no demonstrable donor HLA reactive antibodies in their serum preceding transplantation and who have not been exposed to potential sensitising events since the last serum was tested, it is possible to perform a 'virtual' crossmatch test.[37]

The virtual crossmatch is an active process but does not necessitate any histocompatibility laboratory testing and so can significantly reduce the cold storage time of an organ before transplantation. In turn, in kidney transplantation, there is a greater possibility of immediate function, so avoiding dialysis after transplantation and reducing the length of hospital stay. For heart transplantation a virtual crossmatch can facilitate transplantation for patients who otherwise might not be considered. The essence of a virtual crossmatch is a report from a senior histocompatibility scientist confirming that the recipient's sensitisation profile has been reviewed immediately before transplantation and consequently the planned transplant is of low immunological risk.

There is no convincing evidence that a positive crossmatch should be a veto to liver transplantation.

Whilst some algorithms ignore minimisation of HLA mismatches as a component of the allocation process, others incorporate this as part of the recipient prioritisation process. This choice should be based on evidence that minimising HLA mismatches conveys benefit, other than facilitating a negative crossmatch (**Fig. 4.4**). Clearly a potential recipient who has developed HLA reactive antibodies can only be offered a donor organ that does not carry those antigens if the crossmatch is to be negative.

The UK has adopted a convenient code to summarise the degree of HLA mismatch between a specific donor

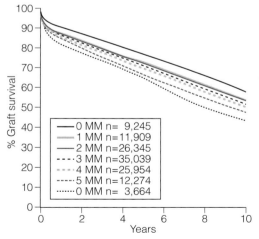

Figure 4.4 • HLA mismatching adversely influences survival after deceased donor kidney transplantation. Source: CTS Collaborative Transplant Study, K-21101-0212. www.ctstransplant.org, accessed 9 February 2012. Reproduced with permission.

and recipient pair. It is important to consider 'mismatch' rather than 'match' since the immune system recognises and reacts to antigenic differences. Since only HLA-A, -B and -DRB1 mismatches are considered in allocation processes, the code is of three digits relating to these three HLA loci respectively. The maximum degree of mismatch at any one locus can be two antigens, one from each chromosome. This occurs when the donor has two HLA antigens that are absent in the recipient; other possibilities are one and zero antigen mismatches. For example, the HLA (-A, -B, -DRB1) mismatch code '010' indicates that the donor carries one HLA-B mismatched antigen but there are no mismatched antigens at both -A and -DRB1. If the donor is homozygous at one HLA locus, as will occur most often with common HLA protein allotypes such as A2, then the maximum mismatch will be one antigen at that locus.

The data available to demonstrate a benefit, or not, to improved survival of organ transplants through avoiding HLA mismatches have been controversial ever since early studies were published in the 1960s. Currently the UK allocation process for kidneys donated after brain death prioritises allocation to recipients when there is no mismatch for HLA-A, -B and -DRB1 ('000') since such transplants have been shown to have the highest survivals at 3 years and more after transplantation. Subsequently, increasing degrees of HLA mismatch ('100', '010', '110', '200', etc.) are permitted but two mismatches for HLA-DRB1 ('002' to '222', etc.) are not, since these transplants perform poorly. For highly sensitised patients, with a calculated reaction frequency exceeding 85%, there comes the point where the degree of acceptable HLA mismatch is limited by the number of HLA protein allotypes to which the patient has developed antibodies. When there is sensitisation to common antigens, such as HLA-A2, then sourcing an HLA compatible organ is a challenge.

Allocation of organs other than kidneys, including combined kidney with pancreas, does not usually require minimisation of HLA mismatches, either because there are few potential recipients waiting for transplantation or because there is no evidence of benefit. When patients are sensitised to HLA protein allotypes then minimising mismatches may be essential to obtain a negative crossmatch and this can be challenging, as in heart transplantation when time available to perform tests in the histocompatibility laboratory is limited by clinical demands. The liver is said to be immunologically privileged and crossmatch positive, HLA mismatched liver transplants are performed with no apparent adverse effect. The mechanisms involved are unclear but may be the result of release of soluble HLA proteins from the donor liver that bind to circulating DSAs.

Allocation of organs for transplantation taking into account HLA mismatching, pre-transplant antibody screening and crossmatching is essentially a risk analysis. This has been summarised effectively by a working group of the British Transplantation Society and the British Society for Histocompatibility and Immunogenetics, and guidelines are available from their websites.[38,39]

Conclusion

Organ, tissue and cell transplantations are highly effective clinical procedures that improve and save many lives each year. The aggressive immune response to alloantigens can be moderated in some patients on some occasions by treatment with an increasingly wide range of immunosuppressants, but these are not without risk. Effective histocompatibility support before, at the time of and after transplantation can ensure transplants survive and work longer. This is not without financial cost, but in contrast to other options of dialysis, long-term medication or perhaps no option at all, this cost is relatively insignificant.

Key points

- Naturally occurring ABO reactive antibodies necessitate ABO blood group identity or compatibility in organ transplantation to avoid immediate humoral rejection.
- HLA proteins are the primary trigger of the alloimmune response.
- Sensitisation to allogeneic HLA proteins occurs through blood transfusion, pregnancy and transplantation, resulting in production of HLA reactive antibodies, and can be increased by infection.

- Conditioning protocols used pre-transplant may remove ABO blood group and/or HLA reactive antibodies to permit antibody incompatible transplantation.
- A pre-transplant crossmatch establishes compatibility, or not, between a donor and a recipient with respect to donor HLA reactive sensitisation.
- HLA reactive antibodies have a significant clinical role pre-, peri- and post-transplantation, making their detection and definition essential.
- Most effective allocation of kidneys from deceased donors uses a policy to minimise HLA protein mismatching.
- The polygenic, polyallelic HLA system has significant variation in HLA protein frequencies within and between ethnic populations.
- Technical developments have resulted in a WHO-recognised HLA nomenclature.
- Laboratory techniques are constantly developing; the current state of the art to identify HLA gene and protein polymorphisms and HLA reactive antibodies is xMAP® Luminex technology.

References

1. Montgomery RA, Locke JE, King KE, et al. ABO incompatible renal transplantation: a paradigm ready for broad implementation. Transplantation 2009;87(8):1246–55.

2. http://hla.alleles.org/nomenclature/index.html; [accessed 6.09.12].

3. Patel R, Terasaki PI. Significance of the positive crossmatch test in kidney transplantation. N Engl J Med 1969;280:735.

4. Kissmeyer-Nielsen F, Olsen S, Petersen VP, et al. Hyperacute rejection of kidney allografts associated with pre-existing humoral antibodies against donor cells. Lancet 1966;2:662.

5. www.luminexcorp.com; [accessed 6.09.12].

6. Horton R, Wilming L, Lovering RC, et al. Gene map of the extended human MHC. Nat Rev Genet 2004;5:889.

7. Collins T, Korman AJ, Wake CT, et al. Immune interferon activates multiple class II major histocompatibility complex genes and the associated invariant chain gene in human endothelial cells and dermal fibroblasts. Proc Natl Acad Sci U S A 1984;81:4917–21.

8. Dunn PPJ. Human leucocyte antigen typing: techniques and technology, a critical appraisal. Int J Immunogenet 2011;38:463–73.

9. Gonzalez-Galarza FF, Christmas S, Middleton D, et al. Allele frequency net: a database and online repository for immune gene frequencies in worldwide populations. Nucleic Acids Res 2011;39:D913–9.

10. Burt C, Cryer C, Fuggle S, et al. HLA-A, -B, -DR allele group frequencies in 7007 kidney transplant list patients in 27 UK centres. Int J Immunogenet 2012;7 Sept. Epub ahead of print.

11. Bodmer WF, Bodmer JG. Evolution and function of the HLA system. Br Med Bull 1978;34:309–16.

12. Claas FHJ, Smeenk RJT, Schmidt R, et al. Alloimmunization against the MHC antigens after platelet transfusions is due to contaminating leukocytes in the platelet suspension. Exp Hematol 1981;9:84–9.

13. Bilgin YM, van de Watering LMG, Brand A. Clinical effects of leucoreduction of blood transfusions. Neth J Med 2011;69:441–50.

14. van de Watering L, Hermans J, Witvliet M, et al. HLA and RBC immunisation after filtered and buffy coat-depleted blood transfusion in cardiac surgery: a randomised controlled trial. Transfusion 2003;43:765–71.

15. Bartel G, Wahrmann M, Exner M, et al. Determinants of the complement-fixing ability of recipient presensitization against HLA antigens. Transplantation 2007;83:727–33.

16. Triulzi D, Kleinman S, Kakaiya R, et al. The effect of previous pregnancy and transfusion on HLA alloimmunisation in blood donors; implications for a transfusion-related acute lung injury risk reduction strategy. Transfusion 2009;49:1825–35.

17. Gill J, Landsberg D, Johnston O, et al. Screening for de novo anti-human leukocyte antigen antibodies in nonsensitised kidney transplant recipients does not predict acute rejection. Transplantation 2010;89:178–84.

18. Ntokou I-S, Iniotaki A, Kontou E, et al. Long-term follow up for anti-HLA donor specific antibodies postrenal transplantation: high immunogenicity of HLA class II graft molecules. Transpl Int 2011;24:1084–93.

19. Marrari M, Duquesnoy R. Detection of donor-specific HLA antibodies before and after removal of a rejected kidney transplant. Transpl Immunol 2010;22:105–9.

20. Fontana M, Moradpour D, Aubert V, et al. Prevalence of anti-HLA antibodies after liver transplantation. Transpl Int 2010;24:858–9.

21. El-Awar N, Lee JH, Tarsitani C, et al. HLA Class I epitopes: recognition of binding sites by mAbs or eluted alloantibody confirmed with single recombinant antigens. Hum Immunol 2007;68:170–80.

22. Duquesnoy RJ. Antibody-reactive epitope determination with HLA Matchmaker and its clinical applications. Tissue Antigens 2011;77:525–34.

23. Zoet Y, Brand-Schaaf S, Roelen D, et al. Challenging the golden standard in defining donor-specific antibodies: does the solid phase assay meet the expectations. Tissue Antigens 2011;77:225–8.

24. Schnaidt M, Weinstock C, Jurisic M. HLA antibody specification using single-antigen beads – A technical solution for the prozone effect. Transplantation 2011;92:510–5.

25. Susal C, Ovens J, Mahmoud K, et al. No association of kidney graft loss with human leukocyte antigen antibodies detected exclusively by sensitive Luminex single-antigen testing: a collaborative transplant study report. Transplantation 2011;91:883–7.

26. Chen G, Sequeira F, Tyan DB. Novel C1q assay reveals a clinically relevant subset of human leukocyte antigen antibodies independent of immunoglobulin G strength on single antigen beads. Hum Immunol 2011;72:849–58.

27. Talbot D, White M, Shenton BK, et al. Flow cytometric crossmatching in renal transplantation- the long term outcome. Transpl Immunol 1995;3:352–5.

28. Howell WM, Harmer A, Briggs D, et al. British Society for Histocompatibility & Immunogenetics and British Transplantation Society Guidelines for the detection and characterisation of clinically relevant antibodies in allotransplantation. Int J Immunogenet 2010;37:435. www.bts.org.uk/transplantation/standards-and-guidelines/; http://www.bshi.org.uk/pdf/BSHI_BTS_guidelines_2010.pdf; [accessed 6.09.12].
This is a consensus statement that includes guidelines for clinical practice based on available published evidence to support effective management of sensitised patients before, at the time of and after organ transplantation.

29. Amico P, Honger G, Mayr M, et al. Clinical relevance of pre-transplant donor-specific HLA antibodies detected by single-antigen flow-beads. Transplantation 2009;87:1681–8.

30. Worthington J, Martin S, Al-Husseini D, et al. Posttransplantation production of donor HLA-specific antibodies as a predictor of renal transplant outcome. Transplantation 2003;75:1034–40.

This is the first substantive report, using modern antibody detection technologies, relating the post-transplant production of donor HLA reactive antibodies to adverse outcomes.

31. Lee Po-C, Zhu L, Terasaki P, et al. HLA-specific antibodies developed in the first year post-transplant are predictive of chronic rejection and renal graft loss. Transplantation 2009;88:568–74.

32. Lachmann N, Terasaki P, Buddle K, et al. Anti-human leukocyte antigen and donor-specific antibodies detected by Luminex post-transplant serve as biomarkers for chronic rejection of renal allografts. Transplantation 2009;87:1505–13.
This study addresses the incidence of donor HLA reactive antibodies after transplantation to the clinically challenging process of chronic glomeruloropathy.

33. Everly M, Everly J, Arend L, et al. Reducing de novo donor-specific antibody levels during acute rejection diminishes renal allograft loss. Am J Transplant 2009;9:1063–71.

34. Dragun D. Humoral responses directed against non-human leukocyte antigens in solid-organ transplantation. Transplantation 2008;86:1019–25.

35. Sigdel T, Li L, Tran T, et al. Non-HLA antibodies to immunogenic epitopes predict the evolution of chronic renal allograft injury. J Am Soc Nephrol 2012;23:1–14.
This study uses high-density protein arrays to identify non-HLA antibodies in kidney transplant patients with chronic allograft injury. This novel approach reveals significant new information to support better understanding of the mechanisms involved and will inform more effective clinical interventions.

36. Breimer ME, Rydberg L, Jackson AM, et al. Multicenter evaluation of a novel endothelial cell crossmatch test in kidney transplantation. Transplantation 2009;87:549–56.

37. Taylor C, Smith S, Morgan C, et al. Selective omission of the donor cross-match before renal transplantation: efficacy, safety and effects on cold storage time. Transplantation 2000;69:719.
This report substantiates the highly clinically relevant process of proceeding to kidney transplantation on the basis of a virtual crossmatch. A defined protocol validated by an outcomes report is included.

38. www.bts.org.uk; [accessed 6.09.12].

39. www.bshi.org.uk; [accessed 6.09.12].

40. Robinson J, Mistry K, McWilliam H, et al. The IMGT/HLA Database. Nucleic Acids Res 2011;39(Suppl. 1):D1171–6.

41. Robinson J, Malik A, Parham P, et al. IMGT/HLA – a sequence database for the human major histocompatibility complex. Tissue Antigens 2000;55:280–7.

5

Immunosuppression with the kidney as paradigm

David Wojciechowski
Gregory Veillette
Flavio Vincenti

Introduction

Unless a transplant is performed between identical twins, recipients of kidney transplants generally require lifelong immunosuppression to maintain a state of low immunoresponsiveness to the allograft. In the 1980s the calcineurin inhibitor[1] ciclosporin was introduced; additional new small molecules and biologicals were successfully introduced in the clinic during the 1990s. Consequently, rejection rates, which were in the 40% range, fell to 10–15%.[2]

In general, immunosuppression can be divided into two phases: induction and maintenance. Additionally, the drugs used in transplantation can be divided into two categories: small molecules and biological agents. During the induction phase (perioperative and early post-transplant period), when immune responses to the allograft are at their highest, immunosuppression regimens are intensified. Induction agents, which include corticosteroids as well as depleting or non-depleting biological therapeutics (such as polyclonal antibodies or murine, chimeric or humanised monoclonal antibodies), act mainly by either depleting or modulating lymphocytes or suppressing proliferation and blunting the effects of T-cell activation. Biological therapeutics target specific cell surface glycoproteins or membrane-bound receptors.

After the induction phase, transplant patients transition to the maintenance phase of immunosuppression.[3] Effective maintenance immunosuppression is the key to preventing rejection throughout the life of the graft. Modern maintenance therapies include a calcineurin inhibitor (CNI) backbone along with antiproliferative agents (mycophenolate mofetil (MMF)/enteric-coated mycophenolate acid, azathioprine, or mammalian target of rapamycin (mTOR) inhibitors such as sirolimus and everolimus) and corticosteroids.

Unfortunately, immunosuppression has significant toxicities and side-effects. One of the goals of the transplant community has been to develop new drugs with higher specificity for their target and a decreased side-effect profile. In this chapter we will describe the commonly used immunosuppressive agents and how their combination and use have evolved in kidney transplantation over the last four decades.

Calcineurin inhibitors

Ciclosporin

The CNIs ciclosporin and tacrolimus are the backbone maintenance agents of current standard immunosuppressive regimens. Through calcineurin inhibition, both agents block downstream signalling, and thus activation, of T lymphocytes. Prior to the mid-1980s, options for immunosuppression following kidney transplantation included whole-body irradiation, polyclonal antilymphocyte antibodies, azathioprine and corticosteroids.[4] With the introduction of ciclosporin, 1-year allograft survival rates improved from 50–60% to 70–80%.[5] When used in combination with an antimetabolite and corticosteroids (triple-drug therapy), 1-year allograft survival rates of 80–90% are achieved.

Ciclosporin was introduced for use in renal transplant recipients in the early 1980s. It is a peptide isolated from the fungus *Tolypacladium inflatum*. Ciclosporin binds to the cytoplasmic protein cyclophilin, which subsequently inhibits calcineurin; this results in early cell cycle arrest from the inhibition of proinflammatory cytokine transcription, namely interleukin (IL)-2 and tumour necrosis factor (TNF)-α. Ciclosporin is available in both oral and intravenous forms. The most widely used oral form of the medication is in a microemulsion formulation (brand names Neoral and Gengraf). The non-microemulsion form is available as capsules (brand name Sandimmune), oral solution and intravenous concentrate. However, the microemulsion form is preferred, given its better bioavailability and more predictable absorption and drug levels. Target drug trough levels are usually 200–300 ng/mL for the first 6 months post-transplant, after which trough levels of 50–150 ng/mL are acceptable.

Ciclosporin is metabolised by the liver cytochrome P450 enzymes. Typically, patients remain stable on a certain dose; however, it is important to monitor drug levels more frequently if there is liver insufficiency, a new medication is started/stopped or if patients experience major stress (illness, surgery, trauma). Common agents that can significantly increase ciclosporin levels include calcium channel blockers (diltiazem, verapamil, nicardipine), antifungals (fluconazole, itraconazole, voriconazole, ketoconazole) and macrolide antibiotics (clarithromycin, erythromycin). Agents that will decrease levels include rifampin, phenytoin, carbamazepine and phenobarbital. Side-effects of ciclosporin include hypertension, sodium retention, nephrotoxicity, headache, tremor, seizures, nausea, vomiting, anorexia, gingival hyperplasia and hirsutism.

In 1984, the sentinel trial was published that supported the safety and efficacy of ciclosporin in renal transplant recipients.[5] In this study, patients who received ciclosporin alone or azathioprine plus corticosteroids were compared. The 4-year allograft survival was 70% in the ciclosporin group and 62% in the azathioprine/steroid group. Over the subsequent 10 years, allograft survival was prolonged further by the use of triple drug therapy with ciclosporin, azathioprine and corticosteroids.

Tacrolimus

Tacrolimus was FDA approved for liver transplant in 1994, and soon after was also being utilised in renal transplant recipients. Formerly known as FK-506, tacrolimus is a macrolide antibiotic isolated from the fungus *Streptomyces tsukubaensis*. It binds to FK-binding protein in the cytoplasm, which, similar to the ciclosporin/cyclophilin complex, blocks the activity of calcineurin, thus preventing proinflammatory cytokine transcription and T-lymphocyte activation.[6] Both oral and intravenous forms of tacrolimus are available. Similar to the microemulsion forms of ciclosporin, the absorption of tacrolimus is not dependent on bile salts. Tacrolimus is a more potent immunosuppressant than ciclosporin; target trough levels range between 4 and 10 ng/mL.

Tacrolimus is also metabolised by the liver P450 system, and drug levels are susceptible to the same agents that alter ciclosporin levels. The side-effects of tacrolimus include hypertension, tremor, headache, seizures, nephrotoxicity, glucose intolerance, nausea, vomiting, anorexia and alopecia.

There have been numerous studies comparing the two CNIs. The first landmark trial was done in 1997 by the FK-506 Kidney Transplant Study Group.[7] This study demonstrated a significant reduction in the incidence of biopsy-proven acute rejection (BPAR) in those recipients treated with tacrolimus-based immunosuppression (30.7% vs. 46.4%; **Fig. 5.1**). In the same year, the European Tacrolimus Multicentre Renal Study Group published similar results, with rates of BPAR in tacrolimus- and ciclosporin-treated groups of 25.9% and 45.7%, respectively (**Fig. 5.2**).[8] In both of these trials, the 1-year allograft and patient survival rates were similar. Furthermore, these trials were both done using the non-microemulsion form of ciclosporin. In 2005, a large meta-analysis based on 30 trials was performed.[9] In this analysis, tacrolimus was associated with improved allograft survival at 6 months and a decreased incidence of acute rejection

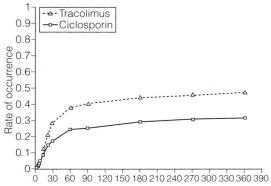

Figure 5.1 • There was a significant reduction in the incidence of biopsy-confirmed acute rejection in the tacrolimus-treated patients (30.7%) compared with the ciclosporin-treated patients (46.4%, $P = 0.001$). Reproduced from Pirsch JD, Miller J, Deierhoi MH et al. A comparison of tacrolimus (FK506) and cyclosporine for immunosuppression after cadaveric renal transplantation. Transplantation 1997; 63(7): 977–83. With permission from Wolters Kluwer Health.

in the first year. However, there are no direct convincing data showing that tacrolimus is associated with better outcomes than ciclosporin except possibly for slightly better renal function.[10] Also, note that an advantage of tacrolimus is that managing drug levels is easier with tacrolimus as trough levels correlate better with the area under the curve (AUC) as compared to ciclosporin.

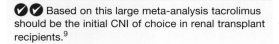

Based on this large meta-analysis tacrolimus should be the initial CNI of choice in renal transplant recipients.[9]

Antimetabolites

The antimetabolites are a class of immunosuppressive medications that act by causing cell cycle arrest in the DNA synthesis (S) phase of lymphocyte proliferation. Specifically, they inhibit the synthesis of the purine nucleotides (adenine and guanine). Since both T- and B-cell lymphoproliferation are dependent on the de novo synthesis of these nucleotides, inhibition precludes lymphocyte activation and proliferation.

The first antimetabolite widely used in kidney transplantation was azathioprine. Prior to the accepted use of ciclosporin, azathioprine along with corticosteroids was the maintenance agent of choice for nearly two decades. Once absorbed, azathioprine is converted to 6-mercaptopurine, which is the active form of the drug. The drug is available in both oral and intravenous forms, with the standard maintenance dosing of 1–3 mg/kg/day. Side-effects include malaise, fevers, nausea, anorexia, hepatotoxicity and leucopenia. Caution must be used in patients also on allopurinol, since the inhibition of xanthine oxidase will allow accumulation of the azathioprine active metabolites.[11]

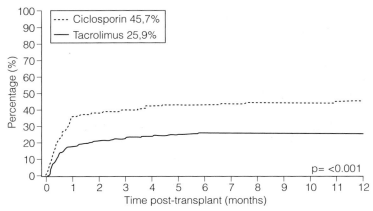

Figure 5.2 • The 12-month Kaplan–Meier estimates of biopsy-proven acute rejection were 25.9% and 45.7% for the tacrolimus and ciclosporin treatment groups, respectively ($P < 0.001$; absolute difference: 19.8%, 95% confidence interval (CI): 10.0–29.6%). Reproduced from Mayer DA, Dmitrewski J, Squifflet JP et al. Multicenter randomized trial comparing tacrolimus (FK506) and cyclosporine in the prevention of renal allograft rejection: a report of the European Tacrolimus Multicenter Renal Study Group. Transplantation 1997; 64(3):436–43. With permission from Wolters Kluwer Health.

MMF and mycophenolate sodium are newer antimetabolite agents used routinely in renal transplant recipients. Both agents are prodrugs and are rapidly metabolised to the active form, mycophenolic acid (MPA). MPA inhibits the enzyme inosine monophosphate dehydrogenase, which plays a key role in purine biosynthesis. MMF is available in both oral and intravenous forms. The typical starting dose for an adult patient is 1000 mg twice daily. Mycophenolate sodium is an enteric-coated formulation and is available only as an oral agent. MMF is teratogenic and is contraindicated in pregnancy.[12]

There remains controversy over the issue of which antimetabolite should be used as first line therapy in renal transplantation. Early studies suggested that MMF was superior to azathioprine since there were fewer acute rejection episodes.[13,14] Arguably, these studies were done before the introduction of ciclosporin microemulsion formulations. In 2004, the Mycophenolate Mofetil versus Azathioprine for Prevention of Acute Rejection in Renal Transplantation (MYSS) trial was published,[15] in which a ciclosporin microemulsion was used, and demonstrated no difference in the incidence of clinical rejection or rates of allograft loss. However, the cost of MMF was over 10-fold more than azathioprine.

Conversely, a recent meta-analysis concluded that MMF, used in combination with any CNI, is superior to azathioprine, resulting in a lower incidence of acute rejection episodes (**Fig. 5.3**) and prolonged allograft survival (**Fig. 5.4**).[16] In general, it is our standard practice to use MMF, in conjunction with tacrolimus. If patients develop gastrointestinal side-effects, we switch to mycophenolate sodium, which is occasionally better tolerated. Also, women who desire to get pregnant should be switched to azathioprine.

mTOR inhibitors

Sirolimus and everolimus are the two FDA-approved, commercially available mammalian target of rapamycin (mTOR) inhibitors currently available. Sirolimus was first discovered in the 1970s from a soil sample containing *Streptomyces hygroscopicus* and was approved for use in 1999. Everolimus is an analogue of sirolimus and was approved for use in the USA in 2010, although it has been available in Europe for the last decade. Similar to tacrolimus, both drugs bind to the FK-binding protein intracellularly. This complex inhibits mTOR, which is a serine-threonine kinase involved in upstream signal transduction. Therefore, unlike the CNIs, which act early in the cell cycle (G-0 to G-1 phase), the mTOR inhibitors prevent cell cycle progression from the G-1 to S phase by blocking the response of B and T cells to cytokine stimulation (mainly IL-2).

Sirolimus and everolimus are both available in oral forms and are metabolised by the liver cytochrome P450 system. Steady-state concentrations occur several days following initiation or alterations in dosing, and target therapeutic trough levels of 5–15 ng/mL are desirable. Similar to the CNIs, any medication that alters the P450 system will require close monitoring and adjustment in dosage. Importantly, dose reduction is required in the setting of hepatic, but not renal, impairment. Sirolimus and everolimus are contraindicated during pregnancy. The side-effects of the mTOR inhibitors include cytopenias, thrombotic microangiopathy, proteinuria, hyperlipidaemia, gastrointestinal upset, interstitial pneumonitis and poor wound healing.

The early studies analysing the efficacy of sirolimus for maintenance therapy in kidney transplantation were done with sirolimus utilised in combination with prednisone and ciclosporin. The comparison groups received ciclosporin and prednisone plus azathioprine,[17] or ciclosporin and prednisone plus placebo.[18] Both of these large studies demonstrated improved efficacy of sirolimus compared to azathioprine or placebo, when used in combination with prednisone and ciclosporin (less BPAR, no difference in allograft or patient survival). Despite this improvement in acute rejection episodes, both studies demonstrated that the sirolimus-treated patients had higher serum creatinine levels at 6 months and 1 year. This raised concern about the combination of sirolimus with full-dose CNI as the cause of worsening allograft function. Other studies have confirmed this apparent negative synergistic nephrotoxic effect of sirolimus with full-dose CNIs.[19–21] Furthermore, the de novo use of sirolimus has been associated with lymphocele formation, prolonged recovery from delayed graft function and poor wound healing.[22–24]

Given these issues, several recent trials have attempted to initiate maintenance therapy with a CNI

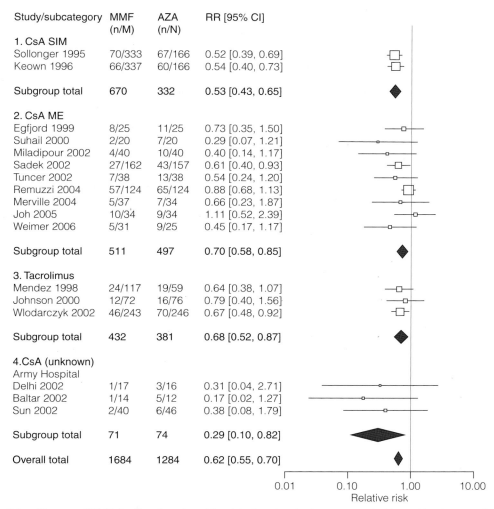

Study/subcategory	MMF (n/M)	AZA (n/N)	RR [95% CI]
1. CsA SIM			
Sollonger 1995	70/333	67/166	0.52 [0.39, 0.69]
Keown 1996	66/337	60/166	0.54 [0.40, 0.73]
Subgroup total	670	332	0.53 [0.43, 0.65]
2. CsA ME			
Egfjord 1999	8/25	11/25	0.73 [0.35, 1.50]
Suhail 2000	2/20	7/20	0.29 [0.07, 1.21]
Miladipour 2002	4/40	10/40	0.40 [0.14, 1.17]
Sadek 2002	27/162	43/157	0.61 [0.40, 0.93]
Tuncer 2002	7/38	13/38	0.54 [0.24, 1.20]
Remuzzi 2004	57/124	65/124	0.88 [0.68, 1.13]
Merville 2004	5/37	7/34	0.66 [0.23, 1.87]
Joh 2005	10/34	9/34	1.11 [0.52, 2.39]
Weimer 2006	5/31	9/25	0.45 [0.17, 1.17]
Subgroup total	511	497	0.70 [0.58, 0.85]
3. Tacrolimus			
Mendez 1998	24/117	19/59	0.64 [0.38, 1.07]
Johnson 2000	12/72	16/76	0.79 [0.40, 1.56]
Wlodarczyk 2002	46/243	70/246	0.67 [0.48, 0.92]
Subgroup total	432	381	0.68 [0.52, 0.87]
4. CsA (unknown)			
Army Hospital Delhi 2002	1/17	3/16	0.31 [0.04, 2.71]
Baltar 2002	1/14	5/12	0.17 [0.02, 1.27]
Sun 2002	2/40	6/46	0.38 [0.08, 1.79]
Subgroup total	71	74	0.29 [0.10, 0.82]
Overall total	1684	1284	0.62 [0.55, 0.70]

Relative risk: 0.01 — 0.10 — 1.00 — 10.00

Figure 5.3 • The use of MMF significantly reduced the risk of acute rejection compared with azathioprine overall (relative risk 0.62; CI 0.55–0.70; $P = 0.0001$) with low heterogeneity ($I^2 = 6.8\%$). Reproduced from Knight SR, Russell NK, Barcena L et al. Mycophenolate mofetil decreases acute rejection and may improve graft survival in renal transplant recipients when compared with azathioprine: a systematic review. Transplantation 2009; 87(6):785–94. With permission from Wolters Kluwer Health.

and subsequently switch to an mTOR inhibitor in an attempt to minimise the long-term nephrotoxicity of CNIs or the combination of calcineurin and mTOR inhibitors. The most recent is the CONVERT trial, a large, randomised trial in which recipients of renal allografts who were 6–120 months post-transplant and receiving tacrolimus or ciclosporin were randomly assigned to continue CNI or convert from CNI to sirolimus.[25] At 12 and 24 months there were no significant treatment differences in glomerular filtration rate (GFR) in the baseline GFR of more than 40 mL/min stratum. On-therapy analysis of this cohort showed significantly higher GFR at 12 and 24 months after sirolimus conversion. Rates of BPAR, graft survival and patient survival were similar between groups. Median urinary protein-to-creatinine ratios were similar at baseline but increased significantly after sirolimus conversion. Post hoc analysis identified a subgroup with baseline GFR more than 40 mL/min and urine protein-to-creatinine ratio less than or equal to 0.11 whose risk–benefit profile was more favourable after conversion than that for the overall sirolimus conversion cohort. The ZEUS trial was a large, randomised trial in which recipients of

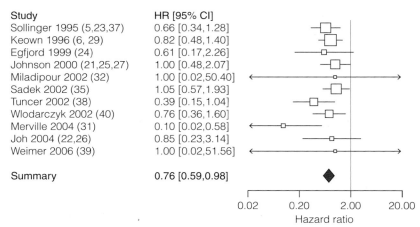

Study	HR [95% CI]
Sollinger 1995 (5,23,37)	0.66 [0.34,1.28]
Keown 1996 (6, 29)	0.82 [0.48,1.40]
Egfjord 1999 (24)	0.61 [0.17,2.26]
Johnson 2000 (21,25,27)	1.00 [0.48,2.07]
Miladipour 2002 (32)	1.00 [0.02,50.40]
Sadek 2002 (35)	1.05 [0.57,1.93]
Tuncer 2002 (38)	0.39 [0.15,1.04]
Wlodarczyk 2002 (40)	0.76 [0.36,1.60]
Merville 2004 (31)	0.10 [0.02,0.58]
Joh 2004 (22,26)	0.85 [0.23,3.14]
Weimer 2006 (39)	1.00 [0.02,51.56]
Summary	0.76 [0.59,0.98]

Figure 5.4 • The hazard of graft loss was significantly reduced in the MMF group (hazard ratio 0.76, CI 0.59–0.98, $P = 0.037$). Reproduced from Knight SR, Russell NK, Barcena L et al. Mycophenolate mofetil decreases acute rejection and may improve graft survival in renal transplant recipients when compared with azathioprine: a systematic review. Transplantation 2009; 87(6):785–94. With permission from Wolters Kluwer Health.

renal allografts were induced with basiliximab (see below) and maintained on three-drug therapy with ciclosporin, prednisone and MMF.[26] At 4.5 months post-transplant, patients were randomised to either continue ciclosporin or switch to everolimus. At 12 months, patients who received everolimus had improved GFRs. However, there was a higher incidence of acute rejection, hyperlipidaemia, anaemia and proteinuria. The Spare-the-Nephron trial was a large, multicentre, randomised trial in which patients were initially maintained on MMF and a CNI and then randomised to either stay on the MMF/CNI combination or switch to MMF plus sirolimus 30–180 days post-transplant.[27] At 12 months, the sirolimus group had significantly better GFRs; however, at 24 months this difference was no longer statistically significant. Also, there was a non-significant trend towards a lower rate of rejection in the sirolimus group.

Currently, mTOR inhibitors are typically not used as part of de novo maintenance therapy following renal transplantation. However, these agents do have proven efficacy and can be utilised in patients who do not tolerate CNIs or develop CNI nephrotoxicity.

> ✓✓ The mTOR inhibitors typically should not be used as part of de novo maintenance immunosuppression following renal transplantation. However, they can be used effectively as part of maintenance immunosuppression in those who do not tolerate CNIs or develop CNI toxicity.[25–27]

Biological agents

New biological agents currently in development have the potential to alter the model of immunosuppression drug design and delivery for organ transplantation. In general, biologicals and antibodies have been relegated to perioperative induction and the treatment of rejection due to their side-effects or an immune response to the agents themselves, limiting long-term efficacy. However, novel biologicals are now being developed for use as maintenance immunosuppression therapy. By selecting specific cell surface targets, new antibodies demonstrate remarkable specificity. This enhanced specificity is ideally suited for long-term immunosuppression as it may alleviate the untoward toxicity seen with daily agents such as CNIs. Technology such as protein humanisation as well as the ability to eliminate long-term immunogenicity has made antibody and fusion protein receptor therapy a present-day reality.[28] The transition, for biological agents, from short-term perioperative induction therapy to chronic maintenance immunosuppression was driven by a desire to eliminate CNIs and their toxicities. Furthermore, the development costs of a biological agent can only be justified when coupled with planned chronic use. The challenge, of course, is to demonstrate the safety of inhibiting a particular pathway with a biological over long periods of time. The prototype of such an endeavour is belatacept.

Depleting antibodies

Depleting antibodies are used as part of induction immunosuppression as well as for the treatment of acute rejection in kidney transplantation. These agents can further be divided into polyclonal or monoclonal preparations. The two available polyclonal agents are equine antithymocyte globulin (E-ATG) and rabbit antithymocyte globulin (R-ATG). The two monoclonal agents are muromonab CD3 (OKT3) and alemtuzumab. OKT3 is no longer being produced but will be discussed briefly in this section to place it in historical context. These four agents will be discussed in the order of approval for use.

Equine antithymocyte globulin

E-ATG, a depletional agent, was first studied in renal transplantation as part of an induction regimen.[29] This important study was an open-label trial that enrolled 358 renal transplant recipients. Patients were randomised to receive E-ATG for 14 days at the time of transplant in addition to standard immunosuppressive therapy, which at the time included azathioprine and prednisone (n = 183), versus standard immunosuppression without E-ATG (n = 175). E-ATG was dosed between 10 and 30 mg/kg/day. The outcomes evaluated were time to first rejection episode, steroid dosage requirements, graft and patient survival. A total of four lots of E-ATG were tested. Results within each lot were analysed separately and the data were also pooled to obtain an overall impression. In the pooled data analysis E-ATG delayed the onset of the first rejection episode during the prescribed treatment period (2 weeks). Concurrently, fewer i.v. corticosteroids were required, but the steroid dosage requirement then rebounded in the 2 weeks after the end of the prescribed treatment period. E-ATG did not significantly improve the proportion of patients alive with functioning grafts 6 months after transplantation, except in one of the four lots.

Later, Shield et al. published their experience using E-ATG for the treatment of acute rejection rather than as part of an induction regimen.[30] A total of 20 patients with rejection were randomised to receive E-ATG 15 mg/kg for 14 days or methylprednisolone 1000 mg i.v. daily for up to 5 days. Maintenance immunosuppression consisted of azathioprine and prednisone in both groups. Both therapies successfully reversed rejection episodes in these 20 patients, with E-ATG reversing rejection on average in 3 days and methylprednisolone in 6 days. Although underpowered to detect true differences in efficacy between these two regimens, these early data were able to demonstrate that E-ATG was at least as effective as methylprednisolone in reversing rejections and E-ATG may achieve that goal more quickly than methylprednisolone.

The intriguing data of Shield et al. prompted an evaluation of E-ATG for the treatment of steroid-resistant rejections in kidney transplant recipients. Hardy et al. evaluated 10 patients who did not respond to their usual treatment of acute rejection, which included methylprednisolone 15 mg/kg/day (not to exceed 750 mg) plus graft irradiation on days 1, 3 and 5 after rejection diagnosis.[31] After failure of usual therapy to reverse acute rejection these 10 patients were treated with E-ATG (15 mg/kg/day for 21 days). Their response to this therapy was then described and compared to that of 10 other patients who were treated with and responded to the typical rejection protocol (control group). Outcomes of interest were return of serum creatinine to baseline, frequency of other rejection episodes following E-ATG treatment, and 1-year patient and graft survival. Seven of the 10 patients in the E-ATG group experienced a return of creatinine to baseline compare to only three of the 10 patients in the control group. Two patients in the E-ATG group experienced a second rejection episode within 1 year and no patient in the E-ATG group experienced a third rejection episode. In contrast, four patients in the control group experienced a second rejection episode and two of these patients experienced rejection a third time within 1 year. Serum creatinine concentrations also were lower in the E-ATG group compared to the control group 1 year later. Graft failure appeared to occur equally among the two groups, with five and four grafts lost in the control and E-ATG groups, respectively, over the 1-year follow-up. There were no deaths in either group during the follow-up period. Later, this same group published their experience with 12 additional patients receiving E-ATG for the treatment of a first acute rejection episode compared to 20 control patients receiving the standard protocol for their first acute rejection.[32] Graft survival at 1 year was 73% and 46.6% for patients treated with E-ATG and standard therapy, respectively. Mortality was 3% and 20% in the E-ATG and standard therapy groups, respectively. Therefore, the data suggested that E-ATG was superior to standard therapy for graft and patient survival for the treatment of a first acute rejection episode.

It should be noted that these studies were small in numbers and not compared against patients on current immunosuppression, which typically includes a CNI. However, the data suggested that E-ATG was effective in preventing acute rejection as part of an induction regimen and for the treatment of acute rejection episodes. It should be noted, however, that since the introduction of R-ATG, E-ATG is no longer used in renal transplantation.

Muromonab CD3

OKT3 was the first monoclonal antibody approved for use in kidney transplantation. It was approved for the treatment of acute rejection in kidney transplant recipients in 1986. Typically, OKT3 was reserved for the treatment of severe rejections or for rejections that are refractory to corticosteroids. OKT3 is a murine monoclonal antibody directed against the cell surface antigen CD3, which is present on mature T lymphocytes. Since it is T-cell specific OKT3 does not result in the depletion of other cellular blood lines, such as platelets. Occasionally the development of human antimurine antibodies was noted and thought to account for the observation of rising CD3-positive T-cell concentrations toward the end of treatment. The most notable side-effect of OKT3 treatment was the cytokine release syndrome. Initial binding of OKT3 to T lymphocytes resulted in transient activation. Subsequently, a release of cytokines such as TNF-α, IL-2, IL-6 and interferon-γ was noted. This cytokine release manifested as a mild, flu-like syndrome and could progress to severe shortness of breath and pulmonary oedema. It was important to ensure patients treated with OKT3 were not significantly volume overloaded and required close monitoring with the initial dose. The availability of R-ATG decreased the need to use OKT3 and in 2009 Ortho Biotech decided to withdraw it from the marketplace.

Rabbit antithymocyte globulin

R-ATG was approved in the USA for the treatment of acute rejection in renal transplant recipients in 1999. R-ATG is extensively used off-label as induction immunosuppression given at the time of transplantation. R-ATG is a polyclonal IgG antibody, produced by immunising rabbits with human T lymphocytes. R-ATG is comprised of multiple different antibodies directed against various T- and B-lymphocyte surface antigens, such as CD2, CD3, CD4, CD8, CD11a, CD18, CD25, human leucocyte antigen (HLA)-DR and HLA class I. R-ATG exerts its antirejection effects by clearing T lymphocytes from peripheral blood and modulation of T-lymphocyte activity. When used for the treatment of acute rejection R-ATG is usually administered in doses of 1.5 mg/kg i.v. daily for 7–14 days. Primary side-effects are related to an infusion syndrome consisting of various signs and symptoms, including fever, chills, rigors, headache, shortness of breath, and hyper- or hypotension. These side-effects can be minimised with the addition of corticosteroid, acetaminophen and antihistamine premedication. Additionally, haematological side-effects can occur; these include leucopenia and thrombocytopenia. These may persist for several weeks after the last infusion of R-ATG. Complete blood counts should be monitored closely during and after therapy. The manufacturer of R-ATG recommends that the dose should be halved if the white blood cell count (WBC) drops to between 2000 and 3000 cells/mm^3 or if the platelet count falls to between 50 000 and 75 000 cells/mm^3. The manufacturer also recommends considering stopping R-ATG treatment if the WBC falls below 2000 cells/mm^3 or the platelet count falls below 50 000 cells/mm^3. Many centres administer R-ATG according to the absolute T-cell count with daily monitoring of this parameter, as individual patient response to the same dose regimen can be very variable.[33]

R-ATG was studied in a double-blind, randomised, multicentre trial compared to E-ATG for the treatment of acute rejection following kidney transplantation.[34] A total of 163 patients were enrolled at 25 transplant centres in the USA. Patients were randomised to receive R-ATG 1.5 mg/kg/day versus E-ATG 15 mg/kg/day, each for a total of 7–14 days. With regard to the primary end-point, reversal of acute rejection rate, R-ATG was superior to E-ATG (88% vs. 76%; $P = 0.027$). Day 30 graft survival (R-ATG 94% and E-ATG 90%; $P = 0.17$), day 30 serum creatinine levels as a percentage of baseline (R-ATG 72% and E-ATG 80%; $P = 0.43$) and improvement in post-treatment biopsy results (R-ATG 65% and E-ATG 50%; $P = 0.15$) were not statistically different. T-cell depletion was maintained more effectively with R-ATG compared to E-ATG both at the end of therapy ($P = 0.001$) and at day 30 ($P = 0.016$). Recurrent rejection at 90 days after therapy occurred less frequently with R-ATG (17%) compared to E-ATG (36%; $P = 0.011$). A similar incidence of adverse events, post-therapy infections, and 1-year patient and graft survival rates was noted in both treatment groups. Overall, R-ATG was found to be superior to E-ATG in reversing acute rejection and preventing recurrent rejection after treatment in renal transplant recipients.

> ✔✔ This trial demonstrated that R-ATG was superior to E-ATG in reversing acute rejection. It also demonstrated that R-ATG was superior at preventing recurrent rejections compared to E-ATG.[34]

R-ATG has also gained common off-label use as an induction agent. R-ATG has been evaluated for this purpose in a randomised, double-blind, single-centre trial versus E-ATG with initial results published in 1999 and 10-year follow-up data published in 2008.[35] The primary end-point was to compare the safety and efficacy of R-ATG to E-ATG as an induction agent in renal transplant recipients. A total of 72 kidney transplant recipients were randomised 2:1 in a double-blinded fashion to receive R-ATG ($n = 48$) at 1.5 mg/kg i.v. or E-ATG ($n = 24$) at 15 mg/kg i.v., intraoperatively, then daily for at least 6 days. By 1 year after transplantation, 4% of R-ATG-treated patients experienced acute rejection compared to 25% of E-ATG-treated patients ($P = 0.014$). Patient survival was not different between the two groups but the composite end-point of freedom from death, graft loss or rejection (the 'event-free survival') was superior with R-ATG (94%) compared with E-ATG (63%; $P = 0.0005$). Fewer adverse events occurred with R-ATG but leucopenia was more common with R-ATG than with E-ATG (56% vs. 4%, respectively; $P < 0.0001$) during induction. The incidence of cytomegalovirus (CMV) disease was less with R-ATG than with E-ATG at 6 months (10% vs. 33%, respectively; $P = 0.025$). At 5 years the event-free survival was 73% and 33% for R-ATG and E-ATG, respectively ($P = 0.047$). Freedom from rejection at 5 years was 92% and 66% for R-ATG

and E-ATG, respectively ($P = 0.007$). No additional cases of CMV disease occurred in either group; however, there were two cases of post-transplant lymphoproliferative disorder (PTLD) with the E-ATG group and none in the R-ATG group. At 10 years the event-free survival was higher with R-ATG than with E-ATG (48% vs. 29%, respectively; $P = 0.011$). Patient and graft survival was 75% and 48%, respectively, for R-ATG-treated patients, and 67% and 50%, respectively, for E-ATG-treated patients. However, the incidence of acute rejection was lower in R-ATG-treated patients compared to E-ATG-treated patients (11% vs. 42%, respectively; $P = 0.004$). There were no new cases of PTLD or CMV in either group compared to the 5-year results.

> ✔✔ When used as an induction agent R-ATG is more effective than E-ATG at preventing acute rejection.[35]

Both R-ATG and E-ATG have been used for the treatment of acute rejection as well as for induction therapy in kidney transplant recipients. R-ATG appears to be more effective at reversing acute rejection compared with E-ATG. R-ATG also appears to be more effective at preventing acute rejection when used as an induction agent compared to E-ATG.

Alemtuzumab

Alemtuzumab was approved for the treatment of B-cell chronic lymphocytic leukaemia in 2001. Alemtuzumab is a humanised monoclonal antibody directed against the CD52 antigen present on malignant and normal B lymphocytes, T lymphocytes, monocytes, macrophages and natural killer cells. Alemtuzumab has been used off-label in renal transplantation as an induction agent and as a treatment for acute rejection. When used as part of an induction regimen, transplant centres were hopeful that alemtuzumab could induce tolerance. Additionally, centres have evaluated the use of alemtuzumab with lowered dosing and exposure of maintenance immunosuppression due to a concern regarding a higher risk of infectious complications.

An evaluation of alemtuzumab versus R-ATG versus daclizumab (a monoclonal antibody directed against the CD25 antigen, to be discussed later), all utilised as induction agents, was undertaken for the first-time renal transplant recipients at a single centre as a randomised clinical trial.[36] Group A received R-ATG at 1 mg/kg/day during the first week postoperatively (a total of seven doses), group B received alemtuzumab 0.3 mg/kg on the day of surgery and again 4 days later (each dose preceded by i.v. methylprednisolone, 500 and 250 mg, respectively), group C received daclizumab 1 mg/kg at surgery and four additional doses once every 2 weeks. In groups A and C maintenance immunosuppression consisted of tacrolimus with an initial target trough of 8–10 ng/mL, MMF 1 g twice daily and methylprednisolone 500 mg i.v. daily for 3 days postoperatively with subsequent weaning to achieve a target maintenance dosing of 0.3 and then 0.15 mg/kg, respectively, at 1 and 3 months (and subsequently) postoperatively. In group B maintenance immunosuppression consisted of tacrolimus with an initial target trough of 4–7 ng/mL at 1 month post-transplant and 4–6 ng/mL at 6 months post-transplant and, thereafter, MMF 500 mg twice daily, and an avoidance of maintenance corticosteroids after the first week postoperatively. A total of 90 patients were enrolled, 30 patients in each group. Patients were followed for a minimum of 27 months. By month 12 there was no difference in biopsy-proven acute rejection (BPAR) between the groups, with 18% in group A, 18% in group B and 19% in group C ($P = 0.99$). There was no difference in graft failure between the groups at 12 months (group A 3%, group B 0% and group C 0%; $P = 0.38$). There was also no difference in renal function as defined by the calculated CrCl between the groups at 12 months (group A 80 mL/min, group B 72.8 mL/min and group C 81 mL/min; $P = 0.63$). In a subsequent report, in which patients had a minimum of 27 months of follow-up, there were six (20%), seven (23%) and seven (23%) patients who experienced BPAR in groups A, B and C, respectively. The long-term report also demonstrated no difference between the three groups in patient or graft survival. Interestingly, however, the death censored graft survival was significantly poorer in group B compared to groups A and C combined ($P = 0.01$), with one, six and one kidney graft failures occurring in groups A, B and C, respectively. Larger, longer-term, multicentre trials need to be performed to better evaluate the role of alemtuzumab as induction immunosuppression. However, it is unlikely that alemtuzumab will undergo clinical trials to pass regulatory approval for use in kidney transplant recipients.

> ✅ The exact role of alemtuzumab in renal transplantation is still to be determined. Thus far there seems to be no advantage in using alemtuzumab over other available induction agents.

Non-depleting antibodies and biologicals

Daclizumab

Daclizumab is a humanised monoclonal IgG antibody approved in 1997 for the prevention of acute rejection in kidney transplant recipients when used with concurrent maintenance immunosuppression. It is directed against the CD25 subunit of the IL-2 receptor present on the surface of activated T cells. In December 2009 daclizumab was withdrawn from the market. Therefore, we will focus on the other currently available IL-2 receptor blocker basiliximab in the next section. However, it is interesting to note that there are currently ongoing trials evaluating the effectiveness of a subcutaneous formulation of daclizumab for the treatment of multiple sclerosis.

Basiliximab

Basiliximab is a chimeric monoclonal antibody targeting the α-subunit of the IL-2 receptor. It was approved for the prevention of renal allograft rejection in 1998. Basiliximab is similar to daclizumab in mechanism of action. Basiliximab is given as a two-dose regimen, with 20 mg given i.v. preoperatively followed by another 20 mg on postoperative day 4. Basiliximab has a terminal half-life of 7.2 ± 3.2 days. When administered as the two-dose regimen it provides a 30-to 45-day blockade of the IL-2 receptor in adults.[37,38]

Basiliximab was studied in two identical randomised, double-blind, placebo-controlled clinical trials, one conducted in the USA and the other conducted in Europe and Canada.[39,40] Each trial evenly randomised patients to receive either basiliximab or placebo as induction treatment on the day of the transplant and 4 days later. Maintenance immunosuppression in each trial consisted of ciclosporin and corticosteroids. The primary end-point of each trial was the 6-month incidence of BPAR. Secondary end-points included the incidence of steroid-resistant acute rejection, patient and graft survival, and graft function.

The European/Canadian trial was first published in 1997.[40] A total of 376 patients were eligible for the intention-to-treat analysis (basiliximab, $n = 190$; placebo, $n = 186$). The incidence of BPAR 6 months after transplantation was 29.8% and 44% in the basiliximab and placebo groups, respectively ($P = 0.012$). This difference persisted at 12 months, with the incidence of BPAR being 37.9% and 54.8% in the basiliximab and placebo groups, respectively ($P = 0.002$). The incidence of steroid-resistant first rejection episodes was significantly lower in the basiliximab group compared to the placebo group (10% vs. 23.1%, respectively; $P < 0.001$). The incidence of graft loss at 12 months was not different between the two groups (basiliximab, 12.1%; placebo, 13.4%; $P = 0.591$). During the first 12 months a total of 14 deaths occurred, nine in the basiliximab group and five in the placebo group ($P = 0.293$).

The US trial was published in 1999[39] and included a total of 346 patients divided equally into the two treatment groups. The incidence of BPAR by 6 months after transplantation was 32.9% and 49.1% in the basiliximab and placebo groups, respectively ($P = 0.017$). This difference persisted at 12 months, with the incidence of BPAR being 35.3% and 49.1% in the basiliximab and placebo groups, respectively ($P = 0.009$). The incidence of steroid-resistant first rejection episodes was significantly lower in the basiliximab group compared to the placebo group (25.4% vs. 41.6%, respectively; $P = 0.001$). A total of five and seven deaths occurred in the basiliximab and placebo groups, respectively.

✔✔ Two trials demonstrate that basiliximab when used as an induction agent is more effective at preventing acute rejection compared to placebo but there was no difference in patient or graft survival. However, maintenance immunosuppression in these trials utilised only two agents: ciclosporin and corticosteroids.[39,40]

Overall, both studies confirmed the effectiveness of basiliximab compared to placebo at preventing BPAR. However, data on the secondary end-points were mixed. There was a decrease in the incidence of steroid-resistant rejections in both studies in basiliximab-treated patients; however, neither study demonstrated a patient or graft survival benefit. Lastly, neither study demonstrated a difference in graft function, with the CrCl in both studies at 1 year ranging from 52 to 58 mL/min.

It is important to note that both the US and the European/Canadian trials utilised maintenance immunosuppression with two agents. By the time both trials were published most centres were utilising triple drug immunosuppression. Consequently, a Phase IV trial was performed to assess whether induction with basiliximab could reduce the incidence of acute rejection in kidney transplant recipients treated with ciclosporin, corticosteroids and azathioprine.[41] A total of 340 patients were randomised to receive either placebo or basiliximab at a dose of 20 mg i.v. on days 0 and 4. All patients received three-drug maintenance immunosuppression with the regimen noted above. The primary end-point was the incidence of acute rejection at 6 months. Secondary end-points included the safety and tolerability of basiliximab and placebo, 1-year patient and graft survival, and significant medical events up to 12 months. Acute rejection occurred during the first 6 months in 20.8% and 34.9% of patients treated with basiliximab and placebo, respectively ($P = 0.005$). Similarly, there was a reduction in BPAR at 6 months in patients receiving basiliximab. One-year patient survival was 97.6% with basiliximab and 97.1% with placebo; graft survival was 91.5% versus 88.4%, respectively ($P = NS$). The adverse event profile of patients treated with basiliximab was indistinguishable from that of patients treated with placebo. The number of patients with infections was similar (65.5% for basiliximab vs. 65.7% for placebo), including CMV infections (17.3% vs. 14.5%; $P = 0.245$). Lastly, nine neoplasms were recorded up to 1 year from transplant, three in the basiliximab group and six in the placebo group.

In the three studies discussed so far, basiliximab was superior to placebo at reducing the incidence of acute rejection. However, as mentioned previously, the maintenance immunosuppression regimen in the first two trials included only two drugs. In the third trial the antiproliferative agent used was azathioprine. By the time of that study's publication, most patients were receiving MMF as their antiproliferative drug with maintenance CNI and corticosteroids. Additionally, the use of R-ATG as induction was becoming more widespread. Therefore, another trial was undertaken to evaluate the effectiveness and safety of R-ATG versus basiliximab in patients at high risk of rejection or delayed graft function and who received a renal transplant from a deceased donor. A total of 278 patients were randomised in a 1:1 manner to receive R-ATG (n = 141) at 1.5 mg/kg i.v. initiated intraoperatively, with subsequent doses given daily through day 4 for a total dose of 7.5 mg/kg versus basiliximab (n = 137) 20 mg i.v. preoperatively and a second infusion on day 4. Maintenance immunosuppression for all patients consisted of ciclosporin, MMF and corticosteroids. The primary end-point was a composite of acute rejection, delayed graft function, graft loss and death. At 12 months the incidence of the primary end-point did not differ significantly between the two groups: 50.4% and 56.2% in patients treated with R-ATG and basiliximab, respectively (P = 0.34). However, there were fewer patients treated with R-ATG versus basiliximab who experienced BPAR (15.6% vs. 25.5%, respectively; P = 0.02). The incidence of graft loss was similar among patients receiving R-ATG (9.2%) and those receiving basiliximab (10.2%), as were the incidences of death (4.3% and 4.4%, respectively). Overall, the incidence of infection was higher in the R-ATG group than in the basiliximab group (85.8% vs. 75.2%, respectively; P = 0.03). There was no significant difference between the two groups in the incidence of cancer, including PTLD. Thus, basiliximab is best when used for low immunological risk patients and R-ATG should be preferentially used in high immunological risk patients.

Belatacept

Belatacept, a fusion protein and selective co-stimulation blocker, was approved in June 2011 by the US Food and Drug Administration for the prophylaxis of organ rejection in adult patients receiving a kidney transplant. The approval of belatacept represented a paradigm shift; biologicals are no longer relegated to the sole purpose of induction immunosuppression and the treatment of acute rejection but now have entered the realm of maintenance immunosuppression. It is given as a 30-minute infusion that can be done either in an infusion centre or in the home. Belatacept was developed to provide effective immunosuppression as an alternative to CNIs and thus avoid the toxicities associated with CNIs.

The CD28/B7 (CD80 and 86) co-stimulation pathway is an essential signal for T-cell activation. After 25 years of research the fusion receptor protein CTLA4-Ig (abatacept), a competitive antagonist for CD28 blocking CD80/CD86 binding, was approved for human use in the treatment of rheumatoid arthritis.[42] Early experiments with co-stimulation blockade in transplantation were mixed. Prolongation of graft survival or induction of tolerance using co-stimulation blockade in rodent transplantation experiments could not be reproduced in non-human primates.[43,44] CTLA4-Ig did not achieve as good affinity to CD86 as compared with CD80 and was the likely cause of failure in a more stringent animal model.[43]

Belatacept, a re-engineered CTLA4-Ig with two amino acid substitutions in the CTLA4 binding domains, binds CD80 twofold better and CD86 fourfold better than CTLA4-Ig and has a 10-fold more potent inhibition of T-cell activation in vitro versus CTLA4-Ig.[45] The in vitro superiority of belatacept in blocking T-cell responses was confirmed by better survival of renal allografts in a non-human primate model.[43] In these experiments, a CNI-free regimen with belatacept and a combination of an anti-IL-2 receptor antibody and maintenance therapy with MMF and steroids resulted in marked prolongation of the survival of renal allografts.[43]

These encouraging data were utilised to design a Phase II multicenter clinical trial comparing the safety and efficacy of two dosing regimens of belatacept versus ciclosporin.[46] In this trial belatacept was found to be non-inferior (with a non-inferior margin set at 20%) to ciclosporin as a means of preventing acute rejection after renal transplantation, with five (7%) and four (6%) patients treated with a more intensive (MI) and less intensive (LI) belatacept regimen, respectively, experiencing acute rejection at 6 months compared to six (8%) ciclosporin-treated patients.

With regard to safety it was also noted that three patients receiving the MI regimen developed PTLD compared to one patient receiving ciclosporin. Two of these developed PTLD after belatacept had been replaced with conventional immunosuppression (tacrolimus, MMF and corticosteroids). Two of the three patients had primary Epstein–Barr virus (EBV) infections while the third received lymphocyte-depleting therapy with muronomab CD3 for acute rejection. In the 5-year long-term extension trial one patient treated with ciclosporin developed PTLD in year 4 after transplantation compared to no patients treated with belatacept.[47]

Given the promising Phase II trial results, two Phase III trials were undertaken. Both trials have provided important data on the role of belatacept as part of a CNI-free regimen in acute rejection prevention.

The first trial, Belatacept Evaluation of Nephroprotection and Efficacy as First-line Immunosuppression Trial (BENEFIT)[48] is a multicentre, randomised, active-controlled, parallel-group Phase III trial. Adult patients receiving a living donor or standard criteria deceased donor kidney were eligible. First-time patients with a panel reactive antibody ≥50%, re-transplants with a panel reactive antibody ≥30%, recipients of prior or concurrent non-renal solid-organ transplants and recipients of extended criteria donor kidneys were excluded. Patients were randomised to one of three regimens for maintenance immunosuppression: a more intensive regimen (MI) of belatacept, and a less intensive regimen (LI) of belatacept or ciclosporin (**Fig. 5.5**). Patients in all treatment arms received basiliximab induction and were maintained on MMF and corticosteroids. Lymphocyte-depleting therapy was permitted in the ciclosporin group for delayed or anticipated delayed graft function. Patients with acute rejection ≥Grade IIB could be treated with T-cell-depleting therapy at the investigator's discretion.

The trial was designed with three co-primary outcomes: composite patient and graft survival; composite renal impairment end-point; and incidence of acute rejection. The non-inferiority margin for patient and graft survival and for acute rejection was set at 10% and 20%, respectively. Protocol biopsies were performed at implantation and at week 52. A total of 527 patients were randomised to three treatment groups, transplanted and completed the initial 12-month treatment phase. Recipient demographics and baseline characteristics as well as donor characteristics were similar between the three groups.

Both belatacept regimens were non-inferior to ciclosporin on the primary end-point of patient and graft survival. At 1 year patients enrolled in the MI, LI and ciclosporin treatment groups had 95%, 97% and 93% graft survival, respectively. The mean measured GFR was 65, 63.4 and 50.4 mL/min/1.73 m² in the MI, LI and ciclosporin-treated patients, respectively ($P < 0.0001$ for both MI and LI vs. ciclosporin). The prevalence of chronic allograft nephropathy on protocol biopsies was lower in belatacept-treated patients compared to ciclosporin-treated patients (18% MI; 24% LI; 32% ciclosporin).

There was a higher incidence of acute rejection at 12 months in the belatacept-treated groups compared with the ciclosporin-treated group (22% MI; 17% LI; 7% ciclosporin). The incidence of

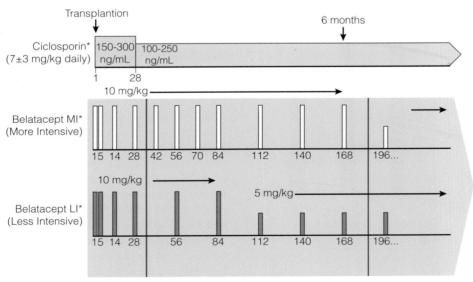

Figure 5.5 • Treatment regimen utilized in the Phase III BENEFIT and BENEFIT-EXT trials.

acute rejection met the non-inferiority cut-off for LI versus ciclosporin groups but not for MI versus ciclosporin groups. Almost 100% of these rejections occurred within the first 6 months post-transplantation. Belatacept-treated patients had more type IIa and IIb rejections compared to ciclosporin-treated patients but were not associated with an increase in donor-specific antibody (DSA). The mean measured GFR at month 12 was higher in belatacept-treated patients with acute rejection compared to ciclosporin-treated patients without acute rejection (**Fig. 5.6**), although it should be noted that in all groups patients with rejection had a lower GFR compared to patients in the same group without rejection.

Belatacept-treated patients had a significantly lower mean blood pressure (MI 133/79 mmHg; LI 131/79 mmHg) compared to ciclosporin-treated patients (139/82 mmHg) ($P \leq 0.0273$ for MI or LI vs. ciclosporin in all comparisons). The mean change in non-high-density-lipoprotein (non-HDL) cholesterol from baseline was significantly different in belatacept-treated patients (MI 8.1 mg/dL; LI 8.0 mg/dL) compared to ciclosporin-treated patients (18.3 mg/dL) ($P = 0.0115$ for MI and $P = 0.0104$ for LI vs. ciclosporin). The incidence of new-onset diabetes mellitus after transplant (NODAT) was not significantly different between the three groups: MI 7%, LI 4% and ciclosporin 10% (P = NS for MI or LI vs. ciclosporin).

Two- and 3-year data are available for BENEFIT.[49,50] Between months 12 and 24 a total of eight patients had an acute rejection episode (MI, n = 4; ciclosporin, n = 4) for a total of 24% (MI) and 9% (ciclosporin) from baseline to month 24.[49] The 3-year data demonstrate that there were no new cases of acute rejection in the belatacept groups from year 2 to 3.[50] However, one patient in the ciclosporin group experienced acute rejection after year 2. By year 3 DSA occurred more commonly in ciclosporin-treated patients (MI, 6%; LI, 5%; ciclosporin, 11%). In patients who had an acute rejection episode by year 3 the proportion of patients with DSA was 12% MI, 8% LI and 19% ciclosporin. With regard to renal function at year 3 the mean ± SD calculated GFR (cGFR) was 65.2 ± 26.3 (MI), 65.8 ± 27.0 (LI) and 44.4 ± 23.6 mL/min/1.73 m² (ciclosporin) ($P < 0.0001$ MI or LI vs. ciclosporin). The mean cGFR in belatacept-treated patients was consistently higher compared to ciclosporin-treated patients throughout the study period.

The issue of PTLD, which was raised in the Phase II trial, also merits a discussion from the Phase III data. By 12 months one, two and one patient(s) in the MI, LI and ciclosporin groups developed PTLD, respectively. Additionally, between years 1 and 2 two additional patients in the MI group developed central nervous system PTLD. Four of the six patients who developed PTLD had known risk factors. One patient had Epstein–Barr virus (EBV)-negative serology pre-transplant, one patient received lymphocyte-depleting therapy as treatment for an acute rejection, and two patients had both EBV-negative serology and received lymphocyte-depleting therapy. Lastly, two patients with EBV-negative serology received transplants from EBV-seropositive donors. No new cases of PTLD were reported in any group between years 2 and 3.[50]

The second Phase III trial, Belatacept Evaluation of Nephroprotection and Efficacy as First-line Immunosuppression Trial- EXTended criteria donors (BENEFIT-EXT),[51] is a randomised, multicentre Phase III trial conducted in patients who received a kidney transplant from an extended criteria donor defined as: ≥60 years old; ≥50 years old and at least two other risk factors (cerebrovascular accident, hypertension, serum creatinine >1.5 mg/dL); anticipated

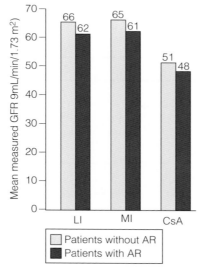

Figure 5.6 • Measured glomerular filtration rate by month 12 in patients with and without rejection in the BENEFIT study.

cold ischaemia time of ≥24 hours; or donation after cardiac death. Patients were treated with basiliximab induction, MMF and corticosteroids. Patients were randomised to receive either belatacept MI, belatacept LI or ciclosporin. Lymphocyte-depleting therapy was allowed for anticipated delayed graft function in ciclosporin-treated patients. Patients with acute rejection ≥Grade IIB could be treated with T-cell-depleting therapy at the investigators' discretion.

The primary outcomes were the composite end-point of patient and graft survival as well as the composite end-point of renal impairment at 12 months. The non-inferiority margin was set at 10% for patient and graft survival. Secondary outcomes included measured GFR, calculated GFR using the modification of diet in renal disease (MDRD) equation, the prevalence of biopsy-proven chronic allograft nephropathy (CAN) and the incidence and severity of biopsy-proven acute rejection. Protocol biopsies were performed at implantation and at week 52. A total of 543 patients were randomised and transplanted (n = 184 MI; n = 175 LI; n = 184 ciclosporin). There were no differences in baseline characteristics between the three groups.

Both belatacept regimens were non-inferior to ciclosporin on the primary end-point of patient and graft survival. Graft loss or death occurred in 14%, 11% and 15% of the patients treated with MI, LI and ciclosporin, respectively. The prevalence of biopsy-proven CAN was similar between the three groups (MI 45%; LI 46%; ciclosporin 52%). The mean measured GFR at 12 months was 52.1, 49.5 and 45.2 mL/min/1.73 m² for the MI-, LI- and ciclosporin-treated groups, respectively. The difference in measured GFR was significantly better in the MI-treated patients versus the ciclosporin-treated patients (P = 0.0083) but was not significantly different for the LI group compared to ciclosporin (P = 0.1039).

Mean systolic and diastolic blood pressure was lower for both belatacept groups compared to the ciclosporin-treated group (MI 141/78 mmHg; LI 141/78 mmHg; ciclosporin 150/82 mmHg). The incidence of NODAT was significantly lower in the MI group compared to the ciclosporin group (MI 2% vs. ciclosporin 9%; P = 0.0308); however, there was not a significant difference in NODAT in the LI group compared to ciclosporin (LI 5%; P = 0.2946). The mean change in non-HDL cholesterol

from baseline was significantly different in the MI (12.6 mg/dL) and LI (11.2 mg/dL) groups compared to ciclosporin (29.3 mg/dL) (P = 0.0016 MI vs. ciclosporin; P = 0.0006 LI vs. ciclosporin).

There was not a significant difference in the incidence of acute rejection between the three groups (MI 17.9%; LI 17.7%; ciclosporin 14.1%). However, more type IIB rejections occurred in belatacept-treated patients compared to ciclosporin-treated patients (MI 9%; LI 5%; ciclosporin 3%). The majority of rejections occurred within the first 3 months (81%) and nearly all occurred within 6 months. The numbers are small but it should be noted that more patients in the MI group (n = 5) experienced more than one episode of acute rejection compared to the LI (n = 1) and ciclosporin (n = 2) groups. The most common treatment for acute rejection was corticosteroids, whereas T-cell-depleting therapy was used in 13, five and four patients in the MI, LI and ciclosporin groups, respectively.

Two- and 3-year data are also available for BENEFIT-EXT.[49,52] Patients surviving with a functioning graft at 3 years were 80%, 82% and 80% in the MI, LI and ciclosporin groups, respectively. By 3 years the rate of acute rejection was 18%, 19% and 16% in the MI, LI and ciclosporin groups, respectively. Similar to what was found in the BENEFIT study, the development of DSA was lower in belatacept-treated patients. The incremental increase in DSA by year 3 was 7%, 6% and 15% in the MI-, LI- and ciclosporin-treated patients, respectively. With regard to renal function the mean cGFR in the intention-to-treat groups was 42.7, 42.2 and 31.5 mL/min/1.73 m² in the MI-, LI- and ciclosporin-treated patients, respectively.

By year 3 PTLD was reported in two MI and three LI patients; four cases involved the CNS and one case (LI) involved the renal allograft and lymph nodes. Four additional cases of PTLD (three LI and one ciclosporin) occurred after 3 years; one case involved the CNS (LI), one involved the renal allograft (LI), one involved the gastrointestinal tract (LI) and the other involved bone marrow (ciclosporin). Seven of the nine patients with PTLD (two MI, four LI and one ciclosporin) died.

Given the issues and concern regarding PTLD in belatacept-treated patients, an integrated safety analysis was performed in 1425 patients (MI 477; LI 472; ciclosporin 476) enrolled in the Phase II trial BENEFIT/BENEFIT-EXT.[53] The frequency of malignancies was 10%, 6% and 7% in the MI-, LI- and ciclosporin-treated patients, respectively. Sixteen cases of PTLD occurred (n = 8 MI; n = 6 LI; n = 2 ciclosporin), including nine cases involving the CNS (n = 6 MI; n = 3 LI). The risk of CNS PTLD was highest in EBV-negative recipients with more CNS PTLD occurring in the MI group. Overall the safety profile favoured the use of the LI over the MI regimen.

✓✓ BENEFIT and BENEFIT-EXT demonstrated that the substitution of belatacept for a CNI resulted in a higher GFR, lower blood pressure and improved lipid profile. The exact role belatacept will play in clinical practice is still to be determined; however, thus far it has shown great promise as part of a CNI sparing regimen.[49–53]

Strategies to lower toxicity

The advent of the CNIs ciclosporin and tacrolimus in the 1980s and 1990s, respectively, in conjunction with enhanced antiproliferative agents such as MMF and the now widespread use of induction agents, have contributed to lower acute rejection rates and improved 1-year allograft survival. However, the improved short-term success has not translated into an appreciable improvement in long-term renal allograft survival.[2] Chronic allograft nephropathy (CAN), although a term that has fallen out of favour, remains the most common cause of late allograft loss,[54] while cardiovascular disease continues to be the leading cause of death with a functioning allograft post-transplantation.[55] The core of most current immunosuppression protocols is CNI therapy with corticosteroids. Reliance on CNIs is a double-edged sword as they have the negative impact of contributing to the progression of CAN and accelerating long-term allograft decline.[56,57] CNIs and corticosteroids also contribute to worsening hypertension, diabetes and dyslipidaemia,[58–60] and thus impart negative effects on the cardiometabolic risk profile. When developing new immunosuppression, 1-year acute rejection rates and short-term graft survival were often used as markers of success. However, a shift in focus has occurred to develop novel immunosuppressive regimens that will maintain low acute rejection rates, excellent short-term outcomes and maximise long-term allograft survival with preserved allograft function and modulation of the cardiometabolic side-effects seen with CNI and corticosteroid protocols.

Corticosteroid-sparing regimens

Since the earliest kidney transplants performed in the 1960s, corticosteroids remain an integral part of immunosuppressive therapy. Corticosteroids are essential during the induction phase of immunosuppression and during episodes of acute rejection. Until recently, steroids have also been routinely used at low levels as part of maintenance therapy. However, given the well-known complications of long-term corticosteroid use (diabetes, bone disease, skin fragility, poor wound healing, infection and hypertension, to name a few), current strategies attempt to minimise, or even eliminate, corticosteroid use as part of maintenance therapy.

The glucocorticoids inhibit multiple facets of the immune response, principally through altering gene expression. Glucocorticoids enter the cell and bind to glucocorticoid receptors in the cytoplasm. This complex is then translocated to the nucleus, where it binds to glucocorticoid response elements within the genome. The consequent alteration in gene expression results in a phenotype of global immune down-regulation. Important features include the inhibition of T lymphocytes, B lymphocytes and antigen-presenting cells (APCs), and of various cytokines critical to the immune response (IL-1, IL-2, IL-4, IL-6, interferon-γ and TNF-α).

The first attempts at eliminating steroids as part of maintenance therapy were made in the 1990s. There were two large trials that looked at outcomes in renal allograft recipients who had prednisone stopped 90 days post-transplant. The first series, published in 1992, compared a maintenance regimen of ciclosporin alone or ciclosporin with prednisone in recipients with well-functioning allografts at 90 days post-transplant. Allograft survival at 5 years was significantly worse in the ciclosporin-alone group compared to those maintained on both ciclosporin and prednisone (73% vs. 85%).[61] Furthermore, there were minimal differences in the side-effect profiles between the two groups. The second series, published in 1999, also compared outcomes in recipients whose prednisone was stopped at 90 days; however, patients were maintained on both ciclosporin and mycophenolate mofetil. This trial was stopped early due to significantly increased rates of acute rejection in those patients whose prednisone was stopped (15% vs. 5%).[62] Again, there were minimal benefits in side-effect profiles in those withdrawn from steroids.

The FREEDOM study group published data from a large randomised, multicentre trial comparing steroid avoidance, steroid withdrawal at post-transplant day 7 and continued steroid therapy.[63] All patients were standard-risk recipients who received induction therapy with basiliximab and were maintained on ciclosporin microemulsion and mycophenolate sodium. Results at 1 year demonstrated higher rates of BPAR in the steroid-free and steroid-withdrawal groups (**Fig. 5.7**). However, allograft function at 1 year was similar and there did appear to be significant benefit to minimising the use of steroids (reduced use of antidiabetic and lipid-lowering medication, lower triglyceride levels and less weight gain).

In October 2008, a landmark paper was published by the Astellas Corticosteroid Withdrawal Study Group.[64] This was a prospective, randomised, double-blind placebo-controlled multicentre trial that compared early steroid withdrawal (post-transplant day 7) and continued low-dose maintenance therapy (prednisone 5 mg per day). There were 386 patients randomised and followed for 5 years. All patients received induction therapy with either basiliximab or thymoglobulin and were maintained on tacrolimus and MMF. At 5 years, there were no differences in allograft loss, episodes of moderate/severe rejection or patient survival. There was an increased rate of BPAR in those taken off steroids by post-transplant day 7. Importantly, post

hoc analysis demonstrated a significant increase in the incidence of chronic allograft nephropathy in the steroid withdrawal group (9.9% vs. 4.1%; $P = 0.028$). Furthermore, minimal benefit in side-effect profiles was gained by early withdrawal of prednisone.

> ✅ Based on the prior two trials[63,64] as well as a large Cochrane review published in 2009 (which included 30 trials with almost 6000 participants), similar conclusions regarding steroid withdrawal have been made: there is no difference in allograft loss or mortality, an increased incidence of acute rejection episodes and minimal benefit in side-effect profiles.

Thus far the prior studies discussed regarding steroid withdrawal or minimisation utilised a CNI regimen. Recently, a randomised, Phase II trial evaluating the effectiveness of belatacept as part of a steroid-avoiding regimen in 89 de novo kidney transplant recipients has been published.[65] Patients received one of the following treatment regimens: belatacept with MMF, belatacept with sirolimus, or tacrolimus with MMF. Thymoglobulin was administered to all treatment arms. Patients received an initial 4-day pulse of corticosteroids that could be extended until day 10 if thymoglobulin infusions continued (then corticosteroid free). The primary efficacy end-point was the incidence of acute rejection by month 6. Secondary end-points included

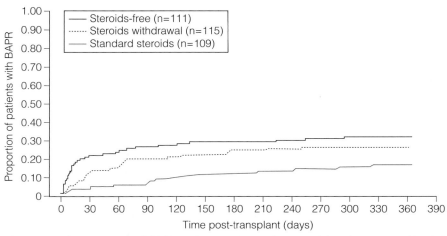

Figure 5.7 • The cumulative incidence of BPAR in patients randomised to steroid-free therapy, steroid withdrawal at day 7, or standard steroids (Kaplan–Meier, intention-to-treat population). Reproduced from Vincenti F, Schena FP, Paraskevas S et al. A randomized, multicenter study of steroid avoidance, early steroid withdrawal or standard steroid therapy in kidney transplant recipients. Am J Transplant 2008; 8:307–16. With permission from John Wiley and Sons.

the incidence and severity of acute rejection, patient and graft survival, and calculated GFR. Cardiovascular and metabolic parameters were also evaluated. Four patients in the belatacept–MMF group (12%), one in the belatacept–sirolimus group (4%) and one in the tacrolimus–MMF group (3%) experienced acute rejection by month 6. By 12 months 91% of the belatacept–MMF group, 92% of the belatacept–sirolimus group and 100% of the tacrolimus–MMF group were alive with functioning grafts. There were more treatment withdrawals in belatacept-treated patients compared to tacrolimus-treated patients (n = 6 belatacept–MMF, n = 5 belatacept–sirolimus versus n = 2 tacrolimus–MMF). The percentages of patients remaining steroid free at month 12 were 73%, 77% and 93%, respectively, in the belatacept–MMF, belatacept–sirolimus and tacrolimus–MMF groups. Most patients were placed on steroids due to adverse events or acute rejection.

At month 12 the mean cGFR was 8–10 mL/min/1.73 m^2 higher in the belatacept groups than in the tacrolimus–MMF group. No significant changes in blood pressure occurred. No clinically relevant differences in lipids or antihyperlipidaemic medication use were noted between the groups. New-onset diabetes occurred in a total of three patients (n = 2 belatacept–sirolimus and n = 1 tacrolimus–MMF). There were no cases of PTLD reported with either belatacept regimen. Overall the use of belatacept as part of a steroid-sparing regimen was well tolerated and was associated with a rejection rate comparable or better to other studies utilising a CNI- or steroid-free regimen. The use of belatacept compared to tacrolimus was associated with improved renal function. The data from this small study should be confirmed in a larger trial.

The issue of steroid withdrawal remains a moving target. Current evidence supports the safety and efficacy of early steroid withdrawal (7 days post-transplant) in low-risk recipients who receive induction therapy and are maintained on a CNI and mycophenolate. The data utilising belatacept are intriguing but need to be evaluated on a larger scale. However, the issue of chronic allograft nephropathy in those taken off of corticosteroids early in the post-transplant period is still a concern and requires further investigation. Currently, complete steroid avoidance and late steroid withdrawal regimens cannot be supported.

CNI minimisation

Like corticosteroids, CNIs are associated with many side-effects. Since the recognition of the untoward effects of CNI maintenance immunosuppression, transplant physicians have attempted to develop protocols that minimise or eliminate CNI exposures. One such study, the Cyclosporine Avoidance Eliminates Serious Adverse Renal Toxicity (CAESAR),[66] randomised 535 first-time renal transplant recipients to receive either standard-dose ciclosporin (trough goal 150–300 ng/mL through month 4, then 100–200 ng/mL thereafter), low-dose ciclosporin (trough goal 50–100 ng/mL) or low-dose ciclosporin (trough goal 50–100 ng/mL) with ciclosporin withdrawal at month 4. MMF and corticosteroids were given to patients in all groups, and patients in the low-dose ciclosporin and ciclosporin withdrawal groups received daclizumab induction therapy. Although no difference between the groups was noted in GFR at 1 year (the primary end-point), significantly more patients experienced at least one episode of BPAR in the ciclosporin withdrawal group. BPAR was experienced by 38% of patients in the ciclosporin withdrawal group, 25.4% in the low-dose ciclosporin group and 27.5% in the standard-dose ciclosporin group. This difference was statistically different between both the ciclosporin withdrawal and low-dose ciclosporin groups (P = 0.027) and the ciclosporin withdrawal and standard-dose ciclosporin groups (P = 0.04). There were no differences between the groups in adverse events overall, and in particular there was no difference in known ciclosporin metabolic side-effects such as hypertension and dyslipidaemia.

An intriguing study attempted to evaluate four different maintenance regimens to determine the effect of an mTOR inhibitor compared to CNIs with a low-dosing strategy in an effort to demonstrate the best regimen to minimise renal toxicity. The Efficacy Limiting Toxicity Elimination (ELITE) Symphony study sought to extend the findings of the CAESAR study by also examining not only low-dose ciclosporin, but low-dose tacrolimus and sirolimus as well. The ELITE Symphony study compared low-dose ciclosporin (goal trough concentrations of 50–100 ng/mL), low-dose tacrolimus (goal trough concentrations of 3–7 ng/mL), low-dose sirolimus (goal trough concentrations of 4–8 ng/mL) and standard-dose ciclosporin (goal trough concentrations of 150–300 ng/mL for 3 months, then

100–200 ng/mL thereafter).[67] All groups received MMF and all groups except for the standard ciclosporin group received daclizumab induction treatment. A total of 1645 patients were randomised in a 1:1:1:1 fashion to one of the four treatment groups and followed for 1 year. The primary end-point was renal function as measured by cGFR. Secondary end-points included BPAR, allograft survival, patient survival and treatment failure. Treatment failure was defined as any of the following: additional immunosuppressive agents needed, discontinuation of study medication for more than 14 consecutive days or 30 total days, allograft loss, or death. GFR at 1 year was better in the low-dose tacrolimus group (65.4 mL/min) compared with low-dose ciclosporin (59.4 mL/min), low-dose sirolimus (56.7 mL/min) and standard-dose ciclosporin (57.1 mL/min) ($P < 0.001$ for all comparisons). Significantly less BPAR was experienced in the low-dose tacrolimus group (15.4%) compared with low-dose ciclosporin (27.2%), low-dose sirolimus (40.2%) and standard-dose ciclosporin (30.1%) groups ($P < 0.001$ for all comparisons). In addition, allograft survival was higher in the low-dose tacrolimus group (94.2%) compared with low-dose sirolimus (89.3%) and standard-dose ciclosporin (89.3%) ($P = 0.007$ for both comparisons). However, there was no difference in allograft survival between the low-dose tacrolimus group and the low-dose ciclosporin group. The low-dose sirolimus group experienced the highest overall rate of side-effects (53%, compared with 43.4–44.3% in other groups; $P < 0.05$ for all comparisons). This group also had the most treatment withdrawals due to side-effects (7.8%, compared with 1.8–3.1% in other groups). The low-dose tacrolimus group experienced more new-onset diabetes (10.6%, compared with 4.7–7.8% in the other groups; $P = 0.02$). This group also experienced more diarrhoea (27.4%, compared with 14.4–24% in the other groups; $P < 0.001$). Overall, opportunistic infections were highest in the standard-dose ciclosporin group (33%, compared with 26.3–28.1% in the other groups; $P = 0.03$). Based on these findings, it appears that when low-dose CNI regimens are used, tacrolimus along with MMF and daclizumab induction therapy results in better renal function and fewer rejection episodes than low-dose ciclosporin along with MMF and daclizumab induction therapy at 1 year. In fact, the low-dose tacrolimus regimen was even superior to the standard-dose ciclosporin

regimen at preventing BPAR, preserving renal function and allograft survival at 1 year. Low-dose tacrolimus was also superior to low-dose sirolimus in preventing rejection episodes, preserving renal function and in tolerability. Longer-term follow-up is necessary to determine if these positive results remain after years of treatment. However, a recent concern has arisen regarding the use of low-dose immunosuppression. A report demonstrated that the majority of late allograft losses are due to immunological/inflammatory lesions rather than CNI nephrotoxicity.[68]

With the recent approval of belatacept we would be remiss if we did not mention data from a randomised Phase II trial evaluating the safety and efficacy of converting from a CNI- to a belatacept-based regimen.[69] In this trial 173 patients 6–36 months post-transplantation were either switched to belatacept ($n = 84$) or remained on a CNI-based regimen ($n = 89$). At month 12 the mean cGFR was 60.5 mL/min/1.73 m^2 in the belatacept group and 56.5 mL/min/1.73 m^2 for the CNI group, increases of 7.0 and 2.1 mL/min/1.73 m^2 from baseline, respectively. No grafts were lost in the first 12 months; however, one patient in the CNI group died with a functioning graft due to a myocardial infarction. Six patients converted to belatacept experienced an episode of acute rejection whereas no patients maintained on a CNI experienced rejection. No episodes of PTLD were reported. Given the long-term negative effects of a CNI on decline in renal allograft function, this study suggests that conversion from a CNI to belatacept results in an improved cGFR at 12 months. If the differences in cGFR persist, the improved renal function seen with belatacept could translate into several additional years of allograft survival. However, the issue of rejection needs to be considered when making the decision for conversion.

Looking ahead

The future of transplant immunosuppression remains bright, with new small molecules and biologicals still to come in the pipeline. The advent of biologicals used as maintenance immunosuppression is an exciting turning point in the field. New drugs to target the inflammatory process of delayed graft function are under investigation. In the future we expect to see drugs with higher specificity for their target receptor with a lower side-effect profile. Ultimately, however, the holy grail goal continues to be the development of a regimen that can be used to induce a state of operational tolerance.

Key points

- The incidence of acute rejection has been lowered dramatically with the introduction of modern immunosuppression.
- Maintenance therapy with three-drug immunosuppression offers the best outcomes for prolonged allograft survival following renal transplantation.
- Induction agents are now used routinely and multiple drug therapy is utilised in maintenance immunosuppression to maximise effectiveness and minimise side-effects.
- The introduction of the biological belatacept exemplifies a paradigm shift in maintenance immunosuppression as this is the first biological agent to be used for that purpose.

References

1. Shiao SL, McNiff JM, Masunaga T, et al. Immunomodulatory properties of FK734, a humanized anti-CD28 monoclonal antibody with agonistic and antagonistic activities. Transplantation 2007;83(3):304–13.

2. Meier-Kriesche HU, Schold JD, Srinivas TR, et al. Lack of improvement in renal allograft survival despite a marked decrease in acute rejection rates over the most recent era. Am J Transplant 2004;4(3):378–83.

3. Halloran PF. Immunosuppressive drugs for kidney transplantation. N Engl J Med 2004;351(26):2715–29.

4. Murray JE, Merrill JP, Harrison JH, et al. Prolonged survival of human-kidney homografts by immunosuppressive drug therapy. N Engl J Med 1963;268:1315–23.

5. Merion RM, White DJ, Thiru S, et al. Cyclosporine: five years' experience in cadaveric renal transplantation. N Engl J Med 1984;310(3):148–54.

6. Prograf® prescribing information. Nutley, NJ; Astellas Inc.

7. Pirsch JD, Miller J, Deierhoi MH, et al. A comparison of tacrolimus (FK506) and cyclosporine for immunosuppression after cadaveric renal transplantation. FK506 Kidney Transplant Study Group. Transplantation 1997;63(7):977–83.

8. Mayer AD, Dmitrewski J, Squifflet JP, et al. Multicenter randomized trial comparing tacrolimus (FK506) and cyclosporine in the prevention of renal allograft rejection: a report of the European Tacrolimus Multicenter Renal Study Group. Transplantation 1997;64(3):436–43.

9. Webster AC, Woodroffe RC, Taylor RS, et al. Tacrolimus versus ciclosporin as primary immunosuppression for kidney transplant recipients: meta-analysis and meta-regression of randomised trial data. Br Med J 2005;331(7520):810.

10. Opelz G, Dohler B. Influence of immunosuppressive regimens on graft survival and secondary outcomes after kidney transplantation. Transplantation 2009;87(6):795–802.

11. Corporation, Imuran package insert. I.p.i.P.

12. Cellcept® prescribing information. Nutley, NJ.

13. The Tricontinental Mycophenolate Mofetil Renal Transplantation Study Group. A blinded, randomized clinical trial of mycophenolate mofetil for the prevention of acute rejection in cadaveric renal transplantation. Transplantation 1996;61(7):1029–37.

14. Sollinger HW. Mycophenolate mofetil for the prevention of acute rejection in primary cadaveric renal allograft recipients. U.S. Renal Transplant Mycophenolate Mofetil Study Group. Transplantation 1995;60(3):225–32.

15. Remuzzi G, Lesti M, Gotti E, et al. Mycophenolate mofetil versus azathioprine for prevention of acute rejection in renal transplantation (MYSS): a randomised trial. Lancet 2004;364(9433):503–12.

16. Knight SR, Russell NK, Barcena L, et al. Mycophenolate mofetil decreases acute rejection and may improve graft survival in renal transplant recipients when compared with azathioprine: a systematic review. Transplantation 2009;87(6):785–94.

17. Kahan BD. Efficacy of sirolimus compared with azathioprine for reduction of acute renal allograft rejection: a randomised multicentre study. The Rapamune US Study Group. Lancet 2000;356(9225):194–202.

18. MacDonald AS. A worldwide, phase III, randomized, controlled, safety and efficacy study of a sirolimus/cyclosporine regimen for prevention of acute rejection in recipients of primary mismatched renal allografts. Transplantation 2001;71(2):271–80.

19. Meier-Kriesche HU, Schold JD, Srinivas TR, et al. Sirolimus in combination with tacrolimus is associated with worse renal allograft survival compared to mycophenolate mofetil combined with tacrolimus. Am J Transplant 2005;5(9):2273–80.

20. Meier-Kriesche HU, Steffen BJ, Chu AH, et al. Sirolimus with neoral versus mycophenolate mofetil with neoral is associated with decreased renal allograft survival. Am J Transplant 2004;4(12):2058–66.

21. Mendez R, Gonwa T, Yang HC, et al. A prospective, randomized trial of tacrolimus in combination

with sirolimus or mycophenolate mofetil in kidney transplantation: results at 1 year. Transplantation 2005;80(3):303–9.

22. Giessing M, Budde K. Sirolimus and lymphocele formation after kidney transplantation: an immunosuppressive medication as co-factor for a surgical problem? Nephrol Dial Transplant 2003;18(2):448–9.

23. Hardinger KL, Koch MJ, Brennan DC. Current and future immunosuppressive strategies in renal transplantation. Pharmacotherapy 2004;24(9):1159–76.

24. McTaggart RA, Gottlieb D, Brooks J, et al. Sirolimus prolongs recovery from delayed graft function after cadaveric renal transplantation. Am J Transplant 2003;3(4):416–23.

25. Schena FP, Pascoe MD, Alberu J, et al. Conversion from calcineurin inhibitors to sirolimus maintenance therapy in renal allograft recipients: 24-month efficacy and safety results from the CONVERT trial. Transplantation 2009;87(2):233–42.

26. Budde K, Becker T, Arns W, et al. Everolimus-based, calcineurin-inhibitor-free regimen in recipients of de-novo kidney transplants: an open-label, randomised, controlled trial. Lancet 2011;377(9768):837–47.

27. Weir MR, Mulgaonkar S, Chan L, et al. Mycophenolate mofetil-based immunosuppression with sirolimus in renal transplantation: a randomized, controlled Spare-the-Nephron trial. Kidney Int 2011;79(8):897–907.

28. Reichert JM. Monoclonal antibodies in the clinic. Nat Biotechnol 2001;19(9):819–22.

29. Wechter WJ, Brodie JA, Morrell RM, et al. Antithymocyte globulin (ATGAM) in renal allograft recipients. Multicenter trials using a 14-dose regimen. Transplantation 1979;28(4):294–302.

30. Shield 3rd CF, Cosimi AB, Tolkoff-Rubin N, et al. Use of antithymocyte globulin for reversal of acute allograft rejection. Transplantation 1979;28(6):461–4.

31. Hardy MA, Nowygrod R, Elberg A, et al. Use of ATG in treatment of steroid-resistant rejection. Transplantation 1980;29(2):162–4.

32. Nowygrod R, Appel G, Hardy MA. Use of ATG for reversal of acute allograft rejection. Transplant Proc 1981;13(1, Pt 1):469–72.

33. Clark KR, Forsythe JL, Shenton BK, et al. Administration of ATG according to the absolute T lymphocyte count during therapy for steroid-resistant rejection. Transpl Int 1993;6(1):18–21.

34. Gaber AO, First MR, Tesi RJ, et al. Results of the double-blind, randomized, multicenter, phase III clinical trial of Thymoglobulin versus Atgam in the treatment of acute graft rejection episodes after renal transplantation. Transplantation 1998;66(1):29–37.

35. Hardinger KL, Rhee S, Buchanan P, et al. A prospective, randomized, double-blinded comparison of thymoglobulin versus Atgam for induction immunosuppressive therapy: 10-year results. Transplantation 2008;86(7):947–52.

36. Ciancio G, Burke GW, Gaynor JJ, et al. A randomized trial of thymoglobulin vs. alemtuzumab (with lower dose maintenance immunosuppression) vs. daclizumab in renal transplantation at 24 months of follow-up. Clin Transplant 2008;22(2):200–10.

37. Amlot PL, Rawlings E, Fernando ON, et al. Prolonged action of a chimeric interleukin-2 receptor (CD25) monoclonal antibody used in cadaveric renal transplantation. Transplantation 1995;60(7):748–56.

38. Kovarik JM, Rawlings E, Sweny P, et al. Prolonged immunosuppressive effect and minimal immunogenicity from chimeric (CD25) monoclonal antibody SDZ CHI 621 in renal transplantation. Transplant Proc 1996;28(2):913–4.

39. Kahan BD, Rajagopalan PR, Hall M. Reduction of the occurrence of acute cellular rejection among renal allograft recipients treated with basiliximab, a chimeric anti-interleukin-2-receptor monoclonal antibody. United States Simulect Renal Study Group. Transplantation 1999;67(2):276–84.

40. Nashan B, Moore R, Amlot P, et al. Randomised trial of basiliximab versus placebo for control of acute cellular rejection in renal allograft recipients. CHIB 201 International Study Group. Lancet 1997;350(9086):1193–8.

41. Ponticelli C, Yussim A, Cambi V, et al. A randomized, double-blind trial of basiliximab immunoprophylaxis plus triple therapy in kidney transplant recipients. Transplantation 2001;72(7):1261–7.

42. Vincenti F. Costimulation blockade in autoimmunity and transplantation. J Allergy Clin Immunol 2008;121(2):299–308.

43. Larsen CP, Pearson TC, Adams AB, et al. Rational development of LEA29Y (belatacept), a high-affinity variant of CTLA4-Ig with potent immunosuppressive properties. Am J Transplant 2005;5(3):443–53.

44. Lenschow DJ, Zeng Y, Thistlethwaite JR, et al. Long-term survival of xenogeneic pancreatic islet grafts induced by CTLA4lg. Science 1992;257(5071):789–92.

45. Latek R, Fleener C, Lamian V, et al. Assessment of belatacept-mediated costimulation blockade through evaluation of CD80/86-receptor saturation. Transplantation 2009;87(6):926–33.

46. Vincenti F, Larsen C, Durrbach A, et al. Costimulation blockade with belatacept in renal transplantation. N Engl J Med 2005;353(8):770–81.

47. Vincenti F, Blancho G, Durrbach A, et al. Five-year safety and efficacy of belatacept in renal transplantation. J Am Soc Nephrol 2010;21(9):1587–96.

48. Vincenti F, Charpentier B, Vanrenterghem Y, et al. A phase III study of belatacept-based immunosuppression regimens versus cyclosporine in renal transplant recipients (BENEFIT study). Am J Transplant 2010;10(3):535–46.

49. Larsen CP, Grinyó J, Medina-Pestana J, et al. Belatacept-based regimens versus a cyclosporine A-based regimen in kidney transplant recipients:

2-year results from the BENEFIT and BENEFIT-EXT studies. Transplantation 2010;90(12):1528–35.

50. Vincenti F, Larsen CP, Alberu J, et al. Three-year outcomes from BENEFIT, a randomized, active-controlled, parallel-group study in adult kidney transplant recipients. Am J Transplant 2012;12(1):210–7.

51. Durrbach A, Pestana JM, Pearson T, et al. A phase III study of belatacept versus cyclosporine in kidney transplants from extended criteria donors (BENEFIT-EXT study). Am J Transplant 2010;10(3):547–57.

52. Pestana JO, Grinyo JM, Vanrenterghem Y, et al. Three-year outcomes from BENEFIT-EXT: a Phase III study of belatacept versus cyclosporine in recipients of extended criteria donor kidneys. Am J Transplant 2012;12(3):630–9.

53. Grinyó J, Charpentier B, Pestana JM, et al. An integrated safety profile analysis of belatacept in kidney transplant recipients. Transplantation 2010;90(12):1521–7.

54. Jevnikar AM, Mannon RB. Late kidney allograft loss: what we know about it, and what we can do about it. Clin J Am Soc Nephrol 2008;3(Suppl. 2):S56–67.

55. USRDS 2008 Annual Data Report. Atlas of Chronic Kidney Disease and End-Stage Renal Disease in the United States, www.usrds.org/adr.htm.

56. Nankivell BJ, Borrows RJ, Fung CL, et al. The natural history of chronic allograft nephropathy. N Engl J Med 2003;349(24):2326–33.

57. Solez K, Vincenti F, Filo RS. Histopathologic findings from 2-year protocol biopsies from a U.S. multicenter kidney transplant trial comparing tarolimus versus cyclosporine: a report of the FK506 Kidney Transplant Study Group. Transplantation 1998;66(12):1736–40.

58. Ducloux D, Motte G, Kribs M, et al. Hypertension in renal transplantation: donor and recipient risk factors. Clin Nephrol 2002;57(6):409–13.

59. Mathis AS, Davé N, Knipp GT, et al. Drug-related dyslipidemia after renal transplantation. Am J Health Syst Pharm 2004;61(6):565–87.

60. Vincenti F, Friman S, Scheuermann E, et al. Results of an international, randomized trial comparing glucose metabolism disorders and outcome with cyclosporine versus tacrolimus. Am J Transplant 2007;7(6):1506–14.

61. Sinclair NR. Low-dose steroid therapy in cyclosporine-treated renal transplant recipients with well-functioning grafts. The Canadian Multicentre Transplant Study Group. CMAJ 1992;147(5):645–57.

62. Ahsan N, Hricik D, Matas A, et al. Prednisone withdrawal in kidney transplant recipients on cyclosporine and mycophenolatemofetil – a prospective randomized study. Steroid Withdrawal Study Group. Transplantation 1999;68(12):1865–74.

63. Vincenti F, Schena FP, Paraskevas S, et al. A randomized, multicenter study of steroid avoidance, early steroid withdrawal or standard steroid therapy in kidney transplant recipients. Am J Transplant 2008;8(2):307–16.

64. Woodle ES, First MR, Pirsch J, et al. A prospective, randomized, double-blind, placebo-controlled multicenter trial comparing early (7 day) corticosteroid cessation versus long-term, low-dose corticosteroid therapy. Ann Surg 2008;248(4):564–77.

65. Ferguson R, Grinyó J, Vincenti F, et al. Immunosuppression with belatacept-based, corticosteroid-avoiding regimens in de novo kidney transplant recipients. Am J Transplant 2011;11(1):66–76.

66. Ekberg H, Grinyó J, Nashan B, et al. Cyclosporine sparing with mycophenolate mofetil, daclizumab and corticosteroids in renal allograft recipients: the CAESAR Study. Am J Transplant 2007;7(3):560–70.

67. Ekberg H, Tedesco-Silva H, Demirbas A, et al. Reduced exposure to calcineurin inhibitors in renal transplantation. N Engl J Med 2007;357(25):2562–75.

68. Sellares J, de Freitas DG, Einecke G, et al. Inflammation lesions in kidney transplant biopsies: association with survival is due to the underlying diseases. Am J Transplant 2011;11(3):489–99.

69. Rostaing L, Massari P, Garcia VD, et al. Switching from calcineurin inhibitor-based regimens to a belatacept-based regimen in renal transplant recipients: a randomized phase II study. Clin J Am Soc Nephrol 2011;6(2):430–9.

6

Preservation and perfusion of abdominal organs for transplantation

John O'Callaghan
Peter Friend
Rutger J. Ploeg

Introduction

Why is organ preservation necessary? At the dawn of clinical transplantation, organ donor and recipient were generally within the same hospital. This allowed the direct transfer of the organ to be transplanted and hence no method of preservation was necessary beyond the flush-out of blood. As programmes have developed into national and even international schemes, the preservation period has become longer in order to allow transport of the organ from the donor to the recipient and also to allow for improved tissue matching. Adequate preservation during this period is essential to ensure that a functional organ with life-sustaining potential is implanted at the end of the preservation period. While it may theoretically be attractive to keep organs in a system as close to their normal physiological state as possible, this was not available in a practical or affordable form at the time. A simple method was therefore adopted, that of rapidly cooling and storing the organ on ice. However, this hypothermic and hypoxic preservation is not without its harmful side-effects, and preservation methods have been designed to counteract these mechanisms of tissue damage. With recent technological advances we have revisited the more complex methods of preservation, and adequate organ preservation has become all the more important given changes in the spectrum of donors we now require to meet the demands of transplant waiting lists.

Despite efforts to increase the number of organs available from the classical donor type (the deceased, heart-beating donors, or donation after brain death (DBD)), transplant waiting lists remain long and in some cases ever-extending. Donation after circulatory death (DCD) has therefore been increasingly used in some countries,[1] as have expanded criteria donors (ECDs).[2] ECDs are, by their definition, associated with reduced graft survival and include all deceased donors over 60 years old, or aged 50–59 years, with at least two of the following conditions: cerebrovascular cause of death, serum creatinine over 1.5 mg/dL, hypertension.[3] Donor comorbidities are associated with a set of problems that need to be addressed by the preservation method in order to improve the outcomes from these organs.

Organs from DCD may be categorised using the Maastricht Criteria (see Table 6.1). They suffer a longer period of warm ischaemia after the withdrawal of supportive treatment in the case of Maastricht Category III donors and an even longer warm ischaemic time (WIT) in the case of the so-called 'uncontrolled' donors of Maastricht Categories I, II and IV.[4] Kidneys from DCD have a higher risk of delayed graft function (DGF) and primary non-function (PNF),[5] and

Table 6.1 • Maastricht categories of deceased donors after cardiac death

Category	Description
I	Dead on arrival at the hospital
II	Unsuccessful resuscitation at the hospital
III	Withdrawal of supportive treatment
IV	Cardiac arrest following establishment of brain death

livers a higher risk of biliary complications and re-transplantation.[6] The tissue injuries associated with this long first warm ischaemic period have prompted the development of new organ preservation techniques to prevent the extension of this damage and to resuscitate the organ if possible.

The spectrum of donors contributing to the DBD organ pool has also changed over the last 30 years, with an increasing number of older individuals becoming donors of this type.[7] Cerebral injury followed by brain death sets in motion a number of inflammatory processes that can directly injure organs, but also prime them to undergo further damage at reperfusion.[8,9] Kidneys from DBD start to undergo a process of damage following ischaemia of the brain; urinary sodium excretion increases, renal tubules undergo necrosis and the arterial intima undergoes fibrous proliferation.[10] There is evidence that brain death increases the immunogenicity of transplanted organs,[11] associated with a higher rejection rate when compared with organs from live donors.[12]

Patient and graft survival has improved since the first transplants were undertaken, making organ transplantation a safe and effective treatment for end-stage organ failure. However, there is still room to improve in the field of organ preservation, in order to reduce the preservation injuries suffered by standard criteria organs, but in particular to help improve outcome in the newer categories of deceased donation that are increasingly used to expand the donor pool.

In this chapter we will introduce the basic methods of organ preservation before taking an organ-specific look at the current state-of-the-art preservation methods of the abdominal organs (kidney, liver, pancreas and intestine). We will also attempt to rank the level of available evidence before moving on to discuss the new developments that will lead to the future of organ preservation and resuscitation.

Development of preservation techniques

If an organ remains at body temperature after circulatory arrest, tissue metabolism will continue at a normal rate for some time. Without a normal circulation to remove metabolites and deliver nutrients and oxygen, catabolic enzymes will be activated and anaerobic metabolism will lead to cellular acidosis and, ultimately, cell death. A simple method to reduce metabolic rate and protect against warm ischaemia is to cool the organ. Metabolism does not cease at low temperatures though, and it has been known for some time that there is a continued, but greatly reduced, oxygen and nutrient requirement during the cold preservation phase.[13] Tissue cooling and hypoxia reduce ATP synthesis, resulting in reduced Na/K-pump activity, with sodium passively entering the cell unopposed. Water subsequently follows the osmotic gradient into the cell, causing cell swelling and lysis. The swelling of endothelial and perivascular cells can cause resistance to blood flow and vessel blockage. Ongoing metabolism in hypoxic conditions leads to an accumulation of lactic acid, causing lysosomal rupture, organelle and membrane damage, and subsequently cell death.[14] See Figure 6.1.

During re-implantation of the organ a second period of warm ischaemia is suffered while vascular anastomoses are fashioned and tissue perfusion is reconstituted. The pre-existing damage accrued in the first warm period and the cold preservation stage now becomes evident. The oxygen-rich blood allows the formation of reactive oxygen species (ROS) that are extremely damaging to cellular organelles and membranes, the so-called 'ischaemia–reperfusion injury' or IRI[15] (see Chapter 3 for more details).

Static cold storage

Surface cooling was first tested as a method to reduce the temperature of renal autografts, with Calne et al. demonstrating that surface cooling could be effective in animals.[16] Surface cooling is slow to achieve low temperatures within the tissues, so a move to perfusion cooling through the abdominal arteries was taken. Initially autologous blood was used, although this was not much quicker, due to increased blood viscosity at lower temperatures. Continuous cold perfusion of the graft became the norm in kidney

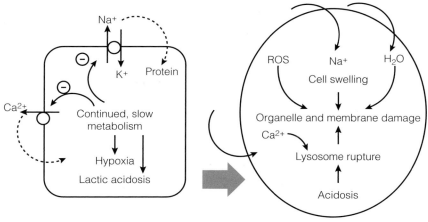

Figure 6.1 • Negative effects of cold ischaemia. Continued but slowed metabolism results in hypoxia, acidosis, reduced ATP synthesis, and activity of sodium and calcium pumps. Resultant sodium influx with water leads to cell swelling. ROS (reactive oxygen species), along with acidosis and lysosomal enzymes, damage cellular organelles and membranes.

transplantation until the development of better preservation solutions for static cold storage (SCS) that demonstrated equivalent results to machine perfusion.[17] This simpler method requires a rapid flushout of blood in situ using the preservation solution and after retrieval the organ is submerged in a sterile bag of the same solution. This bag is then buried in ice in a cool box. SCS is relatively cheap and requires the minimum of input from the retrieval or implant team during the preservation period. See Figure 6.2.

Given the mechanisms of damage mentioned above, preservation fluids were specifically designed to counteract each harmful pathway and preserve the physiological and biochemical conditions of the organ. Of particular importance are the impermeant molecules that prevent the movement of electrolytes and water across the cell membrane. They must remain within the vascular space and/or the interstitium to be effective. Hypertonic solutions were first tested in this capacity. In 1969, Collins et al. developed the first SCS solutions, testing four similar fluids based upon intracellular electrolyte composition, with a high concentration of glucose as an impermeant. The group showed that SCS could be used to preserve kidneys for up to 30 hours.[18] The original Collins solution was later modified by the Eurotransplant Foundation to Eurocollins solution (EC) by the removal of magnesium. A number of impermeant molecules have subsequently been tested, including sucrose,[19,20] mannitol[21] and citrate.[22,23] Colloids such as starches are also very effective impermeant molecules, as they have a large

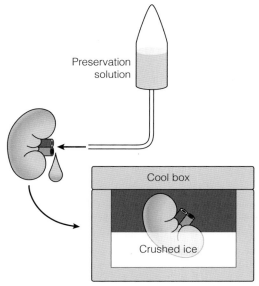

Figure 6.2 • For static cold storage, kidneys are flushed through the renal artery with preservation solution after removal from the donor. Preservation fluid is run until the effluent from the renal vein is clear. The kidney is submerged in the preservation fluid in a sealed bag, which is then packed in a cool box surrounded by crushed ice.

molecular weight and are retained in the vascular compartment. Molecular weight determines the success of extracellular impermeants in preservation solutions, with larger molecules being more successful as impermeant components.[24]

Buffers are also very important constituents that prevent changes in pH and subsequent protein degradation. Examples include bicarbonates, histidine, phosphates and lactobionate. Free radical scavengers have also been tested to counteract ROS, such as glutathione, lactobionate and tryptophan. Nutrients and nutrient precursors have also been included to provide for the ongoing metabolism and also the metabolic surge that follows reperfusion. Examples include adenosine, glutamate and ketoglutarate.

In the past decades a number of preservation solutions have therefore been developed to counteract the detrimental effects of the retrieval process, graft cooling and reperfusion. They specifically target the biochemical and structural changes that occur during this process, yet vary considerably in the type and concentration of their constituents. A few examples of the most commonly used fluids today are described below (details are given in Table 6.2); more organ-specific considerations will be given in the appropriate sections.

University of Wisconsin solution

University of Wisconsin solution (UW, Viaspan®, Bristol-Meyers Squibb, also supplied as SPS-1®, Organ Recovery Systems and Belzer UW Cold Storage Solution®, Bridge to Life) was elegantly designed by Belzer and Southard in the 1980s to counteract the well-known effects of organ retrieval and hypothermic preservation, and showed good results in kidney, liver and pancreas preservation.[25-27] UW has an intracellular-type electrolyte composition, with 120 mM potassium and 30 mM sodium. It contains three impermeant molecules, lactobionate and raffinose, with the colloid hydroxyethyl starch (HES), which in combination are very effective at preventing tissue oedema. Lactobionate, a large anion, also acts as a buffer and free radical scavenger. Glutathione acts a free radical scavenger through its preferential oxidisation, while adenosine is a nutrient precursor. Allopurinol included in UW inhibits xanthine oxidase and hence free radical formation. The addition of the ATP precursor adenosine provides for ongoing metabolism.

> ✔✔ UW is considered the gold standard solution for preservation of abdominal organs given the results of landmark trials demonstrating that it was better, if not equal, to all other available preservation solutions.[28-33]

Some studies have moved on to alter the basic composition of UW slightly to demonstrate that the Na/K ratio could be reversed,[34] and dextran could be substituted for HES.[35]

Histidine–tryptophan–ketoglutarate solution

Histidine–tryptophan–ketoglutarate (HTK, Custodiol®, Dr Franz Kohler Chemie GMBH) was originally used as a cardioplegic solution, but has since been tested in the preservation of kidney, liver and pancreas.[29,30,33] It has been used in the preservation of increasing numbers of kidneys since the early 1990s.[36] HTK contains a much lower concentration of potassium than UW (9 mM). There are several other differences in the composition; the amino acid histidine is the main impermeant molecule, assisted by mannitol. HTK also does not contain a colloid, such as the HES used in UW, and is therefore much less viscous.[37] Histidine also acts as a buffer in the solution while tryptophan and ketoglutarate are free radical scavengers and metabolic precursors, respectively. To achieve the maximal buffering capacity, relatively large flush volumes are recommended (10–15 litres).

Celsior solution

Celsior (Celsior®, Genzyme) was developed initially for cardiac allograft preservation in the early 1990s; it has since proven to be of use in the preservation of kidneys, liver and pancreas.[31,32,38] Unlike UW it has a high sodium content (100 mM) and low potassium content (15 mM), and is relatively low in viscosity. Celsior incorporates lactobionate as an impermeant, which acts through both its molecular weight and negative charge. Histidine is the main buffer and reduced glutathione acts as a scavenger of ROS. It also contains mannitol as a second impermeant and free radical scavenger, along with reduced glutathione as an antioxidant.

Institut-Georges-Lopez-1 solution

The use of polyethylene glycol (PEG) in preservation solutions was prompted by the high viscosity associated

Table 6.2 • Composition of preservation solutions for static cold storage* and hypothermic machine perfusion.

	Celsior	EC	HOC	HTK	IGL-1	UW	Belzer MPS
Colloids (mM)							
HES	–	–	–	–	–	0.25	0.25
PEG	–	–	–	–	0.03	–	–
Impermeants (mM)							
Citrate*	–	–	80	–	–	–	–
Gluconate	–	–	–	–	–	–	85
Glucose	–	195	–	–	–	–	10
Histidine*	30	–	–	198	–	–	–
Lactobionate*	80	–	–	–	100	100	–
Mannitol*	60	–	185	38	–	–	30
Raffinose	–	–	–	–	30	30	–
Ribose	–	–	–	–	–	–	5
Buffers (mM)							
HEPES	–	–	–	–	–	–	10
K_2HPO_4	–	15	–	–	–	–	–
KH_2PO_4	–	43	–	–	25	25	25
$NaHCO_3$	–	10	10	–	–	–	–
Electrolytes (mM)							
Calcium	0.25	–	–	0.0015	–	–	0.5
Chloride	42	15	–	32	20	20	1
Magnesium	13	–	40	4	5	5	5
Potassium	15	115	84	9	25	120	25
Sodium	100	10	84	15	120	30	100
ROS scavengers (mM)							
Allopurinol	–	–	–	–	1	1	–
Glutathione	3	–	–	–	3	3	–
Tryptophan	–	–	–	2	–	–	–
Nutrients (mM)							
Adenine	–	–	–	–	–	–	5
Adenosine	–	–	–	–	5	5	–
Glutamate	20	–	–	–	–	–	–
Ketoglutarate	–	–	–	1	–	–	–
Osmolality (mOsm)	255	406	400	310	320	320	300

*Citrate, histidine and lactobionate also act as buffers. Histidine, lactobionate and mannitol also act as ROS scavengers.
EC, Eurocollins; HEPES, 4-(2-hydroxyethyl)-1-piperazine ethanesulfonic acid; HES, hydroxyethyl starch; HOC, hyperosmolar citrate; HTK, histidine–tryptophan–ketoglutarate; IGL-1, Institut-George Lopez-1; MPS, machine perfusion solution; PEG, polyethylene glycol; UW, University of Wisconsin solution.

with HES, and its tendency to cause red cell aggregation in animal experimental models.[37] This effect has not been demonstrated in humans. PEG has been attributed with the potential to prevent immune interactions by binding to the surface of cells.[39] Institut George Lopez-1 Solution (IGL-1®, Institut Georges Lopez) is similar to UW in the inclusion of raffinose, lactobionate and potassium phosphate; however, it has PEG instead of HES as an impermeant colloid. It has shown potential in the preservation of kidney, liver, pancreas and small bowel.[40–44]

Hypothermic machine preservation

When kidney transplantation programmes were first established, hypothermic machine perfusion (HMP) was used to preserve kidneys and demonstrated good results.[45,46] With the development of better preservation solutions that demonstrated equivalent results at reduced immediate costs, SCS became the prevalent method of storage. Although the new generations of pumps for HMP are lighter and smaller than those used 40 years ago, the principle has not changed; chilled preservation fluid is pumped in a pulsatile or continuous fashion through the renal artery in a recirculating unit. Complete washout of blood and uniform organ cooling is achieved. See Figure 6.3.

> ✅ Recent randomised controlled trials (RCTs) for the preservation of kidneys[47,48] and case series of the preservation of livers[49] have reopened the debate on the use of HMP, particularly for DCD and ECD organs.

A considerable difficulty associated with hypothermic perfusion is that of tissue oedema due to the hydrostatic pressures. In order to overcome this problem a perfusion fluid with strong oncotic pressure is required to retain water in the vascular space. Initially human albumin solution was used for this purpose, and later human cryoprecipitated plasma, allowing the first successful machine preservation of a human kidney for 17 hours.[46] The synthetic perfusate Belzer machine perfusion

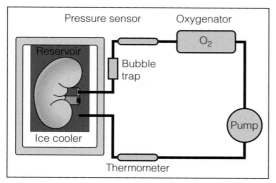

Figure 6.3 • Hypothermic machine perfusion devices maintain the stored kidney in a bath of cooled preservation solution surrounded by ice. The same solution is withdrawn from the bath and pumped (via an oxygenator in some cases) through the renal artery of the kidney. Temperature and flow dynamics can be monitored.

solution (Belzer MPS, KPS-1®, Lifeline Scientific Inc.) was later developed and has since become the most widely used machine perfusion fluid. Attempts to improve upon Belzer MPS through the addition of metabolic substrates, antioxidants and vasodilators (Vasosol®, Procent Technologies LLC) have shown the potential to further reduce DGF following kidney preservation.[50]

Kidney

State of the art

Static cold preservation remains the most commonly used method for preservation of kidneys from deceased donors worldwide, whether they are DCD or DBD. Data from the international Collaborative Transplant Study (CTS) reveal that during the period 1990–2005 SCS was used for approximately 97–98% of all kidneys, with machine preservation making up the remaining 2–3%.[36]

UW solution was established as the gold standard for kidney preservation in the early 1990s following a large international RCT that demonstrated its superiority over the previous gold standard, Eurocollins.[28] This study demonstrated that preservation in UW could deliver reduced rates of DGF, a more rapid fall in serum creatinine and improved graft survival. UW therefore replaced Eurocollins as the dominant solution over the coming years, increasing in use from approximately 46% of deceased donor kidneys in 1990 to 70% by 2002.[36]

In the early 1990s the HTK solution was also shown in a large international RCT to be superior to Eurocollins by reducing DGF,[29] although no impact on graft survival was seen in this study. In the same international RCT, HTK was shown to be equivalent to UW;[29] however, the debate has continued concerning the relative benefits of UW over HTK, with registry analysis demonstrating that HTK was associated with an increased risk of graft loss and PNF.[36,51] The rate of DGF was found to be the same between the two solutions. As cold ischaemic time (CIT) increases, both HTK and UW show a mild increase in graft loss; however, at CIT longer than 24 hours there is a suggestion of an advantage of UW over HTK.[36]

More recently, other solutions have been used for the preservation of kidneys and tested against UW. Celsior has been compared to UW in three large multicentre RCTs, demonstrating comparable rates of DGF and graft survival.[38,52,53] IGL-1 solution has been compared to UW in one small cohort study demonstrating comparable rates of DGF and graft survival.[54] Serum creatinine levels were lower for IGL-1 from days 7 to 14 postoperatively in this study. Overall it would appear that there is good evidence from RCTs that Celsior, HTK and UW are of equal quality for the preservation of standard quality kidneys. There are some concerns raised, however, about the use of HTK, but these arise from retrospective, non-randomised data.

Static cold storage has proven to be a satisfactory method for the preservation of standard organs; however, with an increasing demand, lower quality organs have to be used. In an effort to better preserve these kidneys HMP has been tested. The rate of fluid administration can be either pressure or flow targeted and the electronic systems also allow monitoring of renal vascular resistance. Two recent RCTs using a new generation of pumps have been published; one concentrated on DCD and will be discussed below.

✅✅ In a large multicentre European RCT, overall, and for all types of donors, HMP was found to lower the rate of DGF from approximately 27% to 21% compared to SCS.[47]

In multivariate analysis HMP was found to be independently associated with a significantly reduced risk of DGF. The duration of DGF, when it occurred, was also shorter if following HMP. One-year and 3-year graft survival was also significantly higher following HMP compared to SCS (94% vs. 90% and 91% vs. 87%). In those donor kidneys that developed DGF, 1-year graft survival was 12% lower if cold stored than if machine perfused.[47,55] See Figure 6.4.

Donation after brain death

As the more standard donor type internationally, DBD kidneys have been the focus of most preservation trials, if not a major part of studies in combination with DCD. The preservation solutions for SCS mentioned above were tested in trials largely relying on DBD kidneys, except for the European multicentre comparison of UW with Eurocollins,[28] and HTK with Eurocollins,[29] which used DBD kidneys alone. Despite the already low rate of DGF experienced by

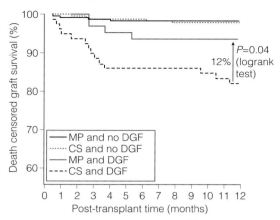

Figure 6.4 • Results from Moers et al.[47] showed that hypothermic machine perfusion was particularly effective in improving graft survival for kidneys with delayed graft function. Delayed graft function following static cold storage was associated with the worst 1-year graft survival.

kidneys from DBD, the European machine preservation trial discussed above showed this rate could be further reduced from 21% to 16%, when compared to SCS.[47]

Controlled donation after circulatory death

The use of kidneys from controlled DCD has risen in response to the falling number of suitable DBD kidneys and comparable long-term outcomes between the two donor types have been demonstrated.[1,56] However, the injury suffered by kidneys from the two donor types differs and it is therefore reasonable to speculate that the best preservation method for each donor type may be different. Kidneys from all four Maastricht classes of DCD donors are used to varying degrees worldwide, but most commonly it is those from classes II and III. Various protocols are in place for the procurement of kidneys from Maastricht class III donors, but by and large the ultimate preservation method used has been SCS in a preservation fluid, as described above for DBD kidneys.

A large meta-analysis of available data on DCD and DBD kidneys shows that DCD kidneys are at a much higher risk of DGF (odds ratio (OR) 3.64) and PNF (OR 2.43). This is believed to be a result of the variable warm ischaemia suffered by the organ following the withdrawal of life-supporting treatment, or pre-hospital cardiac arrest.[56] The potential benefit from a reduction in DGF and PNF is therefore greater for DCD kidneys. It has been speculated that DCD kidneys would receive greater benefit from hypothermic machine perfusion than DBD kidneys. Two recent RCTs have examined the effects of this preservation modality in DCD kidneys. As part of the European multicentre RCT described above, a separately paired RCT was conducted using DCD kidneys.[57] This study showed that the rate of DGF could be decreased in this population from approximately 70% to 54% compared to static cold preservation. One-year graft survival was similar in both groups (94% vs. 95%), as was creatinine clearance at 1 year, although it was better for the first month postoperatively in the machine perfusion group. In contrast to this, the UK multicentre RCT found a similar rate of DGF in the two groups (56% vs. 58%), graft survival at 1 year (93% vs. 98%) and estimated glomerular filtration rate (eGFR) at 1 year.[48] This difference may possibly be explained by the lower rate of DGF in the control arm of the UK trial. The outcomes may also have been influenced by the period of SCS used for kidneys before machine perfusion in the UK trial, whereas in the European trial machine perfusion was used from the point of retrieval until implantation. An experimental model of DCD kidney preservation is supportive of this theory, finding that HMP after a period of static preservation was not beneficial compared to static preservation alone.[58] Kidneys stored statically to begin with had improved renal resistance during the course of the subsequent HMP; however, the renal resistance started at a much higher level than those that went straight on to a pump. Four hours of HMP could not bring the renal resistance back in line with the kidneys that were pumped from the beginning.[58]

Uncontrolled donation after circulatory death

In countries without a legal definition of brain death or an overall shortage of organs, uncontrolled DCD are an important source of kidney allografts. Using strict selection criteria, one centre in Madrid, Spain, has successfully transplanted kidneys from Maastricht categories I, II and IV.[59–61] Following

irreversible cardiac arrest in suitable donors, a femoral arterial and venous catheter is inserted, allowing the maintenance of grafts by extracorporeal membrane oxygenation (ECMO), sometimes called normothermic regional perfusion (NRP) in this context. ECMO systems are widely used in intensive care units to support patients with cardiorespiratory failure. The system circulates the patient's blood through an oxygenator and warmer. In the setting of organ donation it theoretically allows the continued circulation of warm, oxygenated blood through the abdominal organs after cardiac arrest. A double balloon is used to occlude the aorta and prevent recirculation through the brain or heart. This stop-gap allows judicial review and contact with the family while preserving the kidneys for a maximum period of 4 hours. Standard retrieval can then be performed. This method has demonstrated good results, with 1- and 5-year graft survival of approximately 85% and 83%, respectively, compared to 87% and 84% for DBD kidneys at the same institution during the same time period.[61] These kidneys undergo a variable amount of warm ischaemia of up to 2 hours, and the discard rate for retrieved kidneys is therefore high, at approximately 33%. The DGF rate ranges from 68% to 80% and the PNF rate is 6%.[59,60] A series of kidneys from Maastricht I and II DCD in Paris, France, with a longer WIT of up to 150 minutes, demonstrated a higher discard rate (43%) and higher DGF rate (92%), but lower PNF rate (2%).[62] Graft survival was 89% at 6 months. In a small series of Maastricht II and IV donors at one centre in Barcelona, Spain, normothermic ECMO was compared with hypothermic ECMO and with in situ cold perfusion by Eurocollins.[63] The normothermic ECMO group had lower rates of DGF compared to the other groups and less PNF than the in situ group.

Expanded criteria donors

By definition, kidneys from ECDs have worse graft survival than standard criteria donors (SCDs).[64] The potential to improve upon their outcomes through better organ preservation and resuscitation is therefore greater. As part of the European machine perfusion trial, described above, a paired RCT was completed using ECD kidneys.[65] This study showed that the rate of DGF could be decreased in this population from approximately 30% to 22% compared to SCS. One-year graft survival was better following HMP (92% vs. 80%), as was creatinine clearance at 1 year. Particularly striking in this study was the poor 1-year survival of kidneys that had DGF following SCS compared to HMP (41% vs. 85%); there was no significant difference in survival between kidneys with and without DGF following HMP. Rates of PNF were also reduced from 12% to 3% following HMP. Interestingly, in this study the rate of DGF was not significantly different comparing ECD with SCD kidneys. A smaller non-randomised controlled trial in ECD showed a more drastic reduction in DGF rate with HMP compared to SCS (9% vs. 32%).[66]

New developments and the future

The most recent developments in renal preservation have involved the increasing use of more complex mechanisms to preserve, resuscitate and assess organs from donors of increasing age and comorbidity.

Renal resistance during HMP is often used to assess kidney viability and predict both short- and long-term outcomes. The European machine perfusion trial transplanted 302 kidneys with blinding of the surgeons to the machine perfusion parameters. High renal resistance was found to be a predictor of DGF and also 1-year graft loss, but the predictive value was low.[57] Given the multifactorial causation of DGF, renal resistance cannot as yet be used to predict outcome on its own. Several biomarkers measured during HMP have also been implicated in the outcome of kidneys after transplantation, but until recently all evidence was retrospective and subject to selection bias. Six of these biomarkers were recently assessed during the Eurotransplant machine perfusion trial.[67] These included alanine-aminopeptidase (Ala-AP), aspartate aminotransferase (AST), glutathione-S-transferase (GST), heart-type fatty acid binding protein (H-FABP), lactate dehydrogenase (LDH) and N-acetyl-β-D-glucosamine (NAG). Multivariate analysis of perfusates at the end of the preservation period showed that GST, H-FABP and NAG were moderate, independent predictors of DGF.[67] None of the biomarkers were independently associated with PNF or decreased graft survival and should not be used as grounds to discard a kidney. None of the

biomarkers correlated with renal resistance or cold ischaemic time, suggesting that they represent a different aspect of tissue injury.

Future developments in kidney preservation will aim to repair damaged organs by providing mechanisms to support metabolism and remove waste products, counteracting the effects of ischaemia–reperfusion injury. New preservation fluids may allow static storage at normothermic or subnormothermic temperatures and this has been demonstrated in animal studies. AQIX, a non-phosphate-buffered solution, has been used for short-term, subnormothermic, static preservation in a porcine experimental model.[68] Improved outcomes following static cold preservation may also be possible with the development of new solutions. Polysol, a low-viscosity solution, has been tested in porcine autotransplant models, showing improved renal blood flow and tissue oxygenation compared to UW[69] and improved creatinine clearance compared to HTK.[70]

Delivery of oxygen to the graft during the preservation period has been the focus of several studies and various methods, other than the delivery of oxygenated whole blood, have proven to be promising in animal and experimental studies. Persufflation of gaseous oxygen directly through the vasculature of the kidney has been tested as a rescue therapy for ischaemically damaged kidneys. Filtered and humidified gaseous oxygen can be administered through the renal vein and allowed to escape from the surface of the kidney through fine pin-pricks made with a microvascular needle. In animal studies, autotransplanted kidneys displayed better creatinine clearance following oxygen persufflation, rather than cold static or perfusion preservation alone.[71,72] The Groningen and Poitiers groups in collaboration have tested an oxygenated perfusate to preserve kidneys during HMP, and this has been tested in animal models of DCD and in autotransplant models.[73,74] Membrane oxygenators within machine perfusion systems have been shown to promote ATP synthesis, even following 30 minutes of warm ischaemia.[75] Oxygenation of machine perfusates with 100% oxygen to achieve very high oxygen partial pressure has also been tested as an adjunct to machine perfusion, and can recondition kidneys previously stored for 18 hours by SCS.[76] On reperfusion, kidneys previously recirculated with oxygenated perfusate showed improved urine production and creatinine clearance. Oxygen could also be delivered to tissues via soluble oxygen carriers (such as Lifor; see above). The respiratory pigment Hemarina-M101, a large haemoglobin molecule derived from marine invertebrates, has been used to supplement standard preservation fluids in a static cold preservation animal study.[77] Hemarina-M101 improved metabolic activity of preserved cell lines, increased ATP levels, improved creatinine clearance and reduced graft fibrosis following transplantation of preserved whole organs.[77]

Another possible strategy for the in situ protection of organs is the use of ECMO, alternatively known as NRP in the context of organ retrieval. While this technique is used for uncontrolled DCD in some countries (Spain and France, for example), it has not been widely tested in controlled DCD. ECMO provides a possible method by which the acidosis and low venous oxygen levels present after the withdrawal of life-supporting treatment could be reversed in controlled DCD. Following a decision to withdraw treatment on the ICU, family consent for donation is sought, and if agreed a femoral catheter is inserted and supportive treatment withdrawn. Five minutes after cardiac arrest the aortic occlusion balloon is inflated and NRP is initiated. In a case series from Michigan, USA, this method has provided low rates of DGF (8%) and PNF (0%) for Maastricht III DCD.[78] Another group from North Carolina, USA, transplanted a series of kidneys following sub-normothermic (22°C) regional perfusion after controlled DCD.[79] DGF rates were higher in this study (57%). One-year graft survival was 87%. A large case series from Taipei, Taiwan, demonstrated that NRP for kidneys from Maastricht category II, III and IV donors could result in excellent 5-year graft survival rates of approximately 88%.[80] This survival rate is comparable to that for live donor kidneys (89%) and DBD kidneys (83%) transplanted at the same institution during the same time period.

The next logical step would seem to be the combination of normothermic preservation with continuous or pulsatile perfusion to remove metabolites and maintain constant intravascular conditions. Synthetic fluids could possibly be combined with normothermic perfusion. Lifor, a solution incorporating a non-protein oxygen carrier, has been tested for short-term in situ normothermic preservation[81] and in a porcine model of subnormothermic renal perfusion.[82] Lifor demonstrated a better preservation of renal function[81] and reduced renal resistance compared to UW.[82] A haemoglobin-supplemented fluid allowed the resuscitation of kidneys despite 2 hours of

warm ischaemia, providing life-sustaining function.[83] Another option would be to use blood itself and, in an animal study, normothermic perfusion with heparinised whole blood has shown preservation of renal function during 6 hours of perfusion, despite following up to 40 minutes of warm ischaemia.[84]

It is possible that a period of normothermia and oxygenation may be beneficial at the beginning or end of a cold preservation phase. Theoretically, it would offer some degree of ischaemic preconditioning at the beginning of the preservation period, or allow cytoprotective mechanisms to aid the recovery of the organ.

✅ Two hours of normothermic reperfusion with autologous blood after 16 hours of SCS was shown to improve renal blood flow to the level of kidneys statically stored for only 2 hours.[85] This technique was at least equivalent to HMP for 18 hours.[85] Extracorporeal normothermic perfusion has recently been tested in human renal transplantation.[86]

The first published case was that of an ECD declined by six UK centres before being accepted in Leicester. One kidney was perfused at normothermic temperatures with plasma-free, red-cell-based solution for 35 minutes prior to transplantation, while the other kidney was stored by static cold preservation alone. Both kidneys had acute tubular necrosis and rejection on protocol biopsy at 1 week; however, the recipient of the reperfused kidney had primary function, while the recipient of the static cold preserved kidney required dialysis for a further 4 weeks. The Leicester group have moved on to use this method of pre-implantation, normothermic recirculation for a case series of 16 transplants, with promising results so far.[87]

One option in the prevention of ischaemia–reperfusion injury may be 'immune camouflage' whereby selected polymers interact with allograft cell membranes to reduce immune cell invasion of the graft. PEG, a constituent of IGL-1 solution, is one such polymer. Animal studies have suggested that plasma with PEG may have better static preservation effects than IGL-1 or UW with less immune cell infiltration and improved graft survival.[88]

Liver

State of the art

As with kidneys, the static cold storage method, whereby the organ is flushed with chilled preservation solution and then kept on ice, has become the prevalent method for liver allograft preservation. The preservation solutions used for SCS of livers have also followed in the footsteps of those used for kidneys. Currently, primarily UW is used internationally, with an increasing number of livers stored in HTK or Celsior solution.[89] UW was introduced as a preservation fluid for the SCS of livers in the late 1980s and early 1990s, when it demonstrated equal preservation properties to both Eurocollins and Marshall's solution despite longer CIT.[90–92] Like kidneys, the key outcomes of preservation are graft survival and PNF, but additionally primary dysfunction (PDF), where the liver synthetic function is not immediately adequate and also re-transplantation rates.

✅ Several studies have found similar outcomes for preservation in both HTK and UW solutions.[30,93–98] Registry data analysis from the UNOS database, however, including 17 428 transplanted livers, shows that HTK preservation is associated with an increased risk of graft loss, especially with DCD livers and those with a CIT of over 8 hours.[89]

To lower the viscosity of UW and reduce its potassium content, PEG has been substituted for the HES in UW to make Institut Georges-Lopez Solution (IGL-1). It has shown comparable results to UW in one controlled trial of 140 livers.[99]

✅✅ Celsior solution has been tested in comparison with UW for liver preservation in a number of clinical trials. All studies so far have found outcomes such as serum parameters, PNF rates, PDF rates and graft survival up to 3 years to be the same for both UW and Celsior solutions.[32,38,100–102] One study has now completed 5-year follow-up and has not discerned any difference between the graft survival of the two groups.[103] Celsior solution has also been compared to HTK in one RCT, which found no difference in PDF rates, complications or 12-month graft survival.[104] So far it appears that the results of RCTs have not discerned differences in the outcomes of liver transplantation when using any of Celsior, HTK or UW. However, all RCTs have had less than 100 livers in each arm, and are likely underpowered to find an effect on their own.

It is speculated that circulating chilled preservation fluid through the hepatic vasculature makes available the metabolic substrates required for ATP generation, delivers antioxidants and washes out metabolites, thereby reducing ischaemia–reperfusion injury.

✅ Hypothermic machine perfusion of liver allografts remains in the early stages of development and has so far been tested in one case–control study of 20 DBD livers.[49] This study showed that up to 7 hours dual portal and arterial perfusion with chilled Vasosol solution reduced EAD, serum liver enzymes and hospital stay compared to static cold storage in UW.[49]

The same group used tissue samples to characterise the pattern of early phase cytokines implicated in ischaemia–reperfusion injury, demonstrating up-regulation of intercellular adhesion molecule (ICAM)-1, interleukin (IL)-8 and tumour necrosis factor (TNF)-α in the reperfusion biopsies of livers stored statically; this effect was attenuated in the machine-perfused livers.[105] To further improve upon HMP, perfusate solutions have been adapted to address the insult of ischaemia–reperfusion injury. Polysol solution is an adaptation of UW and has been compared to UW in an animal model of DCD, reducing alanine aminotransferase (ALT) and aspartate aminotransferase (AST) release during perfusion, increasing perfusate flow and resulting in higher bile production and cellular ATP.[106]

Controlled donation after circulatory death

Studies of preservation solutions have largely been conducted with DBD livers, given concerns about outcomes from DCD. Retrospective reviews have suggested increased biliary complications following liver transplantation from controlled DCD.[107,108] The particular weakness of DCD is the associated rate of ischaemic-type biliary lesions (ITBLs), with some studies reporting rates as high as 33% at 1 year, compared to 10% for DBD.[108] This complication makes the adequate preservation of DCD livers of particular importance. See Figure 6.5. While controlled DCD livers do present acceptable graft survival rates,[107–109] larger studies have shown reduced graft and patient survival for controlled DCD compared to DBD livers.[108]

Uncontrolled donation after circulatory death

Early experience with uncontrolled DCD for liver transplantation was disappointing, with only 60% of retrieved livers transplantable and only 50%

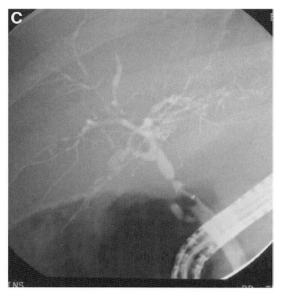

Figure 6.5 • Ischaemic-type biliary lesions (ITBLs) can cause cholestasis in transplanted livers. They are much more common in livers transplanted from donors after circulatory death than donors after brain death, due to the length of warm ischaemia. Most cases can be treated by endoscopic balloon dilatation; however, in the worst cases re-transplantation is necessary.

of these functioning initially.[110] With improved infrastructure and careful donor selection, outcomes have improved; however, uncontrolled DCD livers are still associated with a higher incidence of PNF and biliary complications.[111] More complex methods for liver preservation have therefore been tested, including NRP.

Fondevila and the Barcelona group reported the first case–control study of NRP for uncontrolled DCD liver preservation.[112] The group required strict criteria to accept and transplant organs, resulting in only 10 transplants from 40 donors. Livers were rejected if macroscopically steatotic on inspection, or on the grounds of elevated transaminases or poor perfusion. Donors with prolonged WIT were also excluded. Patient and graft survival were comparable to matched DBD livers transplanted at the same unit, with an average of 23 months' follow-up.

Another case–control series from Spain examined the results of uncontrolled DCD liver allografts.[113] Jimenez-Galanes and the Madrid group had strict criteria for accepting these organs, and donors had to be less than 50 years old, arrest time less than 15 minutes and WIT less than 50 minutes. Maximum acceptable NRP time was 270 minutes. Twenty liver allografts were transplanted from 43 possible donors. The 1-year graft survival was 80% and was comparable to matched DBD livers transplanted at the same unit. PNF rates were also comparable in this small series (10% vs. 5%). Re-transplantation rate, however, was higher for the uncontrolled DCD group (15% vs. 0%), as were the peak AST and ALT levels.

✓ These two studies[112,113] suggest a possible role for NRP in liver preservation from DCD category II donors.

New developments and the future

Hypothermic machine perfusion of the liver has received interest for many years and in the early 1990s it demonstrated the potential for long term preservation in animal studies.[114] The use of HMP as a preferred method for the preservation of livers from DCD donors has been tested in rat models, reducing cellular damage and graft loss in comparison to SCS.[115] HMP has also shown some promise in the preservation of steatotic livers for long preservation times.[106] Bile production, ammonia clearance, urea production, oxygen consumption and ATP levels were significantly higher after HMP compared to SCS.[106] HMP as a resuscitation modality for previously untransplantable livers has since entered pre-clinical testing. Guarerra et al. preserved 10 discarded human livers with pulsatile perfusion for up to 10 hours to test the viability of the technique.[116] Alongside this study the same group preserved porcine livers modelling DCD and completed three transplantations from livers preserved by HMP. All recipients showed initial graft function with reduction in serum enzymes.[116] Vekemans et al. also tested HMP for the rescue of discarded human livers in an experimental model of ischaemia–reperfusion.[117] HMP was used for 4 hours after a period of SCS, which was compared to SCS alone. During normothermic reperfusion with blood after the cold preservation, HMP was associated with reduced AST and LDH release, and reduced mitogen-activated protein kinase (MAPK) levels. Histological examination of liver biopsies from both preservation modalities was similar.[117]

The potential for hypothermic machine perfusion to act as a resuscitation therapy for DCD livers may be further extended by the use of oxygenation of the perfusate during the perfusion period (hypothermic oxygenated perfusion, HOPE). This has been tested in animal models of DCD, using HOPE at the end of a period of SCS to precondition the organs.[118–120] Preconditioning with oxygenated perfusate resulted in reduced cellular damage compared to SCS alone, with reduced necrosis and lipid peroxidation and increased cellular ATP recovery and bile flow.[118–120] HOPE-treated livers also had improved graft survival, although experimental animals did not survive beyond 18 hours whether HOPE was used or not.[119] The use of oxygenated machine perfusate has been further tested using a sanguineous fluid at both normothermic and hypothermic temperatures.[121] HOPE in this format also reversed the microscopic and macroscopic damage present in these livers, reducing AST release, increasing bile flow after reperfusion, reducing serum lactate and improving recipient survival.[121] In this study all experimental animals died within 24 hours if the liver had suffered 120 minutes of warm ischaemia, whether HOPE was used or not.[121]

Future developments in liver preservation will have to address the demands of the transplant waiting list by making previously untransplantable organs viable. It is speculated that the addition of oxygen to preservation modalities may make this possible through maintaining metabolism. Similarly to kidneys, various methods have been tested to deliver increased oxygen concentrations to livers ex vivo. Minor et al. have tested gaseous oxygen persufflation in a pig transplant model. Following 10 hours of SCS, oxygen bubbles are passed into the vena cava for 2 hours prior to implantation.[122] Livers receiving oxygen persufflation had greatly improved 1-week graft survival of 83% (in the control group it was 0%). Histological studies at autopsy showed preserved liver architecture in the study group. Serum liver enzymes and clotting parameters were also all within normal ranges. Post-conditioning with persufflated gaseous oxygen has also been tested in a small series of human livers that were otherwise rejected due to previous warm ischaemic damage.[123] This resuscitation permitted the transplantation of five livers, and all patients were alive and well at 2 years' follow-up, without re-transplantation. There was a significant increase in cellular ATP

levels after oxygen persufflation. Persufflation has also shown positive results as a rescue therapy in experimental models following long periods of SCS (18 hours), reducing serum liver enzymes, LDH and TNF-α, and increasing bile production.[124] The first RCT of resuscitative oxygen persufflation is currently recruiting.[125] When compared with oxygenated HMP, oxygen persufflation has shown slightly more promising results in terms of hepatic enzyme release and bile production in an animal model of DCD.[126] Further adaptations to HMP have included the use of a hyperbaric oxygen chamber to enclose the pump and increase the partial pressure of oxygen within the tissues. In a small experimental series this technique has shown the benefit of increased cellular ATP and bile production and reduced ALT release after reperfusion.[127] The two-layer method, which was developed initially for pancreas preservation, has also been tested in liver preservation. A continuously oxygenated perfluorocarbon layer lies underneath, and in direct contact with the preservation fluid (typically HTK or UW). In liver experimental studies this method improved cellular ATP levels but not cellular morphology.[128]

Normothermic machine perfusion (NMP) provides an intuitive and possibly better alternative to HMP but has associated complexities and technological challenges. Providing a physiological environment for continued metabolism allows assessment of function and recovery of the organ ex vivo. See Figure 6.6. Schön and the Berlin group were the first to demonstrate, in an animal model, that 4 hours of ex vivo normothermic preservation of the liver was safe prior to transplantation.[129] This technique also seemed to have increased benefit when following a period of warm ischaemia if compared to SCS.[129] The Oxford group followed on from this work to show that porcine livers could be preserved for much longer periods of time (72 hours) by NMP with oxygenation of the perfusate.[130] Further development of these experimental models allowed testing of liver synthetic function during a simulated reperfusion phase. They then compared SCS in UW to NMP in this fashion.[131] NMP resulted in increased bile production, glucose production and galactose clearance, with reduced release of hepatic enzymes and histological damage.[131] The same group used a model of DCD liver preservation (60 minutes WIT) to show that NMP could recover function, in comparison

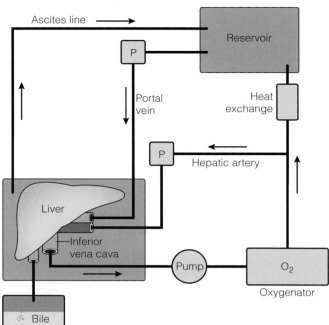

Figure 6.6 • Normothermic machine perfusion of the liver can use dual or single perfusion. The dual perfusion device depicted here provides blood flow into the portal vein as well as the hepatic artery. Ascites fluid is collected and mixed with venous blood in the reservoir. P, pressure sensor.

to SCS, which resulted in no evidence of viability, with no bile production or substrate utilisation.[132] Moving into animal transplantation experiments, NMP has shown the potential to reduce hepatic enzyme release, increase patient survival and improve hepatic histology in experiments mimicking both DBD and DCD.[133] This benefit was consistent only if the preservation period was long (20 hours).[133] The Barcelona group, in collaboration with the Groningen group, have performed animal models of uncontrolled DCD, with long WIT (90 minutes) using NMP. In this study, NMP after a period of ECMO has shown the potential to further improve upon the results obtained by ECMO followed by SCS.[134] Improvements were seen in function, and macroscopic and histological appearances of the livers.[134] Tolboom et al. used animal transplantation studies with long WIT (60 minutes) to show that ischaemically damaged livers preserved with NMP could be transplanted with excellent (92%) 4-week survival.[135] This is comparable to controls receiving healthy livers preserved by SCS or NMP.[135] Animals receiving ischaemically damaged livers preserved by SCS alone all died within 12 hours of transplantation. The same group moved on to examine subnormothermic machine perfusion, again following

60 minutes of WIT.[136] Machine perfusion at both 20 and 30°C recovered ischaemically damaged livers, and all animals survived beyond 1 month.[136] Steatotic livers are particularly susceptible to ischaemia–reperfusion injury, and given that they make up an increasing proportion of the donor pool, their preservation and resuscitation are of increasing importance. NMP has the potential to reduce the level of evident hepatic injury in these livers, which SCS does not.[137]

Pancreas

State of the art

Static cold storage on ice is the predominant method for the preservation of pancreas allografts for whole-organ transplantation. Belzer and Southard, at the University of Wisconsin, developed a potassium–lactobionate solution, later to become the UW solution, which was first tested for the pancreas by Wahlberg et al.[25] See Figure 6.7. It was subsequently used for the other abdominal organs. Since the 1980s both HTK and Celsior solutions have been compared to UW for clinical pancreas preservation, although there have only been three small RCTs published so far.

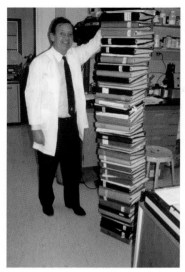

Figure 6.7 • Folkert Belzer in the laboratory at the University of Wisconsin. He is pictured with some of the lab books of researchers working with him on developing methods of organ preservation.

✅ Schneeberger et al. examined the results of 68 pancreas transplants in a recent RCT, finding no difference in 6-month graft survival or graft function between HTK and UW.[138] Boggi and the Pisa group also report an RCT of 105 pancreatic transplants comparing UW with Celsior, finding no difference in early complications or 1-year graft survival.[31] A more recent, smaller RCT of 30 pancreas transplants found UW and Celsior solutions to be equally safe.[139]

A number of retrospective studies have analysed results comparing these three solutions for pancreas preservation. Potdar et al. presented results from the University of Pittsburgh, comparing results between HTK and UW preservation of human allografts, finding comparable early graft function and 1-month graft survival rates, although HTK was associated with more oedema.[140] Becker et al. also presented single-centre data from Hannover, finding comparable early graft function and 1-year graft survival.[141] The largest single-centre case series, from Indianapolis, Indiana, reports on the transplantation of 146 pancreata preserved in HTK and in this study 1-year graft survival was equivalent to a historical control group preserved in UW.[142] A smaller, multi-centre analysis found no difference in outcome apart from a higher rate of rejection in the HTK group

(30% vs. 12%).[143] The largest analysis of the comparison between HTK and UW, however, is the registry data examined by Stewart et al., which looked at a total of 4392 pancreas transplants.[144] Multivariate analysis of these data found that HTK preservation was an independent risk factor for graft loss, especially with CIT >12 h.[144] This analysis found a higher risk of early graft loss with HTK, and it has been suggested by some studies that this may be related to a higher rate of graft pancreatitis following HTK preservation.[145] This association does remain controversial, however, with other, larger single-centre reviews not finding this association,[146] and the volume of HTK used for the flush may be implicated, with higher flush volumes causing more oedema.[145] Retrospective single-centre analysis of 112 pancreatic transplants from Pisa and Parma, Italy, found that 1-year graft survival was equivalent with Celsior and UW preservation.[147] Surgical complications and early graft function were also equivalent. A single-centre analysis of 71 pancreatic transplants from Madrid, Spain, found comparable complication rates and 2-year graft survival.[148]

One small non-randomised study from Sao Paolo, Brazil, demonstrated that Eurocollins could be used as an initial flush before UW was used as the primary preservation fluid.[149] This was done in an attempt to reduce costs through reducing the volume required of the more expensive UW. Flushing with EC first in this way did not appear to have any adverse effects.[149]

Altogether there is good evidence for the use of SCS in pancreas preservation; however, there is not a good foundation for selecting one preservation solution over another. The RCTs so far published are too small, as are the single-centre reviews. It is registry data alone that suggest a benefit of UW over HTK.

New developments and the future

Unfortunately, most work on pancreas preservation was done over 10 years ago. Two studies, one in the Netherlands and one in the UK, will be starting shortly to assess the impact of HMP and normothermic recirculation on pancreas viability and islet isolation. As with other abdominal organs, interest in oxygen delivery to the graft has prompted experimental studies in pancreas preservation, where the two-layer method has probably seen the most activity. Despite early successes in animal studies by the Kobe group in Japan,[150] the method has not seen expansion into clinical testing until the year 2000. The Minnesota group preserved the first 10 human pancreata for transplantation using the two-layer method.[151] They found the technique feasible and at least equivalent to SCS; however, it has seen much more use in studies of pancreatic islet preparation rather than solid-organ preservation. More recent studies have questioned how effective this technique is at delivering oxygen to the deeper tissues of the pancreas, and we may have to look for other methods to achieve this goal.[152]

Intestine

State of the art

The preservation of intestinal grafts for transplantation falls behind that for other abdominal organs given the relatively early stages of this therapy for intestinal failure. A recent review concluded that the available methods are currently adequate, but probably suboptimal for intestinal preservation.[153] Preservation of intestinal grafts encounters the inherent problem of preserving the intestinal mucosa, which is extremely sensitive to ischaemia.[154] Mucosal damage results in the translocation of luminal bacteria, particularly following long CIT (over 9 hours) or when colon is transplanted.[155] This compromises the graft and patient, making adequate preservation of paramount importance; hence CIT must be kept to a minimum for intestinal transplantation. The gold standard in the preservation of other abdominal organs, UW, is the most commonly used preservation fluid for intestinal grafts, and it has been used by the groups performing the largest numbers of intestinal transplants.[156] Animal reperfusion models have been used to compare Celsior, HTK, Polysol and UW solutions.[157] Celsior, HTK and Polysol showed reduced LDH, higher cellular ATP and better histological examination than UW. The best method for the clinical preservation of human intestinal grafts, however, remains controversial. There is some evidence that both the vasculature and lumen of the bowel need to be in contact with the preservation medium, as shown in experimental studies with human tissue.[158] The nutrient content of the luminal preservation solution is also controversial, with some suggestion that it may be beneficial to include

nutrients such as amino acids.[159,160] In small studies amino acid solutions have been at least as effective as UW, but the exact concentrations of nutrients required remain unknown.[159,161] More recent studies have used PEG solution as a luminal flush, with both high and low sodium concentrations.[162] Low-sodium PEG solution gave better mucosal preservation than vascular flush alone; however, it was not compared with UW.[162]

Good comparisons between methods of preservation for human intestinal transplantation are few and small in size. A retrospective review of 57 grafts from Indianapolis compared HTK with UW, finding no difference in function, acute rejection or endoscopic appearances between the two groups.[163] Experimental studies with human bowel to compare UW and Celsior solution for vascular preservation alone have shown equal levels of histological damage with the two solutions.[164] This has been supported by animal studies that have compared Celsior with UW and glutamine-enriched UW as a luminal flush.[165] The same solution was then used as a preservation medium. Celsior decreased LDH levels in comparison to both types of UW; however, the histological appearances in all groups still showed severe mucosal injury.[165]

New developments and the future

As with the other abdominal organs there is interest in increasing the metabolic support for intestinal grafts during the preservation period through oxygenation. There are, however, only a handful of published studies investigating this area. The Kobe group in Japan have experimented with the two-layer method using perfluorocarbon (PFC) to deliver oxygen to small-bowel grafts.[166] The same group progressed to combine the two-layer method with a luminal amino acid-rich solution, showing further reductions in lactate accumulation with the combined techniques.[167] Oxygenated luminal perfusion has been tested in a small number of animals, showing that it may have benefits in the generation of cellular ATP.[168] There is a suggestion that 1 hour of oxygenated perfusion is better than oxygenated perfusion for the whole preservation period. One group in Sao Paolo have looked at the effect of preservation within a hyperbaric oxygen chamber. There was some suggestion that hyperbaric oxygen could reduce mucosal injury.[169]

Evidence in the field of organ preservation and perfusion

It has often been stated that the evidence in this field of organ transplantation is of variable quality and can be confusing and contradictory. It is hoped that the commentary in this chapter contributes to a full interpretation and on this same theme Tables 6.3–6.5 are included, setting out the evidence in different grades in an organ-specific fashion. The grading system used is not consistent throughout surgery or indeed throughout

Table 6.3 • Levels of available evidence for modalities of kidney allograft preservation

Level of evidence	Modality of preservation	References
I	Hypothermic machine preservation if used for whole preservation period	Moers et al.,[47] Watson et al.,[48] Jochmans et al.,[57] Treckmann et al.[65]
	UW, HTK, Celsior, for static cold preservation	Ploeg et al.[28] de Boer et al.,[29] Faenza et al.,[52] Pedotti et al.,[38] Montalti et al.[53]
II-2	ECMO for DCD	Magliocca et al.,[78] Farney et al.,[79] Valero et al.,[63] Lee et al.[80]
	IGL-1 for static cold preservation	Codas et al.[54]
II-3	Hypothermic ECMO for uncontrolled DCD	Alvarez et al.[60]
III	Normothermic resuscitation pre-transplantation	Hosgood and Nicholson[86]

Levels from US Preventive Services Task Force: I, RCT; II-1, non-randomised controlled trial; II-2, cohort or case–control study; II-3, multiple time series or uncontrolled trial; III, opinion/experience or report of committees.

Table 6.4 • Levels of available evidence for modalities of liver allograft preservation

Level of evidence	Modality of preservation	References
I	UW, HTK, Celsior for static cold preservation	Erhard et al.,[30] Meine et al.,[94] Nardo et al.,[100] Lama et al.,[101] Cavallari et al.,[32] Pedotti et al.,[38] Lopez-Andujar et al.,[102] Garcia-Gil et al.[103]
II-1	IGL-1 for static cold preservation	Dondero et al.[99]
II-2	Hypothermic machine preservation for DBD	Guarrera et al.[49]
	ECMO for uncontrolled DCD	Fondevila et al.,[112] Jimenez-Galanes et al.[113]
III	Hypothermic machine preservation for discarded livers	Guarrera et al.,[116] Vekemans et al.[117]
	Normothermic machine preservation for DCD and steatotic livers	Schon et al.,[129] Butler et al.,[130] Imber et al.,[131] St Peter et al.[132]
	Oxygen persufflation for discarded livers	Minor et al.,[122] Treckmann et al.[123]

Levels from US Preventive Services Task Force: I, RCT; II-1, non-randomised controlled trial; II-2, cohort or case–control study; II-3, multiple time series or uncontrolled trial; III, opinion/experience or report of committees.

Table 6.5 • Levels of available evidence for modalities of pancreas and intestine allograft preservation

Level of evidence	Modality of preservation	References
I	Celsior, HTK, UW for pancreas preservation	Schneeberger et al.,[138] Boggi et al.,[31] Nicoluzzi et al.[139]
II-3	HTK, UW for intestinal preservation	Abu-Elmagd et al.,[156] Mangus et al.[163]
	Two-layer method for pancreas preservation	Matsumoto et al.[151]
III	Celsior, IGL-1 for intestinal preservation	DeRoover et al.[164]
	Luminal contact for intestinal preservation	DeRoover et al.,[158] Olson et al.,[159] Fujimoto et al.[160]

Levels from US Preventive Services Task Force: I, RCT; II-1, non-randomised controlled trial; II-2, cohort or case–control study; II-3, multiple time series or uncontrolled trial; III, opinion/experience or report of committees.

this book, but it is offered as an attempt to help interpret the available evidence prior to any clinical implementation.

Conclusion

After an initial active period in the 1960s, when preservation methods were developed and experimental work moved rapidly to clinical practice, the advancement of preservation methods fell almost silent until the late 1980s. Simple static cold storage appeared to be sufficient to allow recovery after preservation and adequate function using standard criteria donors. The current challenges provided by a relative donor shortage and the increasing use of high-risk donors have now prompted a new period of development and the investigation of exciting new strategies. The use of hypothermic machine perfusion, normothermic resuscitation and miniaturised technology, incorporating biochemical and physiological strategies, means that we are now truly entering a new phase of development. The optimal methods for preservation of abdominal organs are not far away, and the resuscitation of organs that would previously have been discarded is achievable.

Key points

- When transplantation first started, organ preservation/perfusion was not required since donor and recipient were in close proximity. With modern complex allocation algorithms and higher risk donors, organ perfusion and preservation has become, once again, a key subject of research.
- Early research objectives were targeted on organ perfusion and were pioneered by individuals such as Dr Belzer. With the determination of successful recipes for preservation solutions, based on the science of cell protection, the economics and logistics of organ donation dictated that static cold storage was entirely satisfactory for most forms of transplantation.
- The era of acute donor organ shortage has necessitated the use of higher risk organs. Top quality preservation and indeed resuscitation of such organs has now become a new objective.
- This area of research has now become one of the most exciting in the field of transplantation. New techniques are likely to transform the way in which organs are perfused, preserved and transported in the future.

References

1. Summers DM, Johnson RJ, Allen J, et al. Analysis of factors that affect outcome after transplantation of kidneys donated after cardiac death in the UK: a cohort study. Lancet 2010;376(9749):1303–11.

2. Kauffman HM, Bennett LE, McBride MA, et al. The expanded donor. Transplant Rev 1997;11(4):165–90.

3. Port FK, Bragg-Gresham JL, Metzger RA, et al. Donor characteristics associated with reduced graft survival: an approach to expanding the pool of kidney donors. Transplantation 2002;74(9):1281–6.

4. Kootstra G, Daemen JH, Oomen AP. Categories of non-heartbeating donors. Transplant Proc 1995;27:2893.

5. Snoeijs MGJ, Winkens B, Heemskerk MBA, et al. Kidney transplantation from donors after cardiac death: a 25-year experience. Transplantation 2010;90(10):1106–12.

6. Bellingham JM, Santhanakrishnan C, Neidlinger N, et al. Donation after cardiac death: a 29-year experience. Surgery 2011;150(4):692–702.

7. Perico N, Ruggenenti P, Scalamogna M, et al. Tackling the shortage of donor kidneys: how to use the best that we have. Am J Nephrol 2003;23(4):245–59.

8. Bos EM, Leuvenink HGD, van Goor H, et al. Kidney grafts from brain dead donors: inferior quality or opportunity for improvement? Kidney Int 2007;72(7):797–805.

9. Nijboer WN, Schuurs TA, van der Hoeven JAB, et al. Effects of brain death on stress and inflammatory response in the human donor kidney. Transplant Proc 2005;37(1):367–9.

10. Nagareda T, Kinoshita Y, Tanaka A, et al. Clinicopathology of kidneys from brain-dead patients treated with vasopressin and epinephrine. Kidney Int 1993;43(6):1363–70.

11. Koo DDH, Welsh KI, McLaren AJ, et al. Cadaver versus living donor kidneys: impact of donor factors on antigen induction before transplantation. Kidney Int 1999;56(4):1551–9.

12. Pratschke J, Wilhelm MJ, Kusaka M, et al. Accelerated rejection of renal allografts from brain-dead donors. Ann Surg 2000;232(2):263–71.

13. Levy MN. Oxygen consumption and blood flow in the hypothermic, perfused kidney. Am J Physiol 1959;197(5):1111–4.

14. Bonventre JV, Cheung JY. Effects of metabolic acidosis on viability of cells exposed to anoxia. Am J Physiol 1985;249(1):C149–59.

15. McCord JM. Oxygen-derived free radicals in postischemic tissue injury. N Engl J Med 1985;312(3):159–63.

16. Calne RY, Pegg DE, Brown FL. Renal preservation by ice cooling. An experimental study relating to kidney transplantation from cadavers. Br Med J 1963;2(5358):651–5.

17. Opelz G, Terasaki P. Advantage of cold storage over machine perfusion for preservation of cadaver kidneys. Transplantation 1982;33(1):64–8.

18. Collins GM, Bravo-Shugarman M, Terasaki P. Kidney preservation for transportation. Initial perfusion and 30 hours' ice storage. Lancet 1969;294(7632):1219–22.

19. Downes G, Hoffman R, Huang J, et al. Mechanism of action of washout solutions for kidney preservation. Transplantation 1973;16(1):46–53.

20. Andrews PM, Coffey AK. Factors that improve the preservation of nephron morphology during cold storage. Lab Invest 1982;46(1):100–20.

21. Sacks SA, Petritsch PH, Kaufmann JJ. Canine kidney preservation using a new perfusate. Lancet 1973;301(7811):1024–8.

22. Ross H, Marshall VC, Escott ML. 72-hour canine kidney preservation using a new perfusate. Transplantation 1976;21:498.

23. Howden B, Rae D, Jablonski P, et al. Studies of renal preservation using a rat kidney transplant model. Evaluation of citrate flushing. Transplantation 1983;35(4):311–4.

24. Sumimoto R, Jamieson NV, Kamada N. Examination of the role of the impermeants lactobionate and raffinose in a modified UW solution. Transplantation 1990;50(4):573–6.

25. Wahlberg JA, Southard JH, Belzer FO. Development of a cold storage solution for pancreas preservation. Cryobiology 1986;23:477–82.

26. Ploeg RJ, Goossens D, McAnulty JF, et al. Successful 72-hour cold storage of dog kidneys with UW solution. Transplantation 1988;46(2):191–6.

27. Jamieson NV, Sundberg R, Lindell S, et al. Preservation of the canine liver for 24–48 hours using simple cold storage with UW solution. Transplantation 1988;46(4):517–22.

28. Ploeg RJ, van Bockel JH, Langendijk PT, et al. Effect of preservation solution on results of cadaveric kidney transplantation. The European Multicentre Study Group. Lancet 1992;340(8812):129–37.

29. De Boer J, De Meester J, Smits JMA, et al. Eurotransplant randomized multicenter kidney graft preservation study comparing HTK with UW and Euro-Collins. Transpl Int 1999;12(6):447–53.

30. Erhard J, Lange R, Scherer R, et al. Comparison of histidine–tryptophan–ketoglutarate (HTK) solution versus University of Wisconsin (UW) solution for organ preservation in human liver transplantation. Transpl Int 1994;7:177–81.

31. Boggi U, Vistoli F, Del Chiaro M, et al. Pancreas preservation with University of Wisconsin and Celsior solutions: a single-centre, prospective, randomized study. Transplantation 2004;77(8):1186–90.

32. Cavallari A, Cillo U, Nardo B, et al. A multicenter pilot prospective study comparing Celsior and University of Wisconsin preserving solutions for use in liver transplantation. Liver Transpl 2003;9(8):814–21.
University of Wisconsin solution remains the ideal preservation solution.

33. Fridell JA, Agarwal A, Milgrom ML, et al. Comparison of histidine–tryptophan–ketoglutarate solution and University of Wisconsin solution for organ preservation in clinical pancreas transplantation. Transplantation 2004;77(8):1304–6.

34. Moen J, Claesson K, Pienaar H, et al. Preservation of dog liver, kidney, and pancreas using the Belzer-UW solution with a high-sodium and low-potassium content. Transplantation 1989;47(6):940–5.

35. Baatard R, Pradier F, Dantal J, et al. Prospective randomized comparison of University of Wisconsin and UW-modified, lacking hydroxyethyl-starch, cold-storage solutions in kidney transplantation. Transplantation 1993;55(1):31–5.

36. Opelz G, Dohler B. Multicenter analysis of kidney preservation. Transplantation 2007;83(3):247–53.

37. van der Plaats A, t'Hart NA, Morariu AM, et al. Effect of University of Wisconsin organ-preservation solution on haemorheology. Transpl Int 2004;17(5):227–33.

38. Pedotti P, Cardillo M, Rigotti P, et al. A comparative prospective study of two available solutions for kidney and liver preservation. Transplantation 2004;77(10):1540–5.

39. Eugene M. Polyethyleneglycols and immuno-camouflage of the cells tissues and organs for transplantation. Cell Mol Biol (Noisy-le-grand) 2004;50(3):209–15.

40. Zheng TL, Lanza RP, Soon-Shiong P. Prolonged pancreas preservation using a simplified UW solution containing polyethylene glycol. Transplantation 1991;51(1):63–6.

41. Itasaka H, Burns W, Wicomb WN, et al. Modification of rejection by polyethylene glycol in small bowel transplantation. Transplantation 1994;57(5):645–8.

42. Ben Abdennebi H, Steghens J-P, Hadj-Aissa A, et al. A preservation solution with polyethylene glycol and calcium: a possible multiorgan liquid. Transpl Int 2002;15(7):348–54.

43. Badet L, Petruzzo P, Lefrancois N, et al. Kidney preservation with IGL-1 solution: a preliminary report. Transplant Proc 2005;37(1):308–11.

44. Ben-Mosbah I, Roselló-Catafau J, Franco-Gou R, et al. Preservation of steatotic livers in IGL-1 solution. Liver Transpl 2006;12(8):1215–23.

45. Belzer F, Ashby BS, Dunphy JE. 24-hour and 72-hour preservation of canine kidneys. Lancet 1967;290(7515):536–9.

46. Belzer FO, Ashby BS, Gulyassy PF, et al. Successful seventeen-hour preservation and transplantation of human-cadaver kidney. N Engl J Med 1968;278(11):608–10.

47. Moers C, Smits JM, Maathuis MHJ, et al. Machine perfusion or cold storage in deceased-donor kidney transplantation. N Engl J Med 2009;360(1):7–19.

48. Watson CJE, Wells AC, Roberts RJ, et al. Cold machine perfusion versus static cold storage of kidneys donated after cardiac death: a UK multicenter randomized controlled trial. Am J Transplant 2010;10(9):1991–9.

49. Guarrera JV, Henry SD, Samstein B, et al. Hypothermic machine preservation in human liver transplantation: the first clinical series. Am J Transplant 2010;10(2):372–81.

50. Guarrera JV, Polyak M, Arrington BO, et al. Pulsatile machine perfusion with Vasosol solution improves early graft function after cadaveric renal transplantation. Transplantation 2004;77(8):1264–8.

51. Stevens RB, Skorupa JY, Rigley TH, et al. Increased primary non-function in transplanted deceased-donor kidneys flushed with histidine–tryptophan–ketoglutarate solution. Am J Transplant 2009;9(5):1055–62.

52. Faenza A, Catena F, Nardo B, et al. Kidney preservation with University of Wisconsin and Celsior solution: a prospective multicenter randomized study. Transplantation 2001;72(7):1274–7.

53. Montalti R, Nardo B, Capocasale E, et al. Kidney transplantation from elderly donors: a prospective randomized study comparing celsior and UW solutions. Transplant Proc 2005;37(6):2454–5.

54. Codas R, Petruzzo P, Morelon E, et al. IGL-1 solution in kidney transplantation: first multi-center study. Clin Transplant 2009;23(3):337–42.

55. Moers C, Pirenne J, Paul A, et al. Machine perfusion or cold storage in deceased-donor kidney transplantation. N Engl J Med 2012;366(8):770–1.

56. Kokkinos C, Antcliffe D, Nanidis T, et al. Outcome of kidney transplantation from nonheart-beating versus heart-beating cadaveric donors. Transplantation 2007;83(9):1193–9.

57. Jochmans I, Moers C, Smits JM, et al. Machine perfusion versus cold storage for the preservation of kidneys donated after cardiac death: a multicenter, randomized, controlled trial. Ann Surg 2010;252(5):756–62.

58. Hosgood SA, Mohamed IH, Bagul A, et al. Hypothermic machine perfusion after static cold storage does not improve the preservation condition in an experimental porcine kidney model. Br J Surg 2011;98:943–50.

59. Alvarez J, del Barrio R, Arias J, et al. Non-heart-beating donors from the streets: an increasing donor pool source. Transplantation 2000;70(2):314–7.

60. Alvarez J, del Barrio MR, Arias J, et al. Five years of experience with non-heart-beating donors coming from the streets. Transplant Proc 2002;34(7):2589–90.

61. Sanchez-Fructuoso AI, Prats D, Torrente J, et al. Renal transplantation from non-heart beating donors: a promising alternative to enlarge the donor pool. J Am Soc Nephrol 2000;11(2):350–8.

62. Fieux F, Losser M-R, Bourgeois E, et al. Kidney retrieval after sudden out of hospital refractory cardiac arrest: a cohort of uncontrolled non heart beating donors. Crit Care 2009;13(4):R141.

63. Valero R, Cabrer C, Oppenheimer F, et al. Normothermic recirculation reduces primary graft dysfunction of kidneys obtained from non-heart-beating donors. Transpl Int 2000;13(4):303–10.

64. Metzger RA, Delmonico FL, Feng S, et al. Expanded criteria donors for kidney transplantation. Am J Transplant 2003;3(Suppl. 4):114–25.

65. Treckmann J, Moers C, Smits J, et al. Machine perfusion versus cold storage for preservation of kidneys from expanded criteria donors after brain death. Transpl Int 2011;24(6):548–54.

66. Abboud I, Antoine C, Gaudez F, et al. Pulsatile perfusion preservation for expanded-criteria donors kidneys: impact on delayed graft function rate. Int J Artif Organs 2011;34(6):513–8.

67. Moers C, Varnav OC, van Heurn E, et al. The value of machine perfusion perfusate biomarkers for predicting kidney transplant outcome. Transplantation 2010;90(9):966–73.

68. Kay MD, Hosgood SA, Harper SJF, et al. Static normothermic preservation of renal allografts using a novel nonphosphate buffered preservation solution. Transpl Int 2007;20(1):88–92.

69. Schreinemachers MC, Doorschodt BM, Florquin S, et al. Improved preservation and microcirculation with POLYSOL after transplantation in a porcine kidney autotransplantation model. Nephrol Dial Transplant 2009;24(3):816–24.

70. Schreinemachers MC, Doorschodt BM, Florquin S, et al. Improved renal function of warm ischemically damaged kidneys using Polysol. Transplant Proc 2009;41(1):32–5.

71. Treckmann JW, Paul A, Saad S, et al. Primary organ function of warm ischaemically damaged porcine kidneys after retrograde oxygen persufflation. Nephrol Dial Transplant 2006;21(7):1803–8.

72. Treckmann J, Nagelschmidt M, Minor T, et al. Function and quality of kidneys after cold storage, machine perfusion, or retrograde oxygen persufflation: results from a porcine autotransplantation model. Cryobiology 2009;59(1):19–23.

73. Manekeller S, Leuvenink H, Sitzia M, et al. Oxygenated machine perfusion preservation of pre-damaged kidneys with HTK and Belzer machine perfusion solution: an experimental study in pigs. Transplant Proc 2005;37(8):3274–5.

74. Maathuis MH, Manekeller S, van der Plaats A, et al. Improved kidney graft function after preservation using a novel hypothermic machine perfusion device. Ann Surg 2007;246(6):982–91.

75. Buchs J-B, Lazeyras F, Ruttimann R, et al. Oxygenated hypothermic pulsatile perfusion versus cold static storage for kidneys from non heart-beating donors tested by in-line ATP resynthesis to establish a strategy of preservation. Perfusion 2011;26(2):159–65.

76. Koetting M, Frotscher C, Minor T. Hypothermic reconditioning after cold storage improves post-ischemic graft function in isolated porcine kidneys. Transpl Int 2010;23(5):538–42.

77. Thuillier R, Dutheil D, Trieu MT, et al. Supplementation with a new therapeutic oxygen carrier reduces chronic fibrosis and organ dysfunction in kidney static preservation. Am J Transplant 2011;11(9):1845–60.

78. Magliocca JF, Magee JC, Rowe SA, et al. Extracorporeal support for organ donation after cardiac death effectively expands the donor pool. J Trauma 2005;58(6):1095–102.

79. Farney AC, Singh RP, Hines MH, et al. Experience in renal and extrarenal transplantation with donation after cardiac death donors with selective use of extracorporeal support. J Am Coll Surg 2008;206(5):1028–37.

80. Lee C-Y, Tsai M-K, Ko W-J, et al. Expanding the donor pool: use of renal transplants from non-heart-beating donors supported with extracorporeal membrane oxygenation. Clin Transplant 2005;19(3):383–90.

81. Regner KR, Nilakantan V, Ryan RP, et al. Protective effect of Lifor solution in experimental renal ischemia–reperfusion injury. J Surg Res 2010;164(2):e291–7.

82. Gage F, Leeser DB, Porterfield NK, et al. Room temperature pulsatile perfusion of renal allografts with Lifor compared with hypothermic machine pump solution. Transplant Proc 2009;41(9):3571–4.

83. Brasile L, Stubenitsky BM, Booster MH, et al. Overcoming severe renal ischemia: the role of ex vivo warm perfusion. Transplantation 2002;73(6):897–901.

84. Harper SJF, Hosgood SA, Waller HL, et al. The effect of warm ischemic time on renal function and injury in the isolated hemoperfused kidney. Transplantation 2008;86(3):445–51.

85. Bagul A, Hosgood SA, Kaushik M, et al. Experimental renal preservation by normothermic resuscitation perfusion with autologous blood. Br J Surg 2008;95(1):111–8.

86. Hosgood SA, Nicholson ML. First in man renal transplantation after ex vivo normothermic perfusion. Transplantation 2011;92(7):735–8.

87. Hosgood SA, Nicholson ML. The first clinical series of normothermic perfusion in marginal donor kidney transplantation. In: 15th Annual Congress of the British Transplantation Society. Glasgow; 2012. p. 80.

88. Thuillier R, Giraud S, Favreau F, et al. Improving long-term outcome in allograft transplantation: role of ionic composition and polyethylene glycol. Transplantation 2011;91(6):605–14.

89. Stewart ZA, Cameron AM, Singer AL, et al. Histidine–Tryptophan–Ketoglutarate (HTK) is associated with reduced graft survival in deceased donor livers, especially those donated after cardiac death. Am J Transplant 2009;9:286–93.

90. Todo S, Nery J, Yanaga K, et al. Extended preservation of human liver grafts with UW solution. JAMA 1989;261(5):711–4.

91. Kalayoglu M, Sollinger HW, Stratta RJ, et al. Extended preservation of the liver for clinical transplantation. Lancet 1988;1(8586):617–9.

92. Badger IL, Michell ID, Buist LJ, et al. Human hepatic preservation using Marshall's solution and University of Wisconsin solution in a controlled, prospective trial. Transplant Proc 1990;22(5):2183–4.

93. Pokorny H, Rasoul-Rockenschaub S, Langer F, et al. Histidine–tryptophan–ketoglutarate solution for organ preservation in human liver transplantation – A prospective multi-centre observation study. Transpl Int 2004;17(5):256–60.

94. Meine MH, Zanotelli ML, Neumann J, et al. Randomized clinical assay for hepatic grafts preservation with University of Wisconsin or histidine–tryptophan–ketoglutarate solutions in liver transplantation. Transplant Proc 2006;38(6):1872–5.

95. Avolio AW, Agnes S, Nure E, et al. Comparative evaluation of two perfusion solutions for liver preservation and transplantation. Transplant Proc 2006;38(4):1066–7.

96. Mangus RS, Tector AJ, Agarwal A, et al. Comparison of histidine–tryptophan–ketoglutarate solution (HTK) and University of Wisconsin solution (UW) in adult liver transplantation. Liver Transpl 2006;12(2):226–30.

97. Mangus RS, Fridell JA, Vianna RM, et al. Comparison of histidine–tryptophan–ketoglutarate solution and University of Wisconsin solution in extended criteria liver donors. Liver Transpl 2008;14(3):365–73.

98. Rayya F, Harms J, Martin AP, et al. Comparison of histidine–tryptophan–ketoglutarate solution and University of Wisconsin solution in adult liver transplantation. Transplant Proc 2008;40(4):891–4.

99. Dondero F, Paugam-Burtz C, Danjou F, et al. A randomized study comparing IGL-1 to the University of Wisconsin preservation solution in liver transplantation. Ann Transplant 2010;15(4):7–14.

100. Nardo B, Catena F, Cavallari G, et al. Randomized clinical study comparing UW and Celsior solution in liver preservation for transplantation: preliminary results. Transplant Proc 2001;33(1–2):870–2.

101. Lama C, Rafecas A, Figueras J, et al. Comparative study of Celsior and Belzer solutions for hepatic graft preservation: preliminary results. Transplant Proc 2002;34(1):54–5.

102. Lopez-Andujar R, Deusa S, Montalva E, et al. Comparative prospective study of two liver graft preservation solutions: University of Wisconsin and Celsior. Liver Transpl 2009;15(12):1709–17.

103. Garcia-Gil FA, Serrano MT, Fuentes-Broto L, et al. Celsior versus University of Wisconsin preserving solutions for liver transplantation: postreperfusion syndrome and outcome of a 5-year prospective randomized controlled study. World J Surg 2011;35(7):1598–607.

104. Nardo B, Bertelli R, Montalti R, et al. Preliminary results of a clinical randomized study comparing Celsior and HTK solutions in liver preservation for transplantation. Transplant Proc 2005;37(1):320–2. **There are very similar results between UW and Celsior for liver transplantation.**

105. Guarrera JV, Henry SD, Chen SWC, et al. Hypothermic machine preservation attenuates ischemia/reperfusion markers after liver transplantation: preliminary results. J Surg Res 2011;167(2):e365–73.

106. Bessems M, Doorschodt BM, van Marle J, et al. Improved machine perfusion preservation of the non-heart-beating donor rat liver using Polysol: a new machine perfusion preservation solution. Liver Transpl 2005;11(11):1379–88.

107. Abt P, Crawford M, Desai N, et al. Liver transplantation from controlled non-heart-beating donors: an increased incidence of biliary complications. Transplantation 2003;75(10):1659–63.

108. Foley DP, Fernandez LA, Leverson G, et al. Donation after cardiac death: the University of Wisconsin experience with liver transplantation. Ann Surg 2005;242(5):724–31.

109. Muiesan P, Girlanda R, Jassem W, et al. Single-center experience with liver transplantation from controlled non-heartbeating donors: a viable source of grafts. Ann Surg 2005;242(5):732–8.

110. Casavilla A, Ramirez C, Shapiro R, et al. Experience with liver and kidney allografts from non-heart-beating donors. Transplant Proc 1995;27(5):2898.

111. Otero A, Gomez-Gutierrez M, Suarez F, et al. Liver transplantation from Maastricht category 2 non-heart-beating donors. Transplantation 2003;76(7):1068–73.

112. Fondevila C, Hessheimer AJ, Ruiz A, et al. Liver transplant using donors after unexpected cardiac death: novel preservation protocol and acceptance criteria. Am J Transplant 2007;7(7):1849–55.

113. Jimenez-Galanes S, Meneu-Diaz MJC, et al. Liver transplantation using uncontrolled non-heart-beating donors under normothermic extracorporeal membrane oxygenation. Liver Transpl 2009;15(9):1110–8.

114. Pienaar BH, Lindell SL, Van Gulik T, et al. Seventy-two-hour preservation of the canine liver by machine perfusion. Transplantation 1990;49(2):258–60.

115. Lee CY, Jain S, Duncan HM, et al. Survival transplantation of preserved non-heart-beating donor rat livers: preservation by hypothermic machine perfusion. Transplantation 2003;76(10):1432–6.

116. Guarrera JV, Estevez J, Boykin J, et al. Hypothermic machine perfusion of liver allografts for transplantation: technical development in human discard and miniature swine models. Transplant Proc 2005;37:323–5.

117. Vekemans K, Van Pelt J, Komuta M, et al. Attempt to rescue discarded human liver grafts by end ischemic hypothermic oxygenated machine perfusion. Transplant Proc 2011;43(9):3455–9.

118. Manekeller S, Minor T. Possibility of conditioning predamaged grafts after cold storage: influences of oxygen and nutritive stimulation. Transpl Int 2006;19:667–74.

119. de Rougemont O, Breitenstein S, Leskosek B, et al. One hour hypothermic oxygenated perfusion (HOPE) protects nonviable liver allografts donated after cardiac death. Ann Surg 2009;250(5):674–83.

120. Luer B, Koetting M, Efferz P, et al. Role of oxygen during hypothermic machine perfusion preservation of the liver. Transpl Int 2010;23(9):944–50.

121. Dutkowski P, Furrer K, Tian Y, et al. Novel short-term hypothermic oxygenated perfusion (HOPE) system prevents injury in rat liver graft from non-heart beating donor. Ann Surg 2006;244(6):968–77.

122. Minor T, Koetting M, Kaiser G, et al. Hypothermic reconditioning by gaseous oxygen improves survival after liver transplantation in the pig. Am J Transplant 2011;11(12):2627–34.

123. Treckmann J, Minor T, Saad S, et al. Retrograde oxygen persufflation preservation of human livers: a pilot study. Liver Transpl 2008;14(3):358–64.

124. Koetting M, Kaiser G, Paul A, et al. Hypothermic reconditioning by gaseous oxygen improves survival after transplantation of marginally preserved livers in the pig. Langenbecks Arch Surg 2011;396(4):578–9.

125. Minor T, Putter C, Gallinat A, et al. Oxygen persufflation as adjunct in liver preservation (OPAL): study protocol for a randomized controlled trial. Trials 2011;12(1):234.

126. Stegemann J, Hirner A, Rauen U, et al. Gaseous oxygen persufflation or oxygenated machine perfusion with Custodiol-N for long-term preservation of ischemic rat livers? Cryobiology 2009;58(1):45–51.

127. Ijichi H, Taketomi A, Soejima Y, et al. Effect of hyperbaric oxygen on cold storage of the liver in rats. Liver Int 2006;26(2):248–53.

128. Odaira M, Aoki T, Miyamoto Y, et al. Cold preservation of the liver with oxygenation by a two-layer method. J Surg Res 2009;152(2):209–17.

129. Schön MR, Kollmar O, Wolf S, et al. Liver transplantation after organ preservation with normothermic extracorporeal perfusion. Ann Surg 2001;233(1):114–23.

130. Butler AJ, Rees MA, Wight DGD, et al. Successful extracorporeal porcine liver perfusion for 72 hr. Transplantation 2002;73(8):1212–8.

131. Imber CJ, St Peter SD, Lopez de Cenarruzabeitia I, et al. Advantages of normothermic perfusion over cold storage in liver preservation. Transplantation 2002;73(5):701–9.

132. St Peter SD, Imber CJ, Lopez I, et al. Extended preservation of non-heart-beating donor livers with normothermic machine perfusion. Br J Surg 2002;89(5):609–16.

133. Brockmann J, Reddy S, Coussios C, et al. Normothermic perfusion: a new paradigm for organ preservation. Ann Surg 2009;250(1):1–6.

134. Fondevila C, Hessheimer AJ, Maathuis MH, et al. Superior preservation of DCD livers with continuous normothermic perfusion. Ann Surg 2011;254(6):1000–7.

135. Tolboom H, Pouw RE, Izamis M-L, et al. Recovery of warm ischemic rat liver grafts by normothermic extracorporeal perfusion. Transplantation 2009;87(2):170–7.

136. Tolboom H, Izamis ML, Sharma N, et al. Subnormothermic machine perfusion at both 20°C and 30°C recovers ischemic rat livers for successful transplantation. J Surg Res 2012;175(1):149–56.

137. Jamieson RW, Zilvetti M, Roy D, et al. Hepatic steatosis and normothermic perfusion – preliminary experiments in a porcine model. Transplantation 2011;92(3):289–95.

138. Schneeberger S, Biebl M, Steurer W, et al. A prospective randomized multicenter trial comparing histidine–tryptophane–ketoglutarate versus University of Wisconsin perfusion solution in clinical pancreas transplantation. Transpl Int 2009;22(2):217–24.

139. Nicoluzzi J, Macri M, Fukushima J, et al. Celsior versus Wisconsin solution in pancreas transplantation. Transplant Proc 2008;40(10):3305–7.

140. Potdar S, Malek S, Eghtesad B, et al. Initial experience using histidine–tryptophan–ketoglutarate solution in clinical pancreas transplantation. Clin Transplant 2004;18(6):661–5.

141. Becker T, Ringe B, Nyibata M, et al. Pancreas transplantation with histidine–tryptophan–ketoglutarate (HTK) solution and University of Wisconsin (UW) solution: is there a difference? JOP 2007;8(3):304–11.

142. Agarwal A, Powelson JA, Goggins WC, et al. Organ preservation with histidine–tryptophan–ketogluatarate solution in clinical pancreas transplantation: an update of the Indiana University experience. Transplant Proc 2008;40(2):498–501.

143. Englesbe MJ, Moyer A, Kim DY, et al. Early pancreas transplant outcomes with histidine–tryptophan–ketoglutarate preservation: a multicenter study. Transplantation 2006;82(1):136–9.

144. Stewart ZA, Cameron AM, Singer AL, et al. Histidine–tryptophan–ketoglutarate (HTK) is associated with reduced graft survival in pancreas transplantation. Am J Transplant 2009;9(1):217–21.

145. Alonso D, Dunn TB, Rigley T, et al. Increased pancreatitis in allografts flushed with histidine–tryptophan–ketoglutarate solution: a cautionary tale. Am J Transplant 2008;8(9):1942–5.

146. Fridell JA, Mangus RS, Powelson JA. Histidine–tryptophan–ketoglutarate for pancreas allograft preservation: the Indiana University experience. Am J Transplant 2010;10(5):1284–9.

147. Boggi U, Coletti L, Vistoli F, et al. Pancreas preservation with University of Wisconsin and Celsior solutions. Transplant Proc 2004;36(3):563–5.

148. Manrique A, Jimenez C, Herrero ML, et al. Pancreas preservation with the University of Wisconsin versus Celsior solutions. Transplant Proc 2006;38(8):2582–4.

149. Gonzalez AM, Filho GJL, Pestana JOM, et al. Effects of Eurocollins solution as aortic flush for the procurement of human pancreas. Transplantation 2005;80(9):1269–74.

150. Kuroda Y, Kawamura T, Suzuki Y, et al. A new, simple method for cold storage of the pancreas using perfluorochemical. Transplantation 1988;46(3):457–60.

151. Matsumoto S, Kandaswamy R, Sutherland DE, et al. Clinical application of the two-layer (University of Wisconsin solution/perfluorochemical plus O_2) method of pancreas preservation before transplantation. Transplantation 2000;70(5):771–4.

152. Papas KK, Hering BJ, Guenther L, et al. Pancreas oxygenation is limited during preservation with the two-layer method. [Erratum appears in Transplant Proc 2006;38(4):1205] Transplant Proc 2005;37(8):3501–4.

153. Roskott AMC, Nieuwenhuijs VB, Dijkstra G, et al. Small bowel preservation for intestinal transplantation: a review. Transpl Int 2011;24(2):107–31.

154. Park PO, Haglund U, Bulkley GB, et al. The sequence of development of intestinal tissue injury after strangulation ischemia and reperfusion. Surgery 1990;107(5):574–80.

155. Cicalese L, Sileri P, Green M, et al. Bacterial translocation in clinical intestinal transplantation. Transplantation 2001;71(10):1414–7.

156. Abu-Elmagd K, Reyes J, Bond G, et al. Clinical intestinal transplantation: a decade of experience at a single center. Ann Surg 2001;234(3):404–17.

157. Wei L, Hata K, Doorschodt BM, et al. Experimental small bowel preservation using Polysol: a new alternative to University of Wisconsin solution, Celsior and histidine–tryptophan–ketoglutarate solution? World J Gastroenterol 2007;13(27):3684–91.

158. DeRoover A, De Leval L, Gilmaire J, et al. Luminal contact with University of Wisconsin solution improves human small bowel preservation. Transplant Proc 2004;36(2):273–5.

159. Olson DW, Jijon H, Madsen KL, et al. Human small bowel storage: the role for luminal preservation solutions. Transplantation 2003;76(4):709–14.

160. Fujimoto Y, Olson DW, Madsen KL, et al. Defining the role of a tailored luminal solution for small bowel preservation. Am J Transplant 2002;2(3):229–36.

161. Salehi P, Zhu L-F, Sigurdson GT, et al. Nutrient-related issues affecting successful experimental orthotopic small bowel transplantation. Transplantation 2005;80(9):1261–8.

162. Oltean M, Joshi M, Herlenius G, et al. Improved intestinal preservation using an intraluminal macromolecular solution: evidence from a rat model. Transplantation 2010;89(3):285–90.

163. Mangus RS, Tector AJ, Fridell JA, et al. Comparison of histidine–tryptophan–ketoglutarate solution and University of Wisconsin solution in intestinal and multivisceral transplantation. Transplantation 2008;86(2):298–302.

164. DeRoover A, de Leval L, Gilmaire J, et al. A new model for human intestinal preservation: comparison of University of Wisconsin and Celsior preservation solutions. Transplant Proc 2004;36(2):270–2.

165. Leuvenink HG, van Dijk A, Freund RL, et al. Luminal preservation of rat small intestine with University of Wisconsin or Celsior solution. Transplant Proc 2005;37(1):445–7.

166. Kuroda Y, Sakai T, Suzuki Y, et al. Small bowel preservation using a cavitary two-layer (University of Wisconsin solution/perfluorochemical) cold storage method. Transplantation 1996;61(3):370–3.

167. Tsujimura T, Salehi P, Walker J, et al. Ameliorating small bowel injury using a cavitary two-layer preservation method with perfluorocarbon and a nutrient-rich solution. Am J Transplant 2004;4(9):1421–8.

168. Zhu JZJ, Castillo EG, Salehi P, et al. A novel technique of hypothermic luminal perfusion for small bowel preservation. Transplantation 2003;76(1):71–6.

169. Guimaraes FAG, Taha MO, Simoes MJ, et al. Use of hyperbaric oxygenation in small bowel preservation for transplant. Transplant Proc 2006;38(6):1796–9.

7

Recent trends in kidney transplantation

Gabriel C. Oniscu

Introduction

The remarkable progress of kidney transplantation over the past five decades has been brought about by surgical refinements, developments in immunosuppression and a better understanding of post-transplant care, with consequent reduction in acute rejection and graft failure rates and a continuous improvement in long-term outcome. Kidney transplantation is now available despite the social and legal realities of various societies worldwide. More recent years have brought new and tougher challenges. A non-exhaustive list includes extended criteria donors, donation after cardiac death (DCD), challenging comorbidity of transplant candidates, more transplant candidates than ever before and complex ethical dilemmas.So have we reached the limit of what is achievable? The answer is far from that. Renal transplantation is on the brink of an evolution/revolution that will translate into better organs, more transplants and better long-term outcome for the recipients.

This chapter will discuss the recent developments in renal transplantation, highlighting current practice and future trends at various stages of the patient's journey.

Demand inflation or supply recession?

Renal transplantation is firmly established as the optimal form of renal replacement therapy. Despite significant improvements in dialysis, transplantation remains superior, both in terms of survival and quality of life.[1] In fact, very few patients will not benefit from transplantation.[2] And herein lies our problem, as nearly every patient who starts dialysis aspires to receive a renal transplant. An escalating demand for transplantation has been evident over the years, patients joining the transplant lists in higher numbers than ever before. The demographic trend to an ageing population in many countries has also led to an increase in the age of patients requiring transplantation. Currently in the UK, one-third of the waiting list patients are aged 60 or over and 25% of the transplants are performed in this age group (**Fig. 7.1**). A similar trend has been seen in the USA, where older patients represent the fastest growing group on the list.

Unfortunately, the rise in demand means that not everybody will become a transplant candidate. Rationing policies (overt or covert) lead to a significant number of patients, particularly of older age, never joining the list. Despite the fact that some of the reasons are clear (comorbidity burden), there remains a wide practice variation in the evaluation of transplant candidacy,[3] which inevitably leads to a well-documented inequity in access. Similarly, those patients who do join the waiting list require a more careful assessment to ensure their suitability for a transplant, in the current context of longer waiting times. Sadly, the increase in waiting time has been associated with an increase in waiting list mortality, which ranges from around 3% per 100 waiting-list years for young patients to around 9% for patients aged 65 or over (US data). These two

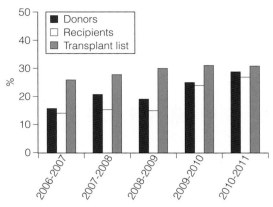

Figure 7.1 • The prevalence of patients aged >60 years old on the transplant waiting list and among transplant recipients in the UK (prevalence amongst donors shown for comparison).

intertwined factors have led to the inevitable question that perhaps the current demand may be artificially too high. Several studies have shown that some groups of patients (e.g. the elderly) will spend a disproportionate amount of time on the list and the chance of transplantation reduces dramatically with increasing waiting times. Furthermore, all patients over 60 years of age currently joining the waiting list have a 50% risk of dying on the list, without a kidney transplant.[4] In an ideal world, these patients may well benefit from transplantation but, in reality, their hopes may be inappropriately raised by a listing decision.[5]

In many countries, the number of available deceased donor organs has reached a peak and despite repeated initiatives to increase donation, and a relaxation of donor acceptance criteria (e.g. extended criteria donors), the gap is ever increasing. Many of the reasons for this trend have been well documented (reduction in trauma death, better neurological care, ageing population). Although an increase in living donation has offered some hope, in many countries even this form of donation has been static over the last few years.

Innovations in living donation

Since the early days of transplantation, living donation has seen a phenomenal expansion. In the UK, this expansion has been more obvious since 2008, with the number of living donor transplants exceeding that of deceased donor kidney transplants

for the last four consecutive years. However, in other countries, such as the USA, living donation has been relatively static since 2004, with around 6000 transplants performed each year.

> ✔ The current trends in renal transplantation focus not so much on rationing the demand (although this is still on the agenda), but more on innovations to improve organ availability and the quality of recovered organs, as well as enhancing the lifespan of every single transplanted organ, by minimising the impact of post-transplant adverse effects such as rejection, medication-related complications or death with a functioning graft.

Changes in surgical techniques (discussed later in the chapter) are considered to be the driving force behind the exponential expansion seen in the late 1990s. However, in order to allow further expansion, new strategies were required.

Altruistic donation (non-directed donation) has seen a surge following the reported success of spousal and unrelated living donor transplantation with 'read across' to stranger donation.[6] This has introduced a whole new level of complexity and ethical dilemmas in the evaluation of the living donor. However, beyond the ethical challenges (motivation, nature of altruism, emotional benefit derived from donation), it is widely accepted that there are benefits in the practice of altruistic donation, as donors gain self-esteem and the society sees an increase in the donor pool. Altruistic donor kidneys are allocated to a matched recipient on the waiting list and this can be carried out by use of one of a number of models of allocation: donor-centric, recipient-centric and socio-centric allocation.[7,8] In the donor-centric setting, the kidney is allocated to the recipient likely to have the best outcome, whilst in the recipient-centric scenario, the kidney is allocated to the patient with the greatest need. The socio-centric model treats the kidney as a national resource and is allocated as per national algorithm as for any deceased donor kidney.

Kidney paired donation was initially proposed in 1986[9] in order to allow two incompatible donor–recipient pairs to exchange kidneys to allow two compatible transplants to take place. Donor–recipient incompatibility accounts for approximately 35–50% of pairs being declined transplantation,[10,11] and represents a significant obstacle for further expansion of living donation.

In order to increase the donor pool and the number of potential matches, several variations of paired donation have been developed. Paired donation may now include a three-way (or higher number) of exchanges, which although logistically more challenging make the finding of a matched pair easier. Another protocol involves the deceased donor waiting list (**list paired donation**), whereby the incompatible living donor donates to a recipient on the list and in return, their incompatible recipient acquires priority on the waiting list for a deceased donor.[12] An alternative paired exchange protocol (**altruistic unbalanced paired kidney exchange**) includes compatible pairs in the match run.[13,14] These pairs may participate in exchange schemes for medical reasons (finding a younger donor or a better match) or altruistic reasons (helping another incompatible pair). Although ethically complex, this approach could lead to a 10% increase in the number of transplants in a paired programme.

Altruistic donation has been combined with the paired exchange programmes in order to increase the flexibility of the paired schemes and increase the potential donor pool for match runs. In a **domino paired donation**, the altruistic kidney donor initiates a chain of matches, by donating the kidney to the first recipient. The recipient's incompatible donor then donates to the next compatible recipient, whose donor donates to the national waiting list, creating a domino effect.[7] This scheme could be extended to include multiple centres and several incompatible pairs before finally transplanting a recipient on the deceased donor list.[15] An alternative arrangement is the **non-simultaneous extended altruistic donor (NEAD) chain**.[16] This consists of domino paired donation segments, except that the last donor in the first segment ('bridge donor') is asked to donate later and trigger another segment of the chain. The NEAD chain is a significant departure from the requirement of simultaneous donation in the paired exchange, but so far no chains have been broken due to a donor's unwillingness to donate, once their incompatible recipient has been transplanted. This new approach raises the prospect of multiple transplants with shorter waiting times, but does require an entirely new level of logistics and cooperation, all within a delicate ethical environment.

Paired exchange and altruistic donation options are summarised in **Fig. 7.2**.

> ✔ Innovative approaches to living donor kidney transplantation must be embraced if maximum use of this modality of treatment is to be attained. In a recent report involving altruistic donor chains and recipient desensitisation, a 13-way exchange was successfully performed.[17]

Incompatible transplantation

The above developments are relatively new and the impact on reducing the number of incompatible pairs that can be transplanted in the paired exchange schemes is yet to be fully understood. It is estimated that around 30% of the incompatible pairs cannot be transplanted in the paired exchange scheme and for these patients, transplantation across blood group or sensitisation barriers is the only option. Despite initial poor results, novel protocols have facilitated transplantation for ABO- and human leucocyte antigen (HLA)-incompatible transplant recipients with better levels of success.

ABO-incompatible transplantation

Successful ABO-incompatible transplantation (ABOi) was developed in the 1980s, but the initial protocols were associated with high morbidity due to the complexity of the immunomodulation therapy, which included splenectomy. Moreover, this approach was not widespread, due to concerns regarding a higher rate of antibody-mediated rejection and initial reports that suggested a poorer outcome when compared with ABO-compatible (ABOc) transplants. However, for these patients, the true survival comparison should be with survival on dialysis and subsequent deceased donor transplantation (assuming a donor becomes available).

Most recent reports suggest that ABOi transplant outcomes are comparable with ABOc transplants and superior to long-term dialysis outcome.

> ✔✔ In a review of the Scientific Registry of Transplant Recipients (SRTR) data in the USA,[18] 738 patients who underwent ABOi transplants had a similar outcome with 3679 matched ABOc patients, making this modality of treatment one that should be considered for a prospective recipient.

The graft loss was higher in the ABOi patients in the first 14 days post-transplant, with no significant difference beyond this time-point (**Fig. 7.3a**),

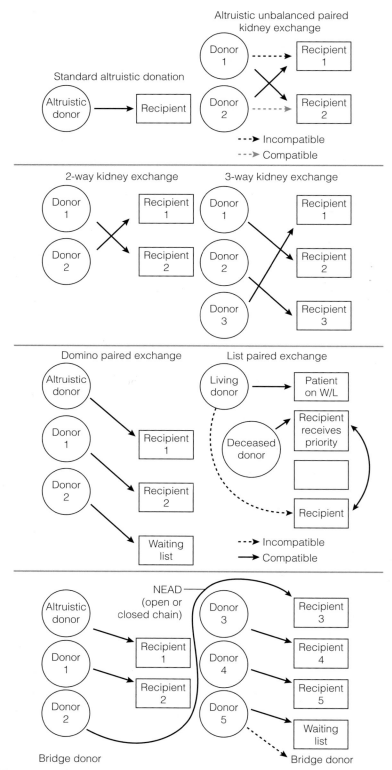

Figure 7.2 • Paired exchange donation and altruistic donation options.

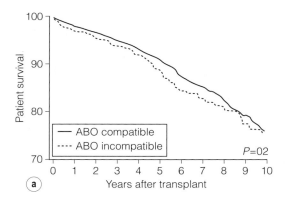

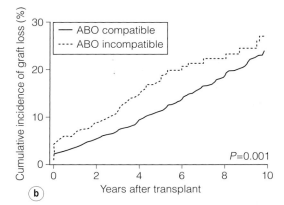

Figure 7.3 • Patient survival **(a)** and graft loss **(b)** after live-donor kidney transplantation, comparing ABO-incompatible (ABOi) recipients (dashed line) with ABO-compatible (ABOc)-matched controls (solid line). Reproduced from Montgomery JR, Berger JC, Warren DS et al. Outcomes of ABO-incompatible kidney transplantation in the United States. Transplantation 2012; 93:603–9. With permission from Wolters Kluwer Health.

This can be achieved via plasmapheresis (PP) or double-filtration plasmapheresis. The latter has a plasma separator for the first filter and a plasma fractionator for the second filter, thus reducing the requirements for fluid replacement. An alternative approach is the use of immunoadsorption, using columns with synthetic ABO antigens. This method has a high capacity for antibody removal but is rather costly.[20]

Plasmapheresis may be required post-transplant to prevent the rebound of anti-A or anti-B titres until accommodation occurs. The number of post-transplant treatments is guided by the initial antibody titres (Table 7.1) and the risk of antibody-mediated rejection (AMR).

Treatment plans are individualised and the number of sessions is detailed after the transplant date is set. A suggested template includes PP performed every other day (with pre- and post-determination of antibody level), immunoglobulin administration with each session of PP and starting tacrolimus and mycophenolate mofetil (MMF) after the first PP session. Induction therapy and standard triple therapy (tacrolimus/MMF/steroids) is continued post-transplant. An alternative is immunoadsorption, intravenous immunoglobulin (IVIG), anti-CD20 and conventional immunosuppression, which achieves comparable results.[20]

One of the main concerns with these approaches is the risk of AMR. This requires careful post-transplant monitoring and prompt treatment. No optimal AMR treatment has emerged, but PP with IVIG and anti-CD20 appears to be favoured.[21]

indicating that a rapid increase in the isohaemagglutin in titres in the immediate postoperative period is likely to lead to graft loss. Interestingly, this study showed no difference in outcome between donor A1 (considered high-risk) and A2 (considered low-risk transplant) subtypes. Throughout the study, patient survival was comparable (**Fig. 7.3b**).

The optimal protocol for immunomodulation is yet to be agreed. What is now generally accepted is that heavy immunosuppressive regimens and splenectomy are not required, as there is no increase in the risk of antibody-mediated rejection and graft loss.[19]

The removal/reduction of circulating antibodies is an essential part of the current protocols and the general aim is to achieve anti-ABO titres <16.

Table 7.1 • Indicative guide for the number of plasmapheresis treatments according to the initial antibody titre

ABO antibody titre	Pre-transplant treatments	Post-transplant treatments
<16	2	2
16	2	2
32	3	3
64	4	3
128	5–6	3
256	7–8	4
512	9–10	4
1024	10–12	4
>1024	>15	5

HLA-incompatible transplantation

Using a similar philosophy, transplantation in HLA-incompatible patients has become increasingly successful. The degree of sensitisation is determined by various methods (see Chapter 4). The single-antigen beads test is the most sensitive analysis and therefore detects the lowest strength antibody, which is usually most easily treated. At the other end of the spectrum, a positive cytotoxic crossmatch (least sensitive assay) identifies the highest antibody strength, which is most difficult to desensitise.

Three approaches to desensitisation have been described. High-dose IVIG (2 g/kg) is effective for patients receiving living or deceased donor kidneys but requires infusion over a 4-month period to ensure good results.[22]

Plasmapheresis with low dose IVIG (with or without rituximab (anti-CD20)) leads to a more consistent desensitisation and lower humoral rejection rates, but is suitable only for living donor recipients.[23]

Finally, a combination of IVIG and rituximab treatment over a 4-week period appears to be effective in desensitising patients and allowing them to receive a living donor or even a deceased donor transplant.[24]

Trends in deceased kidney donation

Traditionally, kidneys are the most commonly donated organs. Allowing for wide international variations, and some potential for development in emerging transplant nations, it is true to say that in many countries the number of donors after brain death (DBDs) has peaked. Changes in population demographics, a reduction in death from trauma and changes in neurosurgical practice have contributed to these trends. Furthermore, changes in population demographics have also meant that donors are more likely to be older and have more comorbid conditions, leading to more marginal organs being accepted for transplantation.

The decrease in DBD organs has been replaced by a resurgence of donation after cardiac death (DCD) and currently, in the UK, one-third of all kidney transplants are from DCD donors. This increase is an under-representation of the upsurge in real activity, as even in the most dynamic DCD programmes,

only approximately 20–25% of referrals proceed to actual donation.[25] The utilisation rate of DCD is highest in the UK (93%) compared with all other European countries.[26]

DCD donation is established in the USA and 10 European countries (Austria, Belgium, Czech Republic, France, Italy, Latvia, the Netherlands, Spain, Switzerland and UK). In six other European countries (Finland, Germany, Greece, Poland, Portugal and Luxembourg), DCD donation is yet to be legalised.

> ✅ The most notable international difference in deceased donation is the utilisation of category II DCD donation in Spain and France; in all other countries programmes are based on DCD III donation.

The recent revival of category II DCD donation is largely due to the success of the Spanish programmes.[27] The fundamental difference between the current Spanish programmes and the earlier category II DCD programmes (such as the ones in Newcastle and Leicester in the UK) is the use of normothermic regional perfusion (NRP) to optimise the function of abdominal organs.

The organisation of a category II DCD programme requires significant logistics and excellent cooperation between donation teams and extra-hospital services (ambulance, legal authorities and police). Close working between the transplant unit and the emergency department is key.

The complex ethical questions facing category II DCD donation have been debated widely,[28] but it is important to reiterate that an open and sensitive discussion, within the legal framework and moral environment of each individual country, is likely to resolve many of these issues and facilitate such programmes. The benefit is likely to be substantial.

> ✅ In the USA alone, it is estimated that although only 7.6% of the out-of-hospital arrests would meet criteria for donation (age <50, cardiopulmonary resuscitation (CPR) started <15 minutes after witnessed collapse and death pronounced <60 minutes after cardiac arrest), potentially there could be 22 000 category II DCD donors per year.[29]

Currently, programmes similar to those in Madrid or Barcelona are being explored in the USA, Scotland, Italy, the Netherlands, Austria and Belgium.

There are several notable differences between category II and III DCD donors. The latter group is primarily represented by patients in intensive care, with extensive irreversible brain injuries (not fulfilling the brain stem death criteria), with various degrees of comorbidity and in whom life support treatment is withdrawn. In contrast, category II DCD donors are usually younger, have fewer comorbid conditions, and death occurs as a consequence of a catastrophic and irreversible cardiac event.

Category III DCD kidneys are subject to a period of warm ischaemia during the agonal phase, which is at its peak between the cessation of cardiorespiratory activity and cold perfusion. This increases the risk of delayed graft function and there has been concern that this would lead to poorer long-term function.

In a study of over 9000 kidney transplants (845 DCD recipients), the 5-year graft survival and function of category III DCD donor kidney transplants was comparable with that of DBD donor transplants.

✔✔ However, a recent UK analysis[30] refuted this theory and showed that delayed graft function and warm ischaemic time had no effect on the outcome of DCD kidney transplants.

The research suggested that DCD kidneys should be transplanted with a short cold ischaemic time, to first transplant recipients matched for age, and HLA matching should only be prioritised for young recipients.

Given the concerns expressed regarding the ischaemic injury, controlled DCD donation has taken place only in the setting of a short and well-controlled time from withdrawal of life support therapy to asystole.[31]

✔ However, recent evidence suggests that the donor pool could be significantly increased by considering donors with a time of withdrawal to asystole of up to 4 hours.[25] This study has shown that the agonal phase parameters (irrespective of their length) do not correlate with the outcome, whilst, as expected, donor age and cold ischaemic time do.

An aggressive policy of pursuing these donors could lead to a 20% increase in transplant activity, but is undoubtedly logistically challenging, and the sensitive nature of discussions must also be acknowledged.

Warm ischaemia is also a concern in category II DCD donors, due to the initial period of no flow between cardiac arrest and initiation of CPR. Furthermore, cardiac massage (even with mechanical devices) achieves a state of low-grade organ perfusion, which increases the risk of further warm ischaemic damage. Most reports in the category II DCD setting highlight a higher rate of delayed graft function, but this does not appear to impact on the long-term outcome of the grafts.[27,32,33]

In order to minimise warm ischaemia, several concepts of in-situ preservation have been used over the years. The initial approach utilised cold in-situ preservation with double balloon isolation of the abdominal organs. The next evolutionary step was the introduction of extracorporeal support, using hypothermic[22] oxygenated blood perfusion. Several studies showed that kidneys recovered in this manner have a lower delayed graft function (DGF) rate and achieve an outcome not too different from DBD kidneys.[34] More recently, normothermic perfusion with oxygenated blood has gained support as a better method to preserve the abdominal organs and to assess their potential function prior to implantation.

✔ A study from Barcelona[35] showed that normothermic preservation is superior to all other methods as it is associated with the lowest rate of delayed graft function and provides an outcome comparable with DBD donors.

Optimising donor organ quality

The current challenges in deceased organ donation have prompted a search for new strategies to preserve, recover and optimise donor kidney function prior to transplantation.

Although organ preservation is discussed in detail elsewhere in this book, it is worth summarising some of the recent trends and areas for future development.

Despite the continued use of simple cold storage, machine preservation (MPS) is gradually becoming the preferred method for organ preservation, particularly for extended criteria kidneys, as it provides a continuous flush of the microcirculation, removes waste products and can sustain a higher metabolic rate. An international trial of 672 kidney recipients showed that hypothermic machine perfusion is superior to cold storage and is associated with a reduced risk of DGF and a better 1-year function.[36]

It has been suggested that the addition of oxygen to the hypothermic machine preservation may have a beneficial effect, but the evidence so far is sparse.

The concept of normothermic preservation has recently been suggested as a better ex-vivo preservation option, allowing restoration of ATP stores and reconditioning of the kidney, despite an initial period of cold storage,[37] but for the moment data to support its wider use are not available.

This is a rapidly changing field in transplantation. Despite the significant progress that has been made in the last decade, the future of preservation, recovery and donor optimisation is likely to hold more promise and allow an increasing number of organs to be transplanted.

Kidney allocation – new principles, same old challenges?

The success of kidney transplantation and the lack of available donor organs have led to a constant gap between demand and supply. This problems is ameliorated by allocation policies that must ensure an equitable and transparent selection of transplant recipients.

Allocation policies are the results of a complex interaction between legislative settings, immunological factors, expected outcomes, organ availability and costs. In many cases, these policies have been developed decades ago and subsequent reiterations tweaked fine details rather than producing a radical redesign of the factors considered in the process. It is now widely accepted that some of the fundamental factors used in allocation (such as HLA matching) do not have the same level of impact as in the past. Others (donor age, time on dialysis,[38] cold ischaemic time[39]) have a cumulative deleterious effect.

Striking a balance between utility, equity and benefit is a tall order and, not surprisingly, new proposals for kidney allocation emerge regularly trying to achieve this feat. Whilst some of the proposals deal with individual factors (e.g. age matching),[40] others employ sophisticated statistics to deal with equity of access or to minimise death with a functioning graft.[41–43]

More recently, the concept of survival benefit offered by transplantation has been proposed as a strategy to rank transplant candidates in the USA.[44] Within this system, kidneys would be allocated according to an estimated number of years of life gained with transplantation (LYFT) as compared with dialysis, thus maximising the outcome from each donated kidney.

Quintessentially utilitarian, this proposal is a significant departure from equity and individual justice and is shifting the emphasis from patient-based allocation to allocation driven by the characteristics of the donor kidney. Beyond the significant question marks regarding the methodology employed to derive these predictions (e.g. factors considered in analysis, time horizon for predictions),[45] such a system would create significant inequities. LYFT has been heavily criticised as 25% of the score comes from the age of the recipient, and as such it is essentially yet another age discriminator, leaving elderly patients with a minimal chance of transplantation. More importantly, by not considering recipient comorbidity, LYFT fails to accurately identify those patients who would truly benefit from transplantation, irrespective of their age or renal disease.

One approach to address these issues is the development of specific allocation policies such as the US ECD donor programme, where transplant candidates indicate their acceptance of a marginal kidney,[46] or the Eurotransplant Senior Program (ESP), where kidneys from donors aged >65 years are allocated to similar aged recipients, regardless of HLA matching.[47] Within this latter programme, the availability of elderly donors has doubled and the waiting time for elderly recipients has decreased. Despite a 5–10% higher rejection rate, the cold ischaemic time and the rate of delayed graft function were lower and survival was comparable with the standard allocation.

The allocation debate is far from over and, with the increasing organ gap, rationing policies will come under even more intense scrutiny in years to come.[48] Nevertheless, efforts should continue to be made to ensure a just system of organ utilisation and reduce organ wastage.

Trends in surgical technique

Donor surgery

The deceased donor surgical procedure has not changed significantly over the last five decades but the living donor surgery technique has seen some remarkable developments. It has evolved from an open procedure with rib resection, via a minimally invasive open nephrectomy (MIDN), to the current standard of care – laparoscopic surgery. Since its introduction in 1995,[49] the laparoscopic approach has had several iterations: full laparoscopic donor nephrectomy (LLN), hand-assisted transperitoneal nephrectomy (HALDN) or hand-assisted retroperitoneal technique (HARP). Whilst technically more demanding and despite longer operating times, laparoscopic approaches result in less intraoperative blood loss, less analgesic requirement, a shorter hospital stay and a quicker recovery and resumption of normal activities compared to open surgery.[50–52]

Several randomised controlled trials and a meta-analysis[52–54] concluded that laparoscopic donor nephrectomy is superior to an open approach and leads to a better quality of life for the donor, with comparable donor safety and recipient outcome.

✔✔ There is no difference between laparoscopic nephrectomy with and without hand assistance,[55] but the role of the retroperitoneal approach needs to be explored further.[56]

Technological innovations have seen the development of robotic-assisted laparoscopic donor nephrectomy (RALDN).[57] Despite several putative advantages over standard laparoscopic surgery (three-dimensional vision, a higher degree of dexterity and precision), robotic surgery remains largely restricted for several centres due to the prohibitive costs of the technology.

Laparo-endoscopic single-site surgery (LESS) is the most recent development in laparoscopic donor surgery, allowing the procedure to be performed via a single umbilical multichannel port. Preliminary reports[58] indicate that the procedure may be associated with a quicker recovery and despite longer warm ischaemic times associated with kidney extraction, transplant outcomes are comparable with standard laparoscopic techniques.

In a quest for improved cosmesis, transvaginal extraction of the kidney (an expansion of natural orifice transluminal surgery – NOTES) has been reported following laparoscopic[59] as well as robotic nephrectomy.[60] It is yet to gain wider acceptance amongst surgeons and patients alike.

With increasing confidence in laparoscopic approaches, several surgical myths, such as higher risks associated with multiple vessels[61] or with the removal of the right kidney,[62] have been dismissed, allowing more judicious utilisation of available living donor kidneys.

Kidney implantation

The technique for retroperitoneal implantation of the kidney has remained virtually unchanged for the past 50 years. It is rather difficult to improve the efficiency of a procedure that provides safe access to the vessels and bladder, whilst allowing peritoneal dialysis continuation (if required) and easy access to the graft for percutaneous interventions, all with reasonable pain control requirements.

Not surprisingly, recipient minimally invasive surgery took a lot longer to develop than donor surgery. A couple of reports on robotic kidney transplantation[63] and laparoscopic kidney transplantation[64] confirm their technical feasibility, but despite potential benefit in morbidly obese patients, wider applicability is for the moment questionable.

Current practice and challenges in immunosuppression

Since the introduction of ciclosporin in clinical practice, kidney transplantation has seen a dramatic reduction in the incidence of acute rejection. However, in recent years, this improvement in acute rejection rates has failed to translate into a sustained improvement in outcome,[65] indicating that other factors (such as death with functioning graft, drug nephrotoxicity, non-adherence, chronic immunological damage) play a significant role in the long-term fate of the transplant. This has triggered a shift in strategy,[66] which has seen recent trials focusing on tailoring treatment options to the individual and optimising the use of currently available drugs, in an attempt to strike a balance between efficacy and side-effect profile. While calcineurin inhibitors (CNIs; tacrolimus and ciclosporin) remain the mainstay of treatment, one of the most popular current immunosuppressive strategies strives to achieve drug minimisation (reduction in CNI exposure or corticosteroids) through the addition of MMF and antibody induction. The results of the ELITE-Symphony trial[67] have crystallised current thinking. This study has shown that induction with low-dose tacrolimus/MMF/steroids leads to better renal function and allograft survival with lower acute rejection rates when compared with standard-dose ciclosporin without induction or two other regimens of low-dose ciclosporin or low-dose sirolimus with induction.

The choice of induction is still a subject of debate, although recent evidence appears to favour lymphocyte-depleting agents such as rabbit anti-thymocyte globulin (R-ATG) or alemtuzumab, particularly as they may allow a reduction in steroid exposure. A recent trial[68] in 139 high-risk and 335 low-risk patients compared alemtuzumab induction with R-ATG (in the high-risk arm) and basiliximab (in the low-risk arm). All patients received tacrolimus and MMF and underwent early steroid withdrawal. The study showed that alemtuzumab is associated with a lower 3-year rejection rate in the low-risk group and a comparable rejection rate in the high-risk group against the index treatment. Despite no difference in the primary end-point in the high-risk group, alemtuzumab was associated with a lower incidence of infective complications than R-ATG.

> ✓✓ The role of alemtuzumab induction has been the subject of a recent meta-analysis[69] that included 10 RCTs with 1223 patients and concluded that alemtuzumab does reduce the risk of acute rejection, but only when compared with basiliximab and not R-ATG.

As the incidence of other outcomes (graft loss, death and delayed graft function) is comparable, the choice of induction should be based on a composite index of safety and cost.

An alternative to the minimisation strategy is complete elimination of CNIs. Although previous attempts have failed to achieve an optimal balance between efficacy and safety,[70,71] recent studies have rekindled the interest in this approach. Three separate reports from the BENEFIT trial (Belatacept Evaluation of Nephroprotectionand Efficacy as First-line Immunosuppression Trial) have suggested that belatacept, a selective co-stimulatory blockade, may be the potential answer to providing adequate immunosuppression whilst avoiding the nephro-toxic effects of CNIs.

> ✓ The 1-year[72] and 3-year[73] reports suggested that belatacept is associated with better renal function and similar patient and graft survival when compared with a ciclosporin-based regimen.

There is, however, a higher early acute rejection rate (in the first year) and a higher incidence of post-transplant lymphoproliferative disorder (which appears to be highest in the first 18 months post-transplant). Similar results were confirmed in an extension of the BENEFIT trial, analysing 543 extended criteria donor kidney recipients.[74]

Over the last few years, several generic drugs have been launched on the immunosuppressive scene as an alternative to branded formulations of tacrolimus, ciclosporin and MMF. Although these drugs are presumed to be bioequivalent (as determined in a healthy population), there is a lack of published data in the transplant population to support clinical equivalence. Given the narrow therapeutic index of these drugs and the multitude of formulations available, concerns have been expressed in different forums[75,76] regarding their liberal use, especially any swapping from one formulation to another. Despite this, the fact that the generic agents are less expensive may drive change.

Conclusion

The successful endeavours of the last few decades have brought new and heightened challenges for renal transplantation. These challenges will require innovative approaches to maintain the upward momentum and see transplantation retain its rightful place at the forefront of scientific and clinical progress. In many ways, renal transplantation is on the brink of an evolutionary step, with potential solutions that will lead, at least in part, to better organ utilisation, wider accessibility and a sustained successful outcome.

Key points

- The increased demand for kidney transplantation has led to longer waiting times, which are associated with a higher waiting-list mortality, particularly in elderly patients.
- There are wider acceptance criteria for category III DCD donors and a growing utilisation of category II DCD donors.

- Innovative paired exchange schemes involving altruistic donors have improved access to transplantation for incompatible pairs.
- ABO-incompatible transplant programmes have achieved a success rate comparable with ABO-compatible transplantation.
- There is a renewed effort to improve organ preservation and organ reconditioning that will lead to increased organ utilisation.
- Kidney allocation continues to be a contentious point in renal transplantation.

References

1. Wolfe RA, Ashby VB, Milford EL, et al. Comparison of mortality in all patients on dialysis, patients on dialysis awaiting transplantation, and recipients of a first cadaveric transplant. N Engl J Med 1999;341(23):1725–30.

2. Oniscu GC, Brown H, Forsythe JL. How great is the survival advantage of transplantation over dialysis in elderly patients? Nephrol Dial Transplant 2004;19:945–51.

3. Akolekar D, Oniscu GC, Forsythe JL. Variations in the assessment practice for renal transplantation across the United Kingdom. Transplantation 2008;85:407–10.

4. Schold J, Srinivas TR, Sehgal AR, et al. Half of kidney transplant candidates who are older than 60 years now placed on the waiting list will die before receiving a deceased-donor transplant. Clin J Am Soc Nephrol 2009;4:1239–45.

5. Stevens KK, Woo YM, Clancy M, et al. Deceased donor transplantation in the elderly – are we creating false hope? Nephrol Dial Transplant 2011;26:2382–6.

6. Terasaki PI, Cecka JM, Gjertson DW, et al. High survival rates of kidney transplants from spousal and living unrelated donors. N Engl J Med 1995;333:333–6.
   A study that confirmed that unrelated living donor transplants have a better outcome than deceased donor transplants.

7. Montgomery RA, Gentry SE, Marks WH, et al. Domino paired kidney donation: a strategy to make best use of live non-directed donation. Lancet 2006;368:419–21.

8. Adams PL, Cohen DJ, Danovitch GM, et al. The non-directed live-kidney donor: ethical considerations and practice guidelines: A National Conference Report. Transplantation 2002;74:582–9.

9. Rapaport FT. The case for a living emotionally related international kidney donor exchange registry. Transplant Proc 1986;18:5–9.

10. Segev DL, Gentry SE, Warren DS, et al. Kidney paired donation and optimizing the use of live donor organs. JAMA 2005;293:1883–90.

11. de Klerk M, Witvliet MD, Haase-Kromwijk BJ, et al. A highly efficient living donor kidney exchange program for both blood type and crossmatch incompatible donor–recipient combinations. Transplantation 2006;82:1616–20.

12. Delmonico FL, Morrissey PE, Lipkowitz GS, et al. Donor kidney exchanges. Am J Transplant 2004;4:1628–34.

13. Gentry SE, Segev DL, Simmerling M, et al. Expanding kidney paired donation through participation by compatible pairs. Am J Transplant 2007;7:2361–70.

14. Ratner LE, Rana A, Ratner ER, et al. The altruistic unbalanced paired kidney exchange: proof of concept and survey of potential donor and recipient attitudes. Transplantation 2010;89:15–22.

15. Lee YJ, Lee SU, Chung SY, et al. Clinical outcomes of multicenter domino kidney paired donation. Am J Transplant 2009;9:2424–8.

16. Rees MA, Kopke JE, Pelletier RP, et al. A nonsimultaneous, extended, altruistic-donor chain. N Engl J Med 2009;360:1096–101.
    First report of a non-simultaneous living donor chain, triggered by altruistic donation.

17. The Washington Times. 13-way kidney transplant sets record, 14 December 2009.

18. Montgomery JR, Berger JC, Warren DS, et al. Outcomes of ABO-incompatible kidney transplantation in the United States. Transplantation 2012;93:603–9.
    Study showing a comparable outcome of ABOi transplants with ABO-compatible transplants, despite a higher risk of graft failure in the first 2 weeks post-transplant.

19. Montgomery RA, Locke JE, King KE, et al. ABO incompatible renal transplantation: a paradigm ready for broad implementation. Transplantation 2009;87:1246–55.

20. Genberg H, Kumlien G, Wennberg L, et al. Long-term results of ABO-incompatible kidney transplantation with antigen-specific immunoadsorption and rituximab. Transplantation 2007;84:S44–7.

21. Lefaucheur C, Nochy D, Andrade J, et al. Comparison of combination plasmapheresis/IVIg/anti-CD20 versus high-dose IVIg in the treatment of antibody-mediated rejection. Am J Transplant 2009;9:1099–107.

22. Jordan SC, Tyan D, Stablein D, et al. Evaluation of intravenous immunoglobulin as an agent to lower allosensitization and improve transplantation in highly sensitized adult patients with end-stage renal disease: report of the NIH IG02 trial. J Am SocNephrol 2004;15:3256–62.

23. Stegall MD, Gloor J, Winters JL, et al. A comparison of plasmapheresis versus high-dose IVIG desensitization in renal allograft recipients with high levels of donor specific alloantibody. Am J Transplant 2006;6:346–51.

24. Vo AA, Lukovsky M, Toyoda M, et al. Rituximab and intravenous immune globulin for desensitization during renal transplantation. N Engl J Med 2008;359:242–51.

25. Reid AW, Harper S, Jackson CH, et al. Expansion of the kidney donor pool by using cardiac death donors with prolonged time to cardiorespiratory arrest. Am J Transplant 2011;11:995–1005.

26. Domínguez-Gil B, Haase-Kromwijk B, Van Leiden H, et al. Current situation of donation after circulatory death in European countries. Transpl Int 2011;24:676–86.

27. Sánchez-Fructuoso AI, Marques M, Prats D, et al. Victims of cardiac arrest occurring outside the hospital: a source of transplantable kidneys. Ann Intern Med 2006;145:157–64.

28. Radcliffe Richards J. The ethics of transplants – why careless thought costs lives. Oxford University Press; 2012.

29. Childress JF, Liverman CT, editors. Institute of Medicine, Committee on Increasing Rates of Organ Donation, Organ donation: opportunities for action. Washington, DC: National Academies Press; 2006.

30. Summers DM, Johnson RJ, Allen J, et al. Analysis of factors that affect outcome after transplantation of kidneys donated after cardiac death in the UK: a cohort study. Lancet 2010;376:1303–11.
    A 9000-patient cohort study demonstrating a comparable 5-year outcome between controlled DCD and DBD kidney transplants. Delayed graft function and warm ischaemic time do not appear to impact on the long-term outcome in DCD kidney recipients.

31. Reich DJ, Mulligan DC, Abt PL, et al. ASTS recommended practice guidelines for controlled donation after cardiac death organ procurement and transplantation. Am J Transplant 2009;9:2004–11.

32. Weber M, Dindo D, Demartines N, et al. Kidney transplantation from donors without a heartbeat. N Engl J Med 2002;347:248–55.

33. Abboud I, Viglietti D, Antoine C, et al. Preliminary results of transplantation with kidneys donated after cardiocirculatory determination of death: a French single-centre experience. Nephrol Dial Transplant 2012;27:2583–7.

34. Farney AC, Singh RP, Hines MH, et al. Experience in renal and extrarenal transplantation with donation after cardiac death donors with selective use of extracorporeal support. J Am Coll Surg 2008;206:1028–37.

35. Valero R, Cabrer C, Oppenheimer F, et al. Normothermic recirculation reduces primary graft dysfunction of kidneys obtained from non-heart-beating donors. Transpl Int 2000;13:303–10.
    Study showing that kidneys retrieved with normothermic extracorporeal support have a low DGF and a comparable outcome with DBD kidneys.

36. Moers C, Smits JM, Maathuis MH, et al. Machine perfusion or cold storage in deceased-donor kidney transplantation. N Engl J Med 2009;360:7–19.
    Randomised controlled trial showing a better outcome for hypothermic machine preservation compared with cold storage.

37. Hosgood SA, Nicholson ML. First in man renal transplantation after ex vivo normothermic perfusion. Transplantation 2011;92:735–8.

38. Meier-Kriesche HU, Kaplan B. Waiting time on dialysis as the strongest modifiable risk factor for renal transplant outcomes: a paired donor kidney analysis. Transplantation 2002;74:1377–81.

39. van der Vliet JA, Warlé MC, Cheung CL, et al. Influence of prolonged cold ischemia in renal transplantation. Clin Transplant 2011;25:E612–6.

40. Meier-Kriesche HU, Schold JD, Gaston RS, et al. Kidneys from deceased donors: maximizing the value of a scarce resource. Am J Transplant 2005;5:1725–30.

41. Johnson RJ, Fuggle SV, Mumford L, et al., Kidney Advisory Group of NHS Blood and Transplant. A New UK 2006 National Kidney Allocation Scheme for deceased heart-beating donor kidneys. Transplantation 2010;89:387–94.

42. Zenios SA, Wein LM, Chertow GM. Evidence-based organ allocation. Am J Med 1999;107:52–61.

43. Oniscu GC, Forsythe JLR. Allocation for transplantation: practical aspects and ethical dilemmas. In: Wiemar W, Bos MA, Bussbach JJ, editors. Organ transplantation: ethical, legal and psychological aspects. Leigerich: Pabst Science Publishers; 2008.

44. Wolfe RA, McCullough KP, Schaubel DE, et al. Calculating life years from transplant (LYFT): methods for kidney and kidney–pancreas candidates. Am J Transplant 2008;8:997–1011.

45. Freeman RB, Matas AT, Henry M, et al. Moving kidney allocation forward: the ASTS perspective. Am J Transplant 2009;9:1501–6.

46. Metzger RA, Delmonico FL, Feng S, et al. Expanded criteria donors for kidney transplantation. Am J Transplant 2003;3(Suppl. 4):114–25.

47. Frei U, Noeldeke J, Machold-Fabrizii V, et al. Prospective age-matching in elderly kidney transplant recipients – a 5-year analysis of the Eurotransplant Senior Program. Am J Transplant 2008;8:50–7.

48. Reese PP, Caplan AL, Bloom RD, et al. How should we use age to ration health care? Lessons from the case of kidney transplantation. J Am Geriatr Soc 2010;58:1980–6.

49. Ratner LE, Ciseck LJ, Moore RG, et al. Laparoscopic live donor nephrectomy. Transplantation 1995;60: 1047–9.

50. Oyen O, Andersen M, Mathisen L, et al. Laparoscopic versus open living-donor nephrectomy: experiences from a prospective, randomized, single-center study focusing on donor safety. Transplantation 2005;79:1236–40.

51. Velidedeoglu E, Williams N, Brayman KL, et al. Comparison of open, laparoscopic, and hand-assisted approaches to live-donor nephrectomy. Transplantation 2002;74:169–72.

52. Kok NF, Lind MY, Hansson BM, et al. Comparison of laparoscopic and mini incision open donor nephrectomy: single blind, randomised controlled clinical trial. Br Med J 2006;333:221.
Randomised controlled trial confirming superiority of laparoscopic approach compared to open nephrectomy.

53. Nanidis TG, Antcliffe D, Kokkinos C, et al. Laparoscopic versus open live donor nephrectomy in renal transplantation: a meta-analysis. Ann Surg 2008;247:58–70.

54. Wolf Jr JS, Merion RM, Leichtman AB, et al. Randomized controlled trial of hand-assisted laparoscopic versus open surgical live donor nephrectomy. Transplantation 2001;72:284–90.

55. Bargman V, Sundaram CP, Bernie J, et al. Randomized trial of laparoscopic donor nephrectomy with and without hand assistance. J Endourol 2006;20:717–22.
Randomised controlled trial showing no difference between the total laparoscopic and hand-assisted laparoscopic approaches.

56. Buell JF, Abreu SC, Hanaway MJ, et al. Right donor nephrectomy: a comparison of hand-assisted transperitoneal and retroperitoneal laparoscopic approaches. Transplantation 2004;77:521–5.

57. Horgan S, Vanuno D, Sileri P, et al. Robotic-assisted laparoscopic donor nephrectomy for kidney transplantation. Transplantation 2002;73:1474–9.

58. Canes D, Berger A, Aron M, et al. Laparo-endoscopic single site (LESS) versus standard laparoscopic left donor nephrectomy: matched-pair comparison. Eur Urol 2010;57:95–101.

59. Allaf ME, Singer A, Shen W, et al. Laparoscopic live donor nephrectomy with vaginal extraction: initial report. Am J Transplant 2010;10:1473–7.

60. Pietrabissa A, Abelli M, Spinillo A, et al. Robotic-assisted laparoscopic donor nephrectomy with transvaginal extraction of the kidney. Am J Transplant 2010;10:2708–11.

61. Hsu TH, Su LM, Ratner LE, et al. Impact of renal artery multiplicity on outcomes of renal donors and recipients in laparoscopic donor nephrectomy. Urology 2003;61:323–7.

62. Minnee RC, Bemelman WA, Maartense S, et al. Left or right kidney in hand-assisted donor nephrectomy? A randomized controlled trial. Transplantation 2008;85:203–8.

63. Giulianotti P, Gorodner V, Sbrana F, et al. Robotic transabdominal kidney transplantation in a morbidly obese patient. Am J Transplant 2010;10:1478–82.

64. Modi P, Rizvi J, Pal B, et al. Laparoscopic kidney transplantation: an initial experience. Am J Transplant 2011;11:1320–4.

65. Meier-Kriesche HU, Schold JD, Srinivas TR, et al. Lack of improvement in renal allograft survival despite a marked decrease in acute rejection rates over the most recent era. Am J Transplant 2004;4: 378–83.

66. Pascual M, Theruvath T, Kawai T, et al. Strategies to improve long-term outcomes after renal transplantation. N Engl J Med 2002;346:580–90.

67. Ekberg H, Tedesco-Silva H, Demirbas A, et al., ELITE-Symphony Study. Reduced exposure to calcineurin inhibitors in renal transplantation. N Engl J Med 2007;357:2562–75.
The largest immunosuppressive study in renal transplantation that showed a superiority of tacrolimus/MMF with induction regimen in preserving renal function and kidney survival with low acute rejection rates.

68. Hanaway MJ, Woodle ES, Mulgaonkar S, et al., INTAC Study Group. Alemtuzumab induction in renal transplantation. N Engl J Med 2011; 364:1909–19.
Prospective randomised controlled study demonstrating superiority of alemtuzumab over basiliximab in low-risk transplant and equivalence with antithymocyte globulin in high-risk patients.

69. Morgan RD, O'Callaghan JM, Knight SR, et al. Alemtuzumab induction therapy in kidney transplantation: a systematic review and meta-analysis. Transplantation 2012;May 31. Epub ahead of print.

70. Vincenti F, Ramos E, Brattstrom C, et al. Multicenter trial exploring calcineurin inhibitors avoidance in renal transplantation. Transplantation 2001;71:1282–7.

71. Larson TS, Dean PG, Stegall MD, et al. Complete avoidance of calcineurin inhibitors in renal transplantation: a randomized trial comparing sirolimus and tacrolimus. Am J Transplant 2006;6:514–22.

72. Vincenti F, Charpentier B, Vanrenterghem Y, et al. A phase III study of belatacept-based immunosuppression regimens versus cyclosporine in renal transplant recipients (BENEFIT study). Am J Transplant 2010;10:535–46.

73. Vincenti F, Larsen CP, Alberu J, et al. Three-year outcomes from BENEFIT, a randomized, active-controlled, parallel-group study in adult kidney transplant recipients. Am J Transplant 2012;12:210–7.

74. Pestana JO, Grinyo JM, Vanrenterghem Y, et al. Three-year outcomes from BENEFIT-EXT: a phase III study of belatacept versus cyclosporine in recipients of extended criteria donor kidneys. Am J Transplant 2012;12:630–9.

75. Sabatini S, Ferguson RM, Helderman JH, et al. Drug substitution in transplantation: a National Kidney Foundation White Paper. Am J Kidney Dis 1999;33:389–97.

76. Harrison JJ, Schiff JR, Coursol CJ, et al. Generic immunosuppression in solid organ transplantation: a Canadian perspective. Transplantation 2012;93:657–65.

8

Liver transplantation

James J. Pomposelli
Mary Ann Simpson
Caroline J. Simon
Elizabeth A. Pomfret

Introduction

Liver transplantation has evolved over the past six decades from a risky procedure with poor outcome to the standard of care for the patient with end-stage liver disease. From the initial attempts of Dr Thomas Starzl in the USA and Sir Roy Calne in the UK, liver transplantation has progressed from a procedure that was experimental, performed on moribund patients with irreversible chronic liver disease with an occasional long-term survival, to a procedure in many centres with 1-year survival exceeding 90% (**Fig. 8.1**).[1–3] Consistent improvements in surgical technique, immunosuppressive regimens and postoperative care, paired with better selection and management of pre-transplant patients, has resulted in an increased number of recipients able to benefit from transplantation. Ironically, these developments combined with the static and/or decreasing number of potential donors in many countries have led to increased waiting-list mortality. In the USA, waiting-list mortality can exceed 20% in many regions and highlights the problem of organ shortage. Although liver transplantation has proven to be a great success in its relatively short history, it should not be considered as either the initial or primary treatment modality for most liver diseases. In this era of organ shortages, it is important to understand the indications and contraindications for liver transplantation, current and future changes in the organ allocation system, and methods for increasing the donor pool, such as split or live donor grafts and using organs from extended criteria and non-heart-beating donors.

At the time of writing, there are nearly 17 000 patients waiting for a liver transplant in the USA. Prior to listing, all patients undergo extensive medical and psychosocial evaluation. Most programmes have adopted a multidisciplinary approach for evaluating potential liver transplant recipients that usually includes representatives from hepatology, surgery, anaesthesia, infectious disease, psychiatry, social work, transplant nursing and finance/insurance. Input from consulting services such as cardiology, pulmonology, neurology, nephrology, etc. is obtained as needed. After all testing and consultations have been obtained, each patient is presented to the multidisciplinary committee and voted on to accept, reject or defer until all information is available, such as an outstanding screening test. In the USA, accepted patients are listed with the United Network for Organ Sharing (UNOS) and prioritised by their Model for End-Stage Liver Disease (MELD) score.[4,5] A comprehensive list of the currently accepted indications for liver transplantation is shown in Box 8.1.

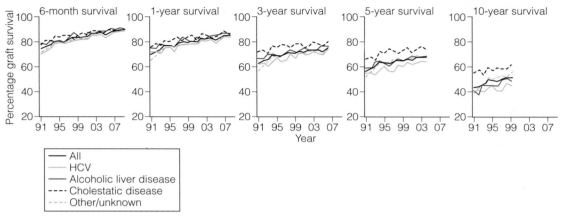

Figure 8.1 • OPTN data shows 6-month to 10-year survival following liver transplantation for various indications. Recipients transplanted for cholestatic liver diseases (PBC, PSC) enjoy improved long-term survival.

A brief review of the MELD score is needed since it has become the main tool used for liver allocation in the USA and in some countries around the world. Initially developed at the Mayo Clinic, the MELD score uses the patient's values for serum bilirubin, serum creatinine and the international normalised ratio for prothrombin time (INR) to predict survival.[6] It is calculated according to the following formula:

$$MELD = 3.78 [Ln \, serum \, bilirubin \, (mg/dL)] + 11.2(Ln \, INR) + 9.57 [Ln \, serum \, creatinine(mg/dL)] + 6.43$$

The Organ Procurement and Transplantation Network/United Network for Organ Sharing (OPTN/UNOS) has made the following modifications to the score:[7]

- If the patient has been dialysed twice within the last 7 days, then the value for serum creatinine used should be 4.0.
- Any value less than 1 is given a value of 1 (i.e. if bilirubin is 0.8, a value of 1.0 is used) to prevent the occurrence of scores below 0 (the natural logarithm of 1 is 0, and any value below 1 would yield a negative result).

Patients with a diagnosis of stage 2 hepatocellular carcinoma (HCC) whose 'natural' MELD score is low are granted exception points to gain additional priority. This is discussed in the HCC section below. The MELD score is used to predict 3-month mortality from the patient's liver disease on a continuous scale:[8]

- 40 or more – 71.3% mortality;
- 30–39 – 52.6% mortality;
- 20–29 – 19.6% mortality;
- 10–19 – 6.0% mortality;
- <9 – 1.9% mortality.

The MELD score was adopted into the liver transplant allocation scheme in 2002 in response to the 'Final Rule', a proclamation issued by the US Department of Health and Human Service. The policy states that the goal of organ allocation would be 'distributing organs over as broad a geographic area as feasible … and in order of decreasing medical urgency'.[9] Many other countries around the world have adopted MELD as the technique to help decide which patient from the waiting list should receive a particular organ. In some countries, an adaptation of MELD has been used based on research from the national database. In the UK, the UKELD (UK model for End-stage Liver Disease) is used with the addition of serum sodium to the mathematical model. A UKELD score >49 predicts a >9% 1-year mortality and is a minimum criterion for entry to the waiting list in the UK.

Of the active patients on the US waiting list, approximately 5000–6000 will receive a liver transplant from either a deceased or living donor this year. Nationally, living donors comprise only about 5% of total recipients but can be as high as 40% in certain programmes such as our own that reside in regions of the country with long waiting lists and limited organ supply. Patient survival nationally for all liver transplant recipients at 1, 3 and 5 years is 87%, 78% and 73%, respectively.[10–12]

Contraindications to liver transplantation include both clinical and psychosocial reasons.[13] Clinically significant reasons to avoid surgery include advanced

Box 8.1 • Indications for liver transplantation

Chronic non-cholestatic liver disorders

- Chronic hepatitis C
- Chronic hepatitis B
- Autoimmune hepatitis
- Alcoholic liver disease

Cholestatic liver disease

- Primary biliary cirrhosis
- Primary sclerosing cholangitis
- Biliary atresia
- Alagille syndrome
- Non-syndromic paucity of intrahepatic bile ducts
- Cystic fibrosis
- Progressive familial intrahepatic cholestasis

Metabolic disorders causing cirrhosis

- Alpha-1-antitrypson deficiency
- Wilson's disease
- Non-alcoholic fatty liver disease (NAFLD) and cryptogenic cirrhosis
- Hereditary haemochromatosis
- Tyrosinaemia
- Glycogen storage disease type IV
- Neonatal haemochromatosis

Metabolic disorders causing severe extrahepatic morbidity

- Amyloidosis
- Hyperoxaluria
- Urea cycle defects
- Disorders of branched chain amino acids

Primary malignancies of the liver

- Hepatocellular carcinoma
- Hepatoblastoma
- Fibrolamellar hepatocellular carcinoma
- Haemangioendothelioma

Fulminant hepatic failure

Miscellaneous conditions

- Budd–Chiari syndrome
- Metastatic neuroendocrine tumours
- Polycystic disease

Retransplantation

Approved indications for liver transplantation adapted from the American Association for Study of Liver Disease Practice Guidelines (www.aasld.org).

cardiopulmonary disease, active sepsis, technical issues such as extensive portal and visceral venous thromboses, and advanced or metastatic malignancy. Relative contraindications are centre specific and include advanced age or acquired immune deficiency syndrome (AIDS), although many programmes decide on a case-by-case basis.

Psychosocial contraindications include poor or absent social support, untreated or uncontrolled psychiatric illness, active drug or alcohol abuse, or inadequate insurance for postoperative medications. Interventions to correct or improve these difficulties can result in appropriate listing after initial denial. Patients with end-stage liver disease who are not qualified for liver transplantation require continuous follow-up for tumour surveillance and management of symptoms such as encephalopathy and portal hypertension if present.

Indications for liver transplantation

Acute fulminant liver failure

The most dramatic patient listed for liver transplantation presents with acute or fulminant liver failure. According to UNOS rules, the patient listed with acute fulminant liver failure (Status 1) must have a life expectancy without liver transplant of 7 days or less. Typical scenarios include, but are not limited to, acute acetaminophen overdose, mushroom poisoning, fulminant hepatitis A or B infection, Wilson's disease, acute Budd–Chiari syndrome or a failed liver transplant (primary graft non-function or hepatic artery thrombosis, HAT).[14] Patients with chronic liver disease cannot be listed as high urgency (Status 1) except after a failed transplant. A more traditional definition of acute liver failure includes the presence of encephalopathy occurring within 8 weeks of the onset of symptoms in a patient with previously normal liver function.

Currently, acute liver failure patients account for about 5–6% of all liver transplants in the USA.[15] Untreated, patient mortality approaches 80% in patients with severe fulminant liver failure or grade IV hepatic encephalopathy. Interestingly, approximately 15% of patients have no identifiable cause for their acute liver failure.[16]

Patients with fulminant liver failure develop rapid onset of multisystem organ failure requiring aggressive supportive therapies including intensive care unit (ICU) admission, ventilatory support and renal replacement therapy. Common causes of subsequent death include cerebral oedema and bacterial and/or fungal sepsis. Lack of gluconeogenesis with the development of hypoglycaemia is an ominous sign and death usually rapidly ensues without immediate transplant. Slight delays in obtaining a replacement organ can result in permanent brain injury even after liver replacement. Measures to monitor and control cerebral pressure may provide additional time while waiting for an organ and improve outcome.[17]

Patients who develop fulminant liver failure as a result of intentional drug overdose such as acetaminophen pose a special ethical dilemma, since organs are scarce and the degree of psychiatric illness is undefined. Fortunately, many of these patients improve spontaneously with supportive measures. Patients with drug overdose resulting from 'impulse decisions' (e.g. fight with a boyfriend or girlfriend) are generally appropriate candidates for liver transplantation and have done well with appropriate treatment postoperatively. Patients with drug overdose and active alcoholism are generally not appropriate candidates but may be evaluated and considered on a case-by-case basis if recovery from the underlying psychiatric illness is likely.

Budd–Chiari syndrome

Budd–Chiari syndrome is a group of disorders caused by acute or gradual occlusion of the hepatic venous outflow of the liver[18] secondary to an underlying hypercoagulable state. Budd–Chiari is a pathological diagnosis since, early in the course of the disease, venous thrombosis is at the sinusoidal level only and the hepatic veins may be patent. Therefore, clinical suspicion of the disease (large tender liver, abnormal 'nutmeg liver' perfusion pattern on imaging and abnormal liver function tests) should prompt a liver biopsy. Other causes of chronic passive congestion such as right heart failure should be ruled out with appropriate testing. Since the liver is engorged with blood, biopsy via the retrohepatic vena cava is preferable to avoid potential life-threatening bleeding via the percutaneous route.

Patients with pathologically proven Budd–Chiari syndrome with intact hepatic architecture may benefit from decompression with side-to-side portocaval shunt to create venous outflow for the liver. Use of prosthetic material to create a functionally equivalent mesocaval shunt should be discouraged due to low patency rates in the setting of a hypercoagulable state. Transjugular intrahepatic portocaval shunts (TIPS; **Fig. 8.2**) are well tolerated and may

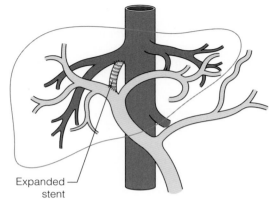

Expanded stent

Figure 8.2 • Transjugular intrahepatic portocaval shunt (TIPS) is a non-selective shunt that relieves portal hypertension by bypassing the liver with an intrahepatic stent. The arrows show augmented flow through shunt. Problems with TIPS include poor 1-year unassisted patency rate (approximately 40–50%) and the development of hepatic encephalopathy in up to one-third of patients. Improper position with the ends of the stent in the right atrium or proximal portal vein can preclude safe transplant.

be helpful in decompressing portal hypertension. However, they do not decompress liver parenchyma adequately and need frequent revisions due to low patency rates.[19] Although the long-term role of TIPS may be limited in this setting, it does not worsen outcome after subsequent liver transplantation.[20]

Patients with advanced fibrosis or cirrhosis are likely to develop decompensated liver failure after major shunt surgery or TIPS and should be considered for transplant initially. Failed shunt procedures may be salvaged with expedited liver transplantation; therefore, it is desirable to manage these patients in a transplant centre. In our experience, technically successful shunt surgery can result in hepatic decompensation and need for salvage liver transplant in up to 25% of patients. Targeted treatment for the underlying cause of Budd–Chiari syndrome should be initiated, although the exact cause of the hypercoaguable state can remain undiagnosed in up to 50% of patients.

Chronic liver disease

General considerations

According to the US Organ Procurement and Transplantation Network (OPTN) and the Scientific Registry of Transplant Recipients (SRTR), between 1999 and 2008, the three most common reasons for liver transplantation were cirrhosis due to hepatitis C virus (HCV) infection, followed by hepatocellular carcinoma (HCC) and alcoholic cirrhosis with or without concomitant infection with HCV.[12] Transplantation of patients with end-stage liver disease and HCC has been somewhat controversial. These patients receive significant priority with the current organ allocation system compared to patients without HCC and enjoy significantly less waiting-list mortality. In 1996, Mazzaferro et al. published a clinical study on a cohort of patients who had undergone liver transplantation for early stage, unresectable HCC (single tumour ≤5 cm and no more than three tumours each ≤3 cm). The authors found a high overall and recurrence-free survival rate at 4 years in patients who had met predetermined criteria for limited stage HCC. These criteria became known as the 'Milan criteria'. The authors concluded that liver transplantation was an effective treatment for early-stage, unresectable hepatocellular carcinoma. Interestingly, the 'Milan criteria' were established on a relatively small study of 48 patients examining explanted livers with incidental tumours, and demonstrated patient and graft survival equivalent to non-tumour patients. This study has been validated with other clinical studies and provides the rationale for the current UNOS allocation scheme for patients with end-stage liver disease and HCC.[21]

Because patients with HCC typically have low calculated MELD scores, they face a higher risk of death on the waiting list due to progression of tumour beyond acceptable transplant criteria (Milan criteria) than due to liver failure. In order to address this issue of waiting list 'drop-out', the OPTN/UNOS developed an organ allocation policy that allows for increased priority for liver transplant candidates with HCC within Milan criteria. The goal was to equate the risk of tumour progression beyond this limit with the risk of death in patients without HCC who have chronic liver disease with comparable MELD scores on the waiting list over a similar period of time. Patients with HCC must meet strict criteria including limited disease stage, meeting Milan criteria, in order to receive a MELD exception score.

When the Milan criteria were first implemented, patients with HCC were given very high priority on the waiting list (29 MELD points) and increases every 3 months as long as the tumour remained within stage 2. Gradually, the number of initial MELD exception points has been reduced, since the excessive priority resulted in HCC patients that were being transplanted at rates above non-HCC patients. Currently, patients with end-stage liver disease and stage 2 HCC are initially awarded 22 MELD points that increase every 3 months by 10% mortality equivalent points. There is consideration to further reduce the initial number of MELD points awarded since the patient with HCC still enjoys a significant advantage with reduced waiting-list mortality compared to non-HCC patients. There is significant geographic variation in the USA (Region 1) regarding waiting-list 'drop-out' rate or death on the waiting list for patients with HCC as compared to non-HCC patients. In some areas of the USA, non-HCC patients are twice as likely either to become too sick for transplant (resulting in removal from the waiting list) or to die on the waiting list, as compared to patients with HCC. Currently the OPTN/UNOS Liver and Intestinal Transplantation Committee is working on development of a calculated continuous HCC priority score for ranking HCC candidates on the waiting list that would incorporate calculated MELD score, alpha fetoprotein (AFP), tumour size and rate of tumour growth.

Less common causes of chronic end-stage liver disease in the USA include primary biliary cirrhosis (PBC), primary sclerosing cholangitis (PSC), non-alcoholic steatohepatitis (NASH), haemochromatosis, alpha-1-antitripsin deficiency, biliary atresia and hepatitis B virus (HBV) infection.

Previously, many transplant centres considered the criterion for inclusion on the waiting list to be appropriate even when the estimated length of a patient's survival in the absence of transplantation was 1 year or less. More recently, a 'natural' or calculated MELD score of 15 points or higher is considered a reasonable threshold to recommend transplant since operative mortality and waiting-list mortality are essentially equivalent. However, patients derive long-term survival benefit with transplant at MELD scores between 10 and 15 points, especially if they have experienced life-threatening events such as spontaneous bacterial peritonitis (SBP) or variceal bleeding.[12] Poor quality of life and the development of other complications of liver disease such as severe ascites, malnutrition or intractable encephalopathy are also indications for transplantation regardless of MELD score.[22] Given the severe organ shortages, most patients in the USA with MELD scores under 20 will not be primarily offered a liver transplant via the UNOS allocation system. These patients may benefit by pursuing living donation or considering less desirable 'import' organs that have been rejected by the primary transplant centre.

Hepatitis C virus (HCV) infection

Approximately 40% of all chronic liver disease in the USA is caused by HCV infection and HCV-associated cirrhosis is the most common indication for liver transplantation among adults.[12,23] It is estimated that 8 million people in the USA are infected and approximately half are unaware that they are infected.

Of every 100 patients with HCV infection, approximately 20% will clear the virus. The remaining 80% will develop chronic active hepatitis, with approximately 20% developing end-stage liver disease. Of these patients, many have concomitant alcohol exposure that accelerates the rate and severity of liver disease.

Post-transplantation, patients with HCV infections invariably develop recurrent viraemia that may range from disease that remains relatively quiescent to development of a more aggressive course with rapid graft dysfunction. HCV reinfection occurs during reperfusion of the graft in the operating room, and viral titres have been shown to reach pre-transplant levels within 72 hours post-transplant.[24] Many factors (such as donor type and age, inflammatory grade of the recipient's explanted liver, viral genotype and viral load, steroid-containing immunosuppression regimens) have all been linked with the rate and extent of HCV reinfection.[25–28]

Eradication of HCV infection prior to liver transplantation is considered the ideal approach, but treatment of patients with decompensated cirrhosis is fraught with difficulty. In this setting, treatment has been associated with exacerbations of encephalopathy, infections and other serious adverse events, and results in low rates of viral clearance.[29–31] Newer medications for the treatment of HCV provide new hope and promise for patients with HCV waiting for liver transplant, or post-transplant recipients.

Post-transplant outcomes of patients with HCV infection rival those of non-HCV patients, especially when younger donors are used.[32] Advanced donor age (>60 years) is associated with poorer patient and graft survival, although outcomes with older donors are still superior to remaining on the waiting list.

Hepatitis B virus (HBV) infection

The risk of development of liver cirrhosis from chronic hepatitis B infection ranges from 4.5% to 36.2%, depending on viral load (HBV-DNA level).[33] Hepatitis B-associated cirrhosis is one of the most common indications for liver transplantation in Asia due to the presence of endemic hepatitis B infection. In the USA, hepatitis B accounts for only 3% of patients on the liver transplant waiting list (SRTR data, waiting list 2010). As with HCV, initial results with liver transplantation for hepatitis B were disappointing due to a high graft reinfection rate.[33] However, outcomes have significantly improved since the introduction of hepatitis B immunoglobulin (HBIG) and nucleoside analogues over the last 20 years to prevent and treat graft reinfection.[34] Current 5-year survival rates for patients transplanted for HBV-related cirrhosis exceed 75%.

Hepatocellular carcinoma (HCC)

Liver transplantation has been established as a viable treatment option for HCC.[21] As previously discussed, the landmark study for this condition established the so-called 'Milan criteria' and demonstrated that when transplantation was restricted to patients with early HCC a 4-year survival rate of 75% could be achieved.[21] Milan criteria are defined as a single lesion less than or equal to 5 cm, up to three separate lesions, none larger than 3 cm, no evidence of gross vascular invasion and no regional nodal or distant metastases. These outcomes are similar to reported and expected survival rates for patients undergoing transplantation for cirrhosis without HCC. Other groups have suggested that these criteria are too strict and should be expanded.

In the UK a consensus meeting to review allocation policies reported in September 2009 and criteria for HCC were expanded as follows:

- A single tumour ≤5 cm in diameter.
- Up to five tumours of ≤3 cm.
- A single tumour >5 cm and ≤7 cm where there is no evidence of tumour progression (volume increase should be <20% over a 6-month period). There should be no extrahepatic spread or new nodule formation.

This last criterion was introduced since there was felt to be some evidence that a relatively indolent tumour may respond well to transplantation as a modality of treatment.

The University of California, San Francisco (UCSF) group have expanded the eligibility indications to include a solitary tumour up to 6.5 cm or three or fewer nodules with the largest tumour up to 4.5 cm and a total tumour diameter of up to 8 cm.[35] Since patients with HCC have significant priority on the waiting list compared to non-HCC patients, it is unlikely that UCSF criteria will be adopted nationally for deceased donor allocation. However, UCSF criteria are used by some programmes performing live donor liver transplantation.

> ✔✔ In these times of donor organ shortage, there is clearly a balance between helping the patient with an HCC versus avoidance of disadvantage to the rest of the patients on the waiting list. It is important that the international community continues to work towards consensus, and two recent reports from such meetings are recommended.[36,37]

Alcoholic liver disease

A population survey of adults suggests that 10% of Americans drink more than two drinks per day, which is defined as 'heavy drinking'.[38] Heavy drinking and its consequences are important public health problems, as 5% of the deaths occurring annually in the USA (approximately 100 000 per year) are either directly or indirectly attributable to alcohol abuse.[38]

Approximately 14 million people in the USA meet the diagnostic criteria for alcohol abuse and, of these, 15% will eventually develop alcoholic liver disease ranging from asymptomatic fatty liver (i.e. steatosis) or abnormalities of liver enzymes to end-stage liver disease and cirrhosis. Women in general show greater susceptibility to alcohol liver damage compared to men, and African Americans show greater susceptibility than Caucasians.

Among heavy drinkers, liver disease is highly prevalent. Thus, 90–100% of heavy drinkers have steatosis, 10–35% have alcohol-induced enzyme abnormalities and 8–20% have alcoholic cirrhosis.[39]

Untreated, the 5- and 10-year survival rates for patients with alcoholic cirrhosis are 23% and 7%, respectively.[39] These rates are significantly worse than survival rates for patients whose cirrhosis was not caused by alcohol.

Liver transplantation is the only definitive treatment for end-stage liver disease caused by alcohol but remains somewhat controversial because of the ever-increasing demand for donor organs combined with concerns that alcoholic patients might relapse to drinking, thereby damaging the transplanted liver. Despite this, in well-selected patients that have been properly screened, outcome after liver transplant for alcoholic cirrhosis is excellent and comparable to those patients with non-alcohol liver disease. To ensure favourable outcome, transplant centres must conduct careful screening procedures that assess patients' coexisting medical problems and psychosocial status to identify those patients who are medically most suited for the procedure and who are most likely to remain abstinent after transplant.

Primary biliary cirrhosis (PBC)

The incidence of liver transplantation for patients with PBC has declined slightly in recent years, possibly reflecting benefits of early treatment.[40] Regardless, liver transplantation remains an important option in patients with progressive disease despite medical therapy. In the USA, the average age of patients undergoing transplantation for PBC is in the range of 53–55 years. Recurrence of disease after liver transplantation can occur in a significant number of patients.[41]

An important clinical question is 'What is the optimal time to perform liver transplantation in the patient with PBC?' In the USA, the MELD score is used by many groups to determine the optimal timing of this event. However, some patients experience significant morbidity from their liver disease that is not reflected by the MELD scores. Patients with evidence of decompensation such as low serum albumin levels (<2.8 g/dL), portal hypertension, encephalopathy, bone fractures or intractable pruritus would benefit from early evaluation and transplantation. However, in areas where livers are allocated at high MELD scores, live donor liver transplantation may be the only realistic opportunity for transplantation for such patients.[42]

Primary sclerosing cholangitis (PSC)

PSC is a chronic cholestatic liver disease of unknown origin that is associated with inflammatory bowel disease (IBD) in the vast majority of cases. The disease is characterised by biliary stricture formation that can occur anywhere in the biliary tree.

Patients with PSC are also at risk of the development of cholangiocarcinoma (CCA), while those with IBD are at risk of colon carcinoma. Colonic resection does not cure the disease or mitigate the progression of liver disease. Although the course of PSC is variable, it frequently is progressive, leading to cirrhosis and end-stage liver disease.

Typically, PSC occurs in men younger than 50 years of age and the clinical course is insidious, typified by a persistent elevation in serum alkaline phosphatase levels. Median survival after diagnosis is approximately 10–15 years, with death usually resulting from complications of portal hypertension, although in some patients recurrent bacterial cholangitis and overwhelming sepsis may be the main clinical problem.

Orthotopic liver transplantation (OLT) has become the only effective therapeutic option for patients with PSC-related complications. Excellent long-term outcome has been reported, with 5-year patient survival rates of approximately 80%. However, PSC recurs in 15–20% after OLT, with significant mortality at 3 years if untreated without re-transplantation.[43] The need for re-transplantation in patients with PSC is more common than in patients with non-obstructive biliary disease.[44]

Non-alcoholic fatty liver disease (NAFLD)

Excessive fat in liver cells in the absence of alcohol consumption is known as non-alcoholic fatty liver disease (NAFLD) and is the most common type of liver disease in the USA, affecting nearly 30% of the general population. In many patients, this fat build-up can lead to inflammation and elevated liver enzymes, which is referred to as steatohepatitis (**Fig. 8.3**). Although the exact aetiology is unknown, risk factors are truncal obesity, insulin resistance and diabetes. As a result of these epidemics in the USA, the proportion of liver transplantations performed for NAFLD cirrhosis rose dramatically from roughly 1% in 1997–2003 to more than 7% in 2010. It is estimated that by 2025 more than 25 million Americans may have NAFLD, with as many as 20% of these cases developing end-stage liver disease.

Despite the high prevalence of diabetes and obesity in NAFLD patients, post-transplantation survival is similar to non-NAFLD patients. Patients undergoing liver transplant for NAFLD-related cirrhosis enjoy excellent outcomes, with 88% 1-year survival, 82% at 3 years and 77% at 5 years. Deaths caused by recurrent disease occurred in roughly 9% of NAFLD patients compared to 17% of patients without NAFLD; this is related to the greater frequency of recurrence of diseases such as HCV and HCC in those without NAFLD.

Liver transplant immunology

Acute cellular rejection occurs in 50–75% of liver allograft recipients and the majority of episodes occur within 90 days of transplant surgery. The targets of activated lymphocytes are donor-derived bile duct epithelial cells and vascular endothelium, whereas direct involvement of hepatocytes is

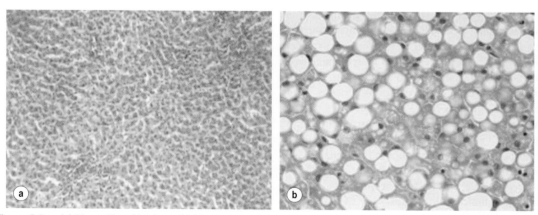

Figure 8.3 • **(a)** Normal liver histology. **(b)** Marked macrovesicular steatosis. Donor liver grafts with greater than 20–30% macrovesicular steatosis are at increased risk of postoperative primary graft non-function. Steatosis can be one of the earliest histological changes seen in patients with liver disease.

uncommon. Chronic rejection, often termed 'duc-topenic rejection', is characterised by ischaemic injury to and paucity of bile ducts; the frequency of chronic rejection has decreased in the past decade and currently occurs in less than 5% of patients. The pharmacological agents used to prevent and treat acute and chronic rejection are covered in Chapter 3. A number of diseases treated by liver transplantation are believed to be autoimmune in origin and, theoretically, any transplanted organ is as susceptible to the autoimmune process as the organ being replaced. In particular, evidence for recurrence of autoimmune hepatitis is supported by most studies, whereas data for recurrence of PSC and PBC (which can be histopathologically indistinguishable from rejection) are controversial. The immunosuppression used to prevent graft rejection is in most cases sufficient to prevent significant autoimmune damage to the allograft, but a proportion of patients may develop graft failure from disease recurrence.

Technical considerations

Organ procurement

Each transplant centre has developed its own technique for organ procurement. Some programmes perform extensive dissection in situ prior to perfusion with preservation solution to minimise cold time and back-table procedure time. Other programmes prefer to place perfusion cannulae early, remove organs en bloc and perform most of the dissection on the back-table. In either case, the procurement surgeon needs to maintain proper etiquette and respect for the deceased patient as well as support personnel at the procurement hospital. Adherence to standard surgical technique and sterility is mandatory.

Donors are typically explored through an incision from the suprasternal notch to the pubic symphysis. When multiple procurement teams are present it is important to maintain open channels of communication for a smooth operation. Thoracic organ procurement teams operate independently of the abdominal organ teams and have to wait for completion of the abdominal organ dissection before cross-clamping can occur. Within the abdomen, the liver is a life-saving organ and has priority in terms of conduct of the operation and

disposition of vessels. For example, with a replaced right hepatic artery, transection of the superior mesenteric artery (SMA) is proximal to the take-off of the replaced right hepatic artery for the liver graft. This results in a much shorter length of SMA for the pancreas graft, if also being procured. Any disagreements regarding conduct of the operation and disposition of vessels etc. should be arbitrated by the organ bank physician or the donor organisation to avoid conflict at the donor operation.

Once organs are flushed and placed in cold storage, they are transported to the recipient hospital for implantation. The back-table procedure at the recipient hospital is important to remove extraneous tissues and to inspect for any procurement damage. At this point, reconstruction of hepatic arterial branches occurs.

Graft implantation

Historically, implantation of the liver allograft was performed with the cavocaval technique with replacement of the entire retrohepatic vena cava (**Fig. 8.4**), often in concert with venovenous bypass (**Fig. 8.5**). Venovenous bypass is a technique that was developed and refined by Dr Tom Starzl to help maintain stable haemodynamics throughout the operation, especially in those patients without extensive collaterals. Some programmes continue to use venovenous bypass today for the same reason, although studies have shown that routine venovenous bypass may not be necessary in many patients, especially in those with significant collaterals that have developed with long-standing portal hypertension.

With the advent of live donor liver transplantation and to avoid the need for venovenous bypass (which has its own complications), many programmes now perform a caval-sparing 'piggyback' technique. Venous outflow for the liver graft can be to right, middle and left hepatic veins, the middle and left only, or as a side-to-side (cava-to-cava) anastomosis. Regardless, the goal is to maintain blood flow through the recipient vena cava to avoid the need for venovenous bypass and to maintain haemodynamic stability.

Some programmes elect to perform hepatic artery reconstruction prior to portal vein reconstruction in an attempt to reperfuse the graft with oxygenated blood. Other groups reperfuse the graft initially with

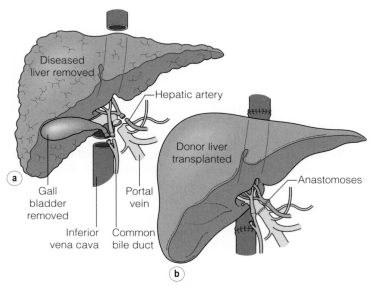

Figure 8.4 • (a) Standard resection of the diseased liver with the retrohepatic vena cava. **(b)** Standard implantation. 'Piggyback' technique removes the diseased liver with the vena cava intact and implantation of the suprahepatic vena cava of the graft into the hepatic vein orifices.

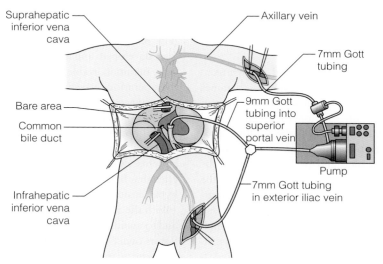

Figure 8.5 • The venovenous bypass circuit removes blood from the splanchnic and lower body systemic circulation with aid of a pump and returns it through a catheter placed in the subclavian vein. Improvements in percutaneous catheter technology have made this procedure easier without the need for 'cut-down', as shown in the figure. Once considered the 'gold standard', many programmes use venovenous bypass selectively. I.V.C, inferior vena cava.

portal blood. It does not appear that either method is markedly superior and choice rests on surgeon preference. Portal vein reconstruction is performed in a standard end-to-end fashion. Complications are relatively low in recipients with 'normal' ultrasounds preoperatively. When intramural clot is encountered,

venous thrombo-endarterectomy can be performed to improve inflow. Extensive clot down to the superior mesenteric vein (SMV)–splenic vein confluence may require venous bypass with iliac vein allograft. Clot extending well into the splenic and SMV may be a contraindication for transplantation.

> ✅ Systemic portal transpositions using the inferior vena cava as inflow for the graft are technically feasible but associated with poor outcome, since hepatotropic factors from the pancreas necessary for liver health (insulin and glucagon) are lacking.[45,46]

Hepatic arterial reconstruction is the most important anastomosis for the short- and long-term viability of the graft. Hepatic artery thrombosis (HAT) occurs in approximately 5% of cases and can result in early graft loss or significant biliary complications. Unfortunately, many cases of HAT are caused by intimal dissection and not amenable to remedial surgery. When HAT occurs at the time of transplant, reconstruction with a jump graft from the supracoeliac or infrarenal aorta is necessary. Iliac artery allograft from a deceased donor is most useful but vein grafts have also been used.

It is recommended that flowmeters are used to determine the flow on the completion of the anastomosis. These can demonstrate an unrecognised problem and also help to find the 'best lie' of the artery to produce good flow. Measurement of the portal venous flow is also useful, particularly if the surgeon is considering tying off a large portosystemic connection such as a splenorenal shunt.

Bile duct reconstruction is most prone to complications, with leak and stricture rates of approximately 5% each in deceased donor liver transplantation and at least double that in live donor transplantation. Efforts to improve on these rates with the use or absence of stents, duct-to-duct versus Roux-en-Y reconstruction have not been definitively proven, although duct-to-duct may have a slight advantage for the avoidance of stricture.

Immunosuppressive agents

There is not a standard immunosuppression regimen for liver transplant recipients. Most protocols employ multiple agents with different mechanisms of action. In general, the most intense levels of immunosuppression are seen immediately after transplantation, with reduction in the dosing and number of agents occurring later in patients with well-functioning grafts and no rejection episode. Aetiology of liver disease sometimes influences selection criteria; for instance, steroids may be maintained in patients with autoimmune liver diseases and agents with antineoplastic activity selected for

patients with hepatocellular carcinoma. Also, HCV has been reported to recur with greater severity in protocols utilising induction agents, so most HCV-positive recipients do not receive induction therapy.[47,48] The individual agents are grouped below according to their most common uses.

Induction agents

The use of induction agents is common in kidney transplantation but less so in liver transplantation.[49] 'Induction agents' are used to induce an acute and powerful but short-lived immunosuppressed state. The original idea behind induction agents was to create a suitable environment for the newly transplanted organ, i.e. one that was minimally able to respond to the foreign tissue. Equally important in liver transplant recipients is the ability to delay or reduce the intensity of calcineurin inhibitor (CNI) exposure in the immediate post-transplant period, when renal function is already impaired due to surgical stressors. The two major groups of induction agents are polyclonal and monoclonal antilymphocyte antibodies. For much greater detail on these agents, please see Chapter 5.

Primary immunosuppressants

CNIs are the mainstay of liver transplant immunosuppression. The introduction of ciclosporin A (CsA) in 1984 (in the USA) provided significant improvement in patient and graft survival for all categories of transplants. Liver transplantation was especially impacted as the drug brought to the procedure the success rates required for it to be seen as an appropriate therapeutic intervention. The earliest formulation of CsA required bile to be present so that the drug could be emulsified and absorbed. This necessitated intravenous administration when bile was externalised through T-tube drainage. A microemulsion formulation was introduced that improved this problem.

The second major drug in this class is tacrolimus (originally called FK506). It became available in the early 1990s and is now the mainstay of maintenance immunosuppression in liver transplant patients. It was not dependent on bile salts for absorption and so provided a more reliable level of immunosuppression for patients with varying degrees of hepatic dysfunction. Both CsA and tacrolimus work by inhibiting the function of calcineurin, a major step in the activation of the genes required for interleukin (IL)-2 production, but do so via different mechanisms. Consequently, they share some side-effects while others are unique to the individual agent. Both are associated with nephrotoxicity, hypertension, dyslipidaemia and electrolyte imbalances. Neurotoxicity is seen in both, but it is significantly more common in patients taking tacrolimus. Alopecia and new-onset diabetes are seen more frequently with tacrolimus, while hirsutism and gingival hyperplasia are associated with CsA.

The major metabolic pathway for both drugs is the cytochrome $P_{450}3A4$ system and non-immunosuppressive drugs commonly used in transplant patients may significantly alter blood levels. In general, enzyme-inducing agents such as phenobarbital, phenytoin or rifampin will lower CNI levels in blood, while enzyme inhibitors such as 'azole' antifungals, erythromycin, diltiazem and grapefruit juice will raise CNI levels.

Adjunct immunosuppressive agents

This refers to one or more immunosuppressive agents prescribed for liver transplant patients in addition to or in place of CNIs. Transplant programmes have developed many individualised protocols so the agents in this section may or may not be used at a specific institution.

Azathioprine

Originally developed as a chemotherapeutic agent, azathioprine was for many years a mainstay of immunosuppression. It is converted to 6-mercaptopurine, a purine analogue that disrupts nucleic acid synthesis and abrogates lymphocyte proliferation. Its side-effects include bone marrow depression, pancreatitis and hepatotoxicity.

Mycophenolic acid

This agent has largely replaced azathioprine in immunosuppression regimens. It also inhibits purine synthesis but uses a mechanism distinct from that of azathioprine. It truncates the de novo purine synthesis pathway in lymphocytes via inhibition of an essential enzyme (inosine monophosphate dehydrogenase, IMDPH) and is associated with similar side-effects. However, pancreatitis and hepatotoxicity

are infrequent, while gastrointestinal complaints (diarrhoea, abdominal cramping, nausea, etc.) are more common.

mTOR Inhibitors

mTOR refers to 'mammalian target of rapamycin', the intracellular molecular complex that regulates ribosomal proteins, initiation of translation and cyclin-dependent kinases. Common side-effects include dyslipidaemia and anaemia. Additional side-effects include impaired wound healing and a concern about increased hepatic artery thrombosis; for these reasons, it is rarely used as initial immunosuppression in liver transplant recipients. However, it is associated with improved renal function compared to CNI-based immunosuppression and it has potent antitumour activity both in vitro and in vivo.[50] This makes it an attractive option for patients with impaired renal function or those transplanted for hepatocellular carcinoma or who develop multiple skin cancers. It does interact with CNIs, CsA in particular, so CNI dose should be reduced or eliminated in patients who are also taking an mTOR.

Corticosteroids

Corticosteroids are potent anti-inflammatory agents that alter lymphocyte function by a variety of mechanisms and are included in many immunosuppression protocols. They are also the most frequently used agents for the treatment of rejection episodes. However, the large number of serious adverse affects associated with prolonged use has led to many groups rapidly reducing or eliminating steroids after the immediate postoperative period. Steroid use is associated with significant hypertension and lipid abnormalities, bone demineralisation, diabetes and psychiatric disorders. This is a particular problem in children, where prolonged steroid use results in poor growth. There is also an economic impact to consider. While steroids are relatively inexpensive, the costs of treating diabetes for the life of the patient or supplying growth hormone until a child achieves acceptable stature are considerable.

Post-transplant complications

The liver occupies a critical role in maintaining homeostasis; therefore, when its function is compromised, a wide range of symptoms may be seen.

Obviously, liver transplantation represents a major disruption in normal hepatic function and is accompanied by multiple hepatotoxic events, including hypotension, hypoxia and ischaemia. The situation may be further complicated by donor factors, including increasing age or hepatic steatosis, and recipient factors such as previous abdominal surgery that increase the complexity of the transplant surgery.[51,52]

Most of the complications discussed below may occur at any time, but the frequency of occurrence varies in relation to the time after transplant. It is convenient to divide the complications in this manner, but in practice it is important to remain aware that individual patients may fall outside these guidelines and to increase the scope of diagnostic testing when indicated.

Perioperative complications (first 30 days)

Preservation/reperfusion injury

Preservation/reperfusion injury obviously occurs at the time of transplantation, but it has the potential to cause complications for the life of the graft. The degree of injury is determined by many factors, but the length of time a graft lacks normal blood flow is directly related to the magnitude of damage incurred. While some period of ischaemia is unavoidable, and improvements in preservation solutions[53] have reduced the impact of reperfusion injury, it remains a major cause of morbidity following liver transplantation. Prolonged cold ischaemia time produces deleterious changes in sinusoidal (mostly endothelial) cells, while warm ischaemia injury primarily affects the hepatocytes.[54] Cold ischaemic injury is also associated with deposition of leucocytes and platelets in the sinusoids and disruption of sinusoidal perfusion. There are reports in both animals and humans of Kupffer cell activation, usually associated with prolonged cold ischaemia. When present, this is significant due to the release of proinflammatory compounds, including IL-8, E-selectin and reactive oxygen species, leading to decreased integrity of sinusoidal architecture and consequently hepatic microcirculation.

Warm ischaemic injury is characterised by distinctive histological changes in hepatocytes, including vacuolisation, chromatin disarray and mitochondrial swelling. These changes are thought to result in the transaminitis noted post-transplantation. Warm ischaemia and reperfusion are also accompanied by activation of the complement cascade. The membrane attack complex is capable of directly damaging most cells that come into contact with it.[55] All of this activity is the likely cause of much of the cellular damage frequently noted on post-perfusion biopsies.

Bile duct cells are particularly susceptible to the effects described above. When these cells are unable to function normally, bilirubin accumulates and this in turn exacerbates preservation injury. A cholestatic picture is produced in the liver function tests.

Primary non-function (PNF)

The exact cause(s) of this life-threatening event is unknown. It is likely that some of the metabolic/immunological events associated with ischaemia/reperfusion injury contribute to PNF in some way, but there is no direct correlation. There is an association with advanced donor age, donor and/or recipient haemodynamic instability and hepatotoxic drugs, but frequently patients with all the risk factors have satisfactory graft function while those with one or none do not. Clinical parameters include profound coagulopathy despite administration of fresh frozen plasma, hepatic encephalopathy and aspartate aminotransferase (AST) values >5000 IU. Biopsy findings include ischaemic cholangiopathy and necrosis. Prostaglandin infusions are sometimes administered in an attempt to improve hepatic microenvironment, but success rates are marginal. Mortality approaches 100% if PNF persists longer than 36–48 hours, and re-transplantation is the only effective treatment.[56]

There is a variant of PNF called primary or initial poor function in which the clinical and laboratory findings are similar to PNF but less extreme. This is often related to rejection, infection or hepatotoxic drugs and resolves when the underlying cause is appropriately treated. Unfortunately, in a significant number of cases, an aetiological agent is not identified and graft function remains suboptimal.[57]

Haemorrhage

Reports of post-liver transplant haemorrhage are common, with some series reaching a 20% incidence. Most occur within the first 48 hours and are diagnosed by some combination of frankly bloody drain output, haemodynamic instability or decreasing haematocrit on serial measurements. Conservative management is sufficient for most cases, but approximately 15% will require surgical exploration. Specific cause is identified in approximately half of these, while most of the remainder will resolve following removal of accumulated clotted blood and abdominal 'washout'.[58]

Hepatic artery thrombosis (HAT)

HAT is the most common vascular complication following liver transplantation, with reported incidence ranging from 1.5% to 25% in different series. The higher incidences are more commonly seen in paediatric series. Early (first 72 hours) and complete thrombosis has a poor prognosis. Untreated, it is strongly associated with graft necrosis and loss, and patient death is common unless re-transplanted. Diagnosis may be made with Doppler ultrasound, selective arteriogram or more commonly nowadays by helical computed tomography (CT) scan. Definitive treatment involves thrombectomy; success with both surgical and radiological intervention has been reported. Intra-arterial thrombolysis has also been reported but success rates are inferior compared to the interventional procedures. HAT that develops at a later time is associated with biliary complications and varying degrees of graft dysfunction. Approximately 50–75% of patients diagnosed with HAT eventually require either emergent or elective re-transplantation.[59–62] Early-onset HAT has biopsy changes consisting of centrolobular coagulative necrosis and ballooning degeneration, while late-onset HAT has poorly described histological changes with bile duct necrosis and bile ductular reactions cited most frequently.[54]

Portal vein thrombosis (PVT)

PVT is an infrequent but serious complication following liver transplantation, with an incidence of 2–3%. It is associated with pre-existing portal hypertension, especially when surgical decompression has been attempted, and also with pre-transplant PVT, even when this has been successfully treated. There are some reports of it occurring more frequently after live donor liver transplantation.[63] When present in the immediate post-transplant period, it frequently presents as encephalopathy, refractory ascites and/or graft failure, and surgical intervention is generally needed. PVT that develops at a later time point is accompanied by signs of portal hypertension and is sometimes amenable to percutaneous dilatation. Liver biopsies from patients with PVT show portal fibrosis, hepatocyte atrophy and sinusoidal dilatation.[54]

Biliary complications: bile leaks

Bile leaks occur when normal bile drainage systems are not intact; the reported incidence varies between 2% and 25%. The higher incidences are seen more frequently in paediatric and live donor (LD) populations as opposed to adult recipients of deceased donor livers. Leaks from the bile duct anastomosis are the most common cause of biliary leaks in the early post-transplant period, but the leak may also emanate from the cystic duct remnant, the T-tube tract or, in the case of LD recipients, the cut surface of the graft.[64] They may be suspected when drain output changes and are confirmed by imaging studies (biloma or abdominal collections). Conservative management such as T-tube drainage with antibiotic coverage may suffice for some individuals, but most will require radiological or endoscopic procedures and up to 10–20% will need surgical intervention.[65] Biliary leaks are uncommon after the first 3 months following transplantation. However, they are an independent risk factor for the development of biliary strictures, and so should be treated to resolution whenever possible.[66]

Early (first 6 months) complications

Biliary strictures

Ischaemic biliary strictures (**Fig. 8.6**) account for approximately 40% of all biliary complications following liver transplantation. Early strictures

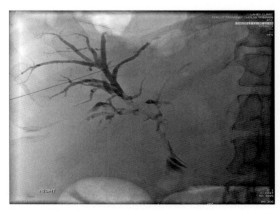

Figure 8.6 • Ischaemic cholangiopathy is commonly seen after hepatic artery thrombosis or prolonged ischaemic time that results in diffuse 'thumb-printing' pattern on cholangiogram as seen in this figure. Re-transplantation is usually indicated.

are usually anastomotic and the result of technical problems related to the transplant surgery. Size mismatch between donor and recipient bile ducts is frequently cited as a cause of anastomotic strictures, as are prior bile leaks and ischaemic insults.[66] Treatment generally consists of multiple endoscopic dilatation and stenting procedures. The majority (70–100%) of patients will be successfully treated initially by this method; however, there is a high rate of recurrence, with approximately 18% of deceased donor recipients and up to 33% of live donor recipients experiencing a recurrence.[64,67] Some patients with anastomotic strictures and appropriate anatomy may be considered for conversion from direct duct-to-duct anastomosis to a Roux-en-Y hepaticojejunostomy.

Acute rejection

Acute cellular rejection, characterised by biopsy findings of mixed portal inflammation, endothelialitis, bile duct damage and occasional eosinophils in portal tracts, is accompanied by varying degrees of hepatic dysfunction. It occurs most commonly in the first 4–8 weeks post-transplantation, but is also common during the first year. Reported rates vary widely, with some series indicating up to 65%. Choice and dose of immunosuppression and whether or not an induction regimen was used significantly affect the actual occurrence, as does autoimmune aetiology of primary liver disease. Patient compliance and existence of comorbid conditions affecting immunosuppression absorption also contribute to the incidence. Modern immunosuppression regimens result in most acute cellular rejection episodes being successfully reversed, usually following administration of increased steroid doses, addition of a second agent or occasionally lymphocytotoxic antibodies.[68–70]

Liver allografts are alone among transplanted organs in that they are not subject to hyperacute rejection episodes. This form of rejection is mediated by preformed antibodies to either human leucocyte antigen (HLA) or ABO antigens and is characterised by complement activation, rapid destruction of parenchymal structures, infiltration of neutrophils and other inflammatory cellular components, and irreversible loss of graft function. The reasons for the liver's immunity from this type of rejection are unclear. Low density of HLA and ABO antigens on hepatocytes and endothelial cells and hepatic

production of soluble HLAs have been suggested as explanations, but remain unproven at this time. There is, however, increasing evidence that antibodies to donor-specific HLAs are associated with inferior long-term outcomes and may play a role in the development of ductopenia.[71,72]

Infections

The need for lifelong immunosuppression following transplantation makes infectious complications a major source of morbidity for recipients. Infections may arise from agents present in the transplanted organ or from blood transfusions, from reactivation of latent viruses in the recipient or from bacteria present within the recipient or his/her environment. Perioperative infections are related to amount of blood products required, duration of intubation/ICU stay and comorbid conditions such as renal failure or diabetes. They are usually bacterial, with *Pseudomonas* and *Klebsiella* isolates commonly reported.[73] There is general agreement that antibiotic therapy should be employed perioperatively, but consensus is lacking regarding the duration. Cephalosporin derivatives are commonly employed for this, but there is concern that this practice may increase the incidence of methicillin-resistant *Staphylococcus aureus*.

Cytomegalovirus (CMV) infection (**Fig. 8.7**) is found in up to 50% of liver transplant patients.[74,75] Infection refers to demonstration of active viral replication and may or may not be accompanied by symptomatic disease. CMV disease refers to an infection that causes significant clinical sequelae, including increased graft loss and patient death.

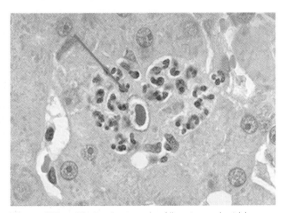

Figure 8.7 • Photomicrograph of liver transplant biopsy showing typical CMV viral inclusion body (arrow).

Risk factors for development of CMV diseases include donor-positive/recipient-negative serological combinations, use of antilymphocyte induction and multiple transfusions. Antiviral prophylaxis with agents such as oral valganciclovir is well accepted by most liver transplant programmes for high-risk recipients; use in lower risk recipients varies. A common practice is to develop programme-specific protocols in conjunction with input from infectious disease.

Epstein–Barr virus (EBV) infection following liver transplantation is associated with a wide spectrum of clinical manifestations. Like CMV, it is a member of the herpes virus family and is characterised by latency that means that immunosuppressed patients are at risk for both reactivation of endogenous virus and de novo infection with exogenous strains. The virus preferentially infects B lymphocytes but other cell types including T cells and nasopharyngeal epithelium may also be involved. The virus drives lymphocyte proliferation that is normally controlled by specific cytotoxic T cells. In an immunosuppressed patient, that control is lacking or impaired, and the proliferation continues in an uncontrolled manner and is referred to as post-transplant lymphoproliferative disorder (PTLD). Patients may present with a mild flu-like illness or a full-blown lymphoma. The disease may be seen as an isolated CNS tumour or an allograft mass (**Fig. 8.8**), as well as a more traditional lymphoma with lymph node involvement. The diagnosis and treatment of PTLD is covered in Chapter 12 and outlined in **Fig. 8.9**. In some cases, reduction in immunosuppression will result in the re-establishment of normal immune surveillance and the tumours will regress. For a few patients with a solitary mass, surgical excision is curative. However, many patients will require standard lymphoma chemotherapy. The addition of rituximab, a monoclonal antibody targeting the CD20 antigen on B cells, to treatment regimens has increased success rates.[76,77]

Liver transplant recipients are also at risk of opportunistic fungal and bacterial infections during this period. *Pneumocystis*, *Candida*, *Aspergillus* and *Cryptococcus* species are the most frequent fungal infections encountered, while *Mycobacteria*, *Nocardia* and *Listeria* species are the most common bacterial ones. Presenting symptoms vary with the site of infection, and in general these infections are associated with heavy immunosuppression, a generalised debilitated state or presence of comorbid conditions, including diabetes. Prognosis and treatment success varies widely, but in general early detection and lower levels of immunosuppression are associated with better outcomes.[78,79]

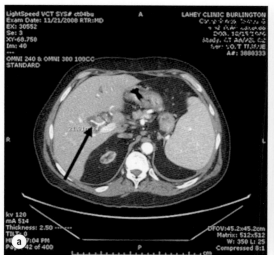
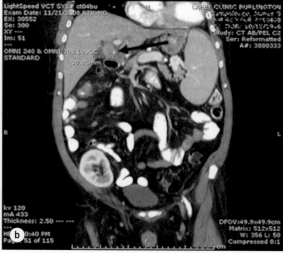

Figure 8.8 • CT scan showing PTLD in liver allograft (arrow). Mass was originally reported as 'suspicious for cholangiocarcinoma'. The mass was resected and biliary tree reconstructed with Roux-en-Y hepaticojejunostomy. Biopsy demonstrated polymorphic PTLD with Epstein–Barr virus (EBV) positivity that responded to lowering the level of immunosuppression and antiviral therapy only. The patient remains disease free 4 years post-resection. Monoclonal PTLD has a poor prognosis without chemotherapy.

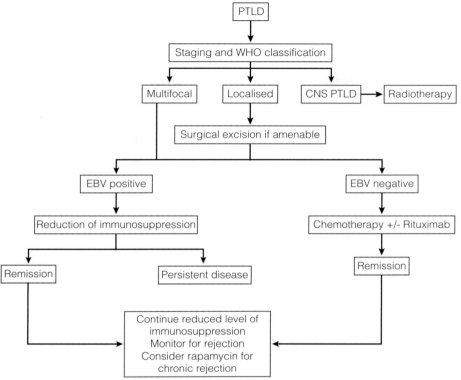

Figure 8.9 • The recommended algorithm for the work-up and treatment of a lymphocyte predominant lesion in organ transplant recipient. Knowledge of Epstein–Barr virus (EBV) status is important since a percentage of EBV-positive cases will respond to reduction immunosuppression alone, but most will require additional intervention such as antiviral therapy. Monoclonal PTLD without EBV has worse prognosis and requires chemotherapy to improve outcome.

Late complications (>6 months)

Malignancy

Between 5% and 15% of transplant recipients will develop a de novo tumour; this is approximately twice the incidence found in age-matched controls in the general population.[80] Kaposi's sarcoma and PTLD are seen earliest relative to time of transplant, with non-melanoma skin cancers and cancers of the vulva and peritoneum developing at later time points. The most significant risk factors for development of malignancy are EBV-negative serology, significant sun exposure, smoking and increasing age. Skin cancers and lymphomas develop with 10-fold greater frequency in transplant patients compared to age-matched controls. Lung, head and neck, and colorectal cancers also occur more frequently in liver transplant patients than the general population, but at a lower rate than lymphoma and skin cancers. Prostate and breast cancers do not appear to occur at increased rates compared to non-transplant patients.[81] Most liver transplant programmes recommend avoidance of behaviours known to increase risk, as well as regular screening protocols to aid in early detection.

Late surgical complications

Incisional hernia is the most common late surgical complication following liver transplantation. The reported incidence ranges between 5% and 25%, and is observed more frequently in conjunction with obesity, sirolimus immunosuppression and rejection episodes treated with steroid boluses. Bowel obstructions are also relatively common; these are associated with adhesions, various types of hernias, PTLD with bowel involvement and Roux-en-Y biliary reconstruction. This latter group may lack usual radiological evidence of bowel obstruction and a CT scan can be useful to diagnose the condition.[81]

Biliary strictures

Biliary strictures that develop later in the post-transplant course may be either anastomotic or non-anastomotic and are frequently associated with vascular insufficiency (**Fig. 8.6**). HAT is reported in 25–50% of patients with late strictures.[82,83] Non-anastomotic strictures that develop despite adequate blood supply are termed ischaemic-type biliary lesions (ITBLs) and are associated with prolonged ischaemia times, older donors and viscous preservation solutions.[84] Immune destruction of bile duct epithelium has been implicated as a possible cause in some reports, but there is not yet definitive proof of this.

Vascular complications

Late vascular complications are relatively uncommon (1–5%) following liver transplantation. Late HAT is associated with prothrombotic conditions or severe rejections. This is difficult to treat and often requires re-transplantation. It is associated with bile leaks and strictures, and often recurrent cholangitis. Re-transplantation has a 50% mortality rate; this is likely related to biliary sepsis, frequently observed in these patients.

Aneurysms or pseudoaneurysms of the hepatic artery are rare occurrences with high mortality rates. Development is associated with procedures such as stent placement or biopsy, and fungal infections are frequently implicated. Coil embolisation is recommended in stable patients; however, operative intervention is needed for those with symptoms of haemorrhagic shock. Hepatic artery aneurysms are fatal in approximately 50% of cases.[85]

Chronic rejection

Literature from the 1980s describes chronic rejection of liver allografts as occurring in 15–20% of recipients. The current literature suggests the rate is now between 2% and 5% and suggests that improved immunosuppression along with better preservation techniques is responsible for the improvement. Histological features include bile duct atrophy and portal tract loss with concomitant arteriopathy or obliterative arteritis. There may or may not be mononuclear cell infiltration. An association with prior acute rejection episodes is suggested but not confirmed. Chronic rejection does not usually respond to increases in immunosuppression.[86,87] Patients are frequently asymptomatic in the early stages, demonstrating only slightly abnormal liver function tests, and may continue to function well for an extended period of time.

Recent publications have suggested involvement of donor-specific HLA antibodies in the pathogenesis of chronic liver allograft rejection and reported that antibody-depleting therapy (plasmapheresis, intravenous immunoglobulin, rituximab) can salvage 'at-risk' grafts that had not responded to increases in traditional immunosuppression.[71]

> ✅ As in other forms of organ transplantation, there is now a suggestion that long-term graft damage may be an antibody-mediated phenomenon (see Chapter 13 for further details). Further research in this area is required.

Kaneku et al. have recently published data showing that donor-specific antibodies of the IgG3 subclass were associated with significant biopsy and clinical findings of chronic allograft rejection while those patients with donor-specific antibodies of other IgG subclasses did not develop chronic rejection.[88] Together, these reports suggest that effective treatment may be available for a subset of recipients with chronic rejection.

Conclusion

Liver transplantation is a relatively recent surgical innovation that has seen rapid development and growth from the pioneering days of Starzl and Calne. Those early procedures had questionable efficacy and only the occasional long-term survivor. Today, liver transplant recipients enjoy excellent patient and graft survival and the procedure has become routine in many centres.

Living donor liver transplantation has emerged as a viable option for patients with end-stage liver disease. It is seen most frequently in areas where deceased donors are in short supply or where societal, political or religious objections to the concept of brain death exist. Ethical questions regarding donor safety are balanced by very high waiting-list mortality that exceeds 20% in many regions.

Advances in surgical technique, immunosuppression, and pre- and postoperative management have not only reduced operative morbidity and mortality, but have also significantly improved the quality of life for the recipient. A successful liver transplant programme requires a multidisciplinary team approach of dedicated individuals with a common purpose. Favourable outcomes require sound judgment, technical acumen and attention to detail.

Key points

- Liver transplantation has developed rapidly from a heroic operation carried out with a low risk of success to a standard therapy with excellent patient and graft survival offering the only hope of rescue for patients with liver failure.
- Continued scrutiny is required for HCC as an indication in liver transplantation. Often this therapy provides the best chance for a particular patient with HCC but any particular decision may not be fair on other patients on the waiting list. Scrutiny of modern results continues to be required.
- Modern methods of preservation and perfusion may offer improvement for liver transplant results in the future (see Chapter 6).
- Rejection is less of a problem in liver transplantation than some other grafts. Nevertheless, advances in immunosuppression are also impacting on results in liver transplantation.
- There is some evidence that chronic liver allograft damage may represent antibody-mediated inflammation (see Chapter 13).

References

1. Starzl TE, Groth CG, Brettschneider L, et al. Extended survival in 3 cases of orthotopic homotransplantation of the human liver. Surgery 1968;63(4):549–63.

2. Calne RY, Williams R. Liver transplantation in man. I. Observations on technique and organization in five cases. Br Med J 1968;4(5630):535–40.

3. Pomposelli JJ, Verbesey J, Simpson MA, et al. Improved survival after live donor adult liver transplantation (LDALT) using right lobe grafts: program experience and lessons learned. Am J Transplant 2006;6(3):589–98.

4. Wiesner RH, McDiarmid SV, Kamath PS, et al. MELD and PELD: application of survival models to liver allocation. Liver Transpl 2001;7(7):567–80.

5. Edwards EB, Harper AM. The impact of MELD on OPTN liver allocation: preliminary results. Clin Transpl 2002;21–8.

6. Kamath PS, Wiesner RH, Malinchoc M, et al. A model to predict survival in patients with end-stage liver disease. Hepatology 2001;33(2):464–70.

7. Wiesner R, Edwards E, Freeman R, et al. Model for end-stage liver disease (MELD) and allocation of donor livers. Gastroenterology 2003;124(1):91–6.

8. Habib S, Berk B, Chang CC, et al. MELD and prediction of post-liver transplantation survival. Liver Transpl 2006;12(3):440–7.

9. Trotter JF, Osgood MJ. MELD scores of liver transplant recipients according to size of waiting list: impact of organ allocation and patient outcomes. JAMA 2004;291(15):1871–4.

10. Thuluvath PJ, Guidinger MK, Fung JJ, et al. Liver transplantation in the United States, 1999–2008. Am J Transplant 2010;10(4, Pt 2):1003–19.

11. Gillespie BW, Merion RM, Ortiz-Rios E, et al. Database comparison of the adult-to-adult living donor liver transplantation cohort study (A2ALL) and the SRTR U.S Transplant Registry. Am J Transplant 2010;10(7):1621–33.

12. Merion RM. 2009 SRTR report on the state of transplantation. Am J Transplant 2010;10(4, Pt 2):959–60.

13. O'Leary JG, Lepe R, Davis GL. Indications for liver transplantation. Gastroenterology 2008;134(6):1764–76.

14. Campbell Jr DA, Ham JM, McCurry KR, et al. Liver transplant for fulminant hepatic failure. Am Surg 1991;57(8):546–9.

15. Bower WA, Johns M, Margolis HS, et al. Population-based surveillance for acute liver failure. Am J Gastroenterol 2007;102(11):2459–63.

16. Ostapowicz G, Fontana RJ, Schiodt FV, et al. Results of a prospective study of acute liver failure at 17 tertiary care centers in the United States. Ann Intern Med 2002;137(12):947–54.

17. Dhiman RK, Jain S, Maheshwari U, et al. Early indicators of prognosis in fulminant hepatic failure: an assessment of the Model for End-Stage Liver Disease (MELD) and King's College Hospital criteria. Liver Transpl 2007;13(6):814–21.

18. Zimmerman MA, Cameron AM. Ghobrial RM. Budd–Chiari syndrome. Clin Liver Dis 2006;10(2):259–73, viii.

19. Zahn A, Gotthardt D, Weiss KH, et al. Budd–Chiari syndrome: long term success via hepatic decompression using transjugular intrahepatic porto-systemic shunt. BMC Gastroenterol 2010;10:25.

20. Segev DL, Nguyen GC, Locke JE, et al. Twenty years of liver transplantation for Budd–Chiari syndrome: a national registry analysis. Liver Transpl 2007;13(9):1285–94.

21. Mazzaferro V, Regalia E, Doci R, et al. Liver transplantation for the treatment of small hepatocellular carcinomas in patients with cirrhosis. N Engl J Med 1996;334(11):693–9.

22. Gines P, Jimenez W, Arroyo V, et al. Atrial natriuretic factor in cirrhosis with ascites: plasma levels, cardiac release and splanchnic extraction. Hepatology 1988;8(3):636–42.

23. Verna EC, Brown Jr RS. Hepatitis C virus and liver transplantation. Clin Liver Dis 2006;10(4):919–40.

24. Garcia-Retortillo M, Forns X, Feliu A, et al. Hepatitis C virus kinetics during and immediately after liver transplantation. Hepatology 2002;35(3):680–7.

25. Charlton M, Seaberg E, Wiesner R, et al. Predictors of patient and graft survival following liver transplantation for hepatitis C. Hepatology 1998;28(3):823–30.

26. Gordon FD, Poterucha JJ, Germer J, et al. Relationship between hepatitis C genotype and severity of recurrent hepatitis C after liver transplantation. Transplantation 1997;63(10):1419–23.

27. Gane EJ, Portmann BC, Naoumov NV, et al. Long-term outcome of hepatitis C infection after liver transplantation. N Engl J Med 1996;334(13):815–20.

28. Zhou S, Terrault NA, Ferrell L, et al. Severity of liver disease in liver transplantation recipients with hepatitis C virus infection: relationship to genotype and level of viremia. Hepatology 1996;24(5):1041–6.

29. Carrion JA, Fernandez-Varo G, Bruguera M, et al. Serum fibrosis markers identify patients with mild and progressive hepatitis C recurrence after liver transplantation. Gastroenterology 2010;138(1):147–58 e1.

30. Van Wagner LB, Baker T, Ahya SN, et al. Outcomes of patients with hepatitis C undergoing simultaneous liver–kidney transplantation. J Hepatol 2009;51(5):874–80.

31. Everson GT. Treatment of chronic hepatitis C in patients with decompensated cirrhosis. Rev Gastroenterol Disord 2004;4(Suppl. 1):S31–8.

32. Khapra AP, Agarwal K, Fiel MI, et al. Impact of donor age on survival and fibrosis progression in patients with hepatitis C undergoing liver transplantation using HCV+ allografts. Liver Transpl 2006;12(10):1496–503.

33. Iloeje UH, Yang HI, Su J, et al. Predicting cirrhosis risk based on the level of circulating hepatitis B viral load. Gastroenterology 2006;130(3):678–86.

34. Kim WR, Poterucha JJ, Kremers WK, et al. Outcome of liver transplantation for hepatitis B in the United States. Liver Transpl 2004;10(8):968–74.

35. Yao FY, Ferrell L, Bass NM, et al. Liver transplantation for hepatocellular carcinoma: expansion of the tumor size limits does not adversely impact survival. Hepatology 2001;33(6):1394–403.

36. Pomfret EA, Washburn K, Wald C, et al. Report of a national conference on liver allocation in patients with hepatocellular carcinoma in the United States. Liver Transpl 2010;16(3):262–78.

37. Clavien PA, Lesurtel M, Bossuyt PM, et al. OLT for HCC consensus group. Lancet Oncol 2012;13(1):E11–22.
   HCC as an indication for liver transplantation continues to undergo scrutiny, with international conferences attempting to strike the balance between treatment for the patient with HCC balanced against the needs of the rest of the patients on a waiting list for liver transplant.

38. Hoofnagle JH, Kresina T, Fuller RK, et al. Liver transplantation for alcoholic liver disease: executive statement and recommendations. Summary of a National Institutes of Health workshop held December 6–7, 1996, Bethesda, Maryland. Liver Transpl Surg 1997;3(3):347–50.

39. McCullough AJ, Falck-Ytter Y. Body composition and hepatic steatosis as precursors for fibrotic liver disease. Hepatology 1999;29(4):1328–30.

40. Kuiper EM, Hansen BE, Metselaar HJ, et al. Trends in liver transplantation for primary biliary cirrhosis in the Netherlands 1988–2008. BMC Gastroenterol 2010;10:144.

41. Khettry U, Anand N, Faul PN, et al. Liver transplantation for primary biliary cirrhosis: a long-term pathologic study. Liver Transpl 2003;9(1):87–96.

42. Kashyap R, Safadjou S, Chen R, et al. Living donor and deceased donor liver transplantation for autoimmune and cholestatic liver diseases – an analysis of the UNOS database. J Gastrointest Surg 2010;14(9):1362–9.

43. Campsen J, Zimmerman MA, Trotter JF, et al. Clinically recurrent primary sclerosing cholangitis following liver transplantation: a time course. Liver Transpl 2008;14(2):181–5.

44. Brandsaeter B, Friman S, Broome U, et al. Outcome following liver transplantation for primary sclerosing cholangitis in the Nordic countries. Scand J Gastroenterol 2003;38(11):1176–83.

45. Tzakis AG, Kirkegaard P, Pinna AD, et al. Liver transplantation with cavoportal hemitransposition in the presence of diffuse portal vein thrombosis. Transplantation 1998;65(5):619–24.

46. Starzl TE, Porter KA, Kashiwagi N, et al. The effect of diabetes mellitus on portal blood hepatotrophic factors in dogs. Surg Gynecol Obstet 1975;140(4):549–62.

47. Marcos A, Eghtesad B, Fung JJ, et al. Use of alemtuzumab and tacrolimus monotherapy for cadaveric liver transplantation: with particular reference to hepatitis C virus. Transplantation 2004;78(7):966–71.

48. Levitsky J, Thudi K, Ison MG, et al. Alemtuzumab induction in non-hepatitis C positive liver transplant recipients. Liver Transpl 2011;17(1):32–7.

49. Wiesner RH, Fung JJ. Present state of immunosuppressive therapy in liver transplant recipients. Liver Transpl 2011;17(Suppl. 3):S1–9.

50. Schnitzbauer AA, Scherer MN, Rochon J, et al. Study protocol: a pilot study to determine the safety and efficacy of induction-therapy, de novo MPA and delayed mTOR-inhibition in liver transplant recipients with impaired renal function PATRON-study. BMC Nephrol 2010;11:24.

51. Murray KF, Carithers Jr RL; AASLD. AASLD practice guidelines; evaluation of the patient for liver transplantation. Hepatology 2005;41(6):1407–32.

52. Cho JY, Suh KS, Lee HW, et al. Hepatic steatosis is associated with intrahepatic cholestasis and transient hyperbilirubinemia during regeneration after living donor liver transplantation. Transplant Int 2006;19(10):807–13.

53. Garcia-Gil FA, Serrano MT, Fuentes-Broto L, et al. Celsior versus University of Wisconsin preserving solutions for liver transplantation: postreperfusion syndrome and outcome of a 5-year prospective randomized controlled study. World J Surg 2011;35(7):1598–607.

54. Washington K. Update on post-liver transplantation infections, malignancies, and surgical complications. Adv Anat Pathol 2005;12(4):221–6.

55. Kissel JT, Mendell JR, Rammohan KW. Microvascular deposition of complement membrane attack complex in dermatomyositis. N Engl J Med 1986;314(6):329–34.

56. Lewis MB, Howdle PD. Neurologic complications of liver transplantation in adults. Neurology 2003;61(9):1174–8.

57. Chen H, Peng CH, Shen BY, et al. Multi-factor analysis of initial poor graft function after orthotopic liver transplantation. Hepatobiliary Pancreat Dis Int 2007;6(2):141–6.

58. Motschman TL, Taswell HF, Brecher ME, et al. Intraoperative blood loss and patient and graft survival in orthotopic liver transplantation: their relationship to clinical and laboratory data. Mayo Clinic Proc 1989;64(3):346–55.

59. Mazariegos GV, Molmenti EP, Kramer DJ. Early complications after orthotopic liver transplantation. Surg Clin North Am 1999;79(1):109–29.

60. Pastacaldi S, Teixeira R, Montalto P, et al. Hepatic artery thrombosis after orthotopic liver transplantation: a review of nonsurgical causes. Liver Transpl 2001;7(2):75–81.

61. Vivarelli M, Cucchetti A, La Barba G, et al. Ischemic arterial complications after liver transplantation in the adult: multivariate analysis of risk factors. Arch Surg 2004;139(10):1069–74.

62. Oh CK, Pelletier SJ, Sawyer RG, et al. Uni- and multi-variate analysis of risk factors for early and late hepatic artery thrombosis after liver transplantation. Transplantation 2001;71(6):767–72.

63. Ponziani FR, Zocco MA, Campanale C, et al. Portal vein thrombosis: insight into physiopathology, diagnosis, and treatment. World J Gastroenterol 2010;16(2):143–55.

64. Balderramo D, Navasa M, Cardenas A. Current management of biliary complications after liver transplantation: emphasis on endoscopic therapy. Gastroenterol Hepatol 2011;34(2):107–15.

65. Moreno R, Berenguer M. Post-liver transplantation medical complications. Ann Hepatol 2006;5(2):77–85.

66. Welling TH, Heidt DG, Englesbe MJ, et al. Biliary complications following liver transplantation in the model for end-stage liver disease era: effect of donor, recipient, and technical factors. Liver Transpl 2008;14(1):73–80.

67. Verdonk RC, Buis CI, Porte RJ, et al. Anastomotic biliary strictures after liver transplantation: causes and consequences. Liver Transpl 2006;12(5):726–35.

68. Corbani A, Burroughs AK. Intrahepatic cholestasis after liver transplantation. Clin Liver Dis 2008;12(1):111–29, ix.

69. Berlakovich GA, Imhof M, Karner-Hanusch J, et al. The importance of the effect of underlying disease on rejection outcomes following orthotopic liver transplantation. Transplantation 1996;61(4):554–60.

70. Varotti G, Grazi GL, Vetrone G, et al. Causes of early acute graft failure after liver transplantation: analysis of a 17-year single-centre experience. Clin Transplant 2005;19(4):492–500.

71. Musat AI, Agni RM, Wai PY, et al. The significance of donor-specific HLA antibodies in rejection and ductopenia development in ABO compatible liver transplantation. Am J Transplant 2011;11(3):500–10.

72. Sakashita H, Haga H, Ashihara E, et al. Significance of C4d staining in ABO-identical/compatible liver transplantation. Mod Pathol 2007;20(6):676–84.

73. Singh N, Wagener MM, Obman A, et al. Bacteremias in liver transplant recipients: shift toward Gram-negative bacteria as predominant pathogens. Liver Transpl 2004;10(7):844–9.

74. Singh N, Wagener MM. Strategies to prevent organ disease by cytomegalovirus in solid organ transplant recipients. Ann Intern Med 2006;144(6):456–7.

75. Seehofer D, Rayes N, Tullius SG, et al. CMV hepatitis after liver transplantation: incidence, clinical course, and long-term follow-up. Liver Transpl 2002;8(12):1138–46.

76. Nourse JP, Jones K, Gandhi MK. Epstein–Barr virus-related post-transplant lymphoproliferative disorders: pathogenetic insights for targeted therapy. Am J Transplant 2011;11(5):888–95.

77. Evens AM, Roy R, Sterrenberg D, et al. Post-transplantation lymphoproliferative disorders: diagnosis, prognosis, and current approaches to therapy. Curr Oncol Rep 2010;12(6):383–94.

78. Singh N. The current management of infectious diseases in the liver transplant recipient. Clin Liver Dis 2000;4(3):657–73, ix.

79. Losada I, Cuervas-Mons V, Millan I, et al. Early infection in liver transplant recipients: incidence, severity, risk factors and antibiotic sensitivity of bacterial isolates[in Spanish]. Enferm Infecc Microbiol Clin 2002;20(9):422–30.

80. Benlloch S, Berenguer M, Prieto M, et al. De novo internal neoplasms after liver transplantation: increased risk and aggressive behavior in recent years? Am J Transplant 2004;4(4):596–604.

81. Herrero JI. De novo malignancies following liver transplantation: impact and recommendations. Liver Transpl 2009;15(Suppl. 2):S90–4.

82. Margarit C, Lazaro JL, Hidalgo E, et al. Cross-clamping of the three hepatic veins in the piggyback technique is a safe and well tolerated procedure. Transplant Int 1998;11(Suppl. 1):S248–50.

83. Verdonk RC, Buis CI, Porte RJ, et al. Biliary complications after liver transplantation: a review. Scand J Gastroenterol 2006;(Suppl. 243):89–101.

84. Buis CI, Hoekstra H, Verdonk RC, et al. Causes and consequences of ischemic-type biliary lesions after liver transplantation. J Hepatobiliary Pancreat Surg 2006;13(6):517–24.

85. Porrett PM, Hsu J, Shaked A. Late surgical complications following liver transplantation. Liver Transpl 2009;15(Suppl. 2):S12–8.

86. Ben-Ari Z, Pappo O, Mor E. Intrahepatic cholestasis after liver transplantation. Liver Transpl 2003;9(10):1005–18.

87. Quaglia AF, Del Vecchio Blanco G, Greaves R, et al. Development of ductopaenic liver allograft rejection includes a "hepatitic" phase prior to duct loss. J Hepatol 2000;33(5):773–80.

88. Kaneku H, O'Leary JG, Taniguchi M, et al. Donor-specific human leukocyte antigen antibodies of the immunoglobulin G3 subclass are associated with chronic rejection and graft loss after liver transplantation. Liver Transpl 2012;18(8):984–92.

9

Pancreas transplantation

Murat Akyol

Introduction

Transplantation of the pancreas is the only treatment currently available that reliably offers long-term insulin independence and normal glucose metabolism for patients with type I diabetes mellitus.

The first pancreas transplant was performed in the University of Minnesota in 1966.[1] Early experience with pancreatic transplantation was disappointing. This remained so for many years. Difficulties were related to the management of the exocrine secretions and septic complications, a high incidence of thrombosis, acute rejection and pancreatitis. For the first half of its 45-year history, less than 1200 pancreas transplants were performed worldwide. Even after the introduction of ciclosporin, in 1983, 1-year patient and graft survival rates were only 75% and 37%, respectively. Understandably, in the 1970s and 1980s enthusiasm for pancreas transplantation was scarce; the predominant sentiment was scepticism.

Throughout the 1990s significant changes occurred. These came about as a consequence of improvements in organ retrieval and preservation methods, refinements in surgical techniques, advances in immunosuppression, advances in the prophylaxis and treatment of infection, and the experience gained in donor and recipient selection. Success rates following pancreas transplantation are now comparable with other forms of organ transplantation. Around 40 000 pancreas transplants have been performed worldwide. Interestingly, pancreas transplantation has never been compared with insulin therapy in a prospective controlled trial. It is very unlikely that such a trial will ever be performed. However, considerable experience and a substantial body of evidence has accumulated, which now favours the viewpoint of the enthusiasts rather than the sceptics.

Indications for pancreas transplantation

Pancreas transplantation for type II diabetes

Pancreas transplantation aims to provide patients with type I diabetes with an alternative source of insulin. In 1998, Sasaki et al. reported a small number of patients with insulin-requiring type II diabetes who had received pancreas transplants with short-term success.[2] This and a few other single-centre retrospective reports focused on small numbers of patients thought to have type I diabetes at the time of transplant, which were subsequently classified as type II. Whilst short-term outcomes after pancreas transplantation for type II diabetics appeared similar to those with type I diabetes, concern existed about the effect of older age of onset, metabolic syndrome, insulin resistance, higher prevalence of obesity and cardiovascular comorbidity in such patients. It also became clear that no clinical or biochemical test exists that can reliably distinguish type I from type II diabetes mellitus. Neither fasting nor stimulated serum C peptide levels predict insulin production, especially in the presence of renal failure and impaired excretion.[3] Type II diabetes can present at a young age with signs of autoimmunity whereas some with type I diabetes can present later in life with no evidence of an autoimmune disorder. There are in fact reasonable grounds to question the validity of the view that type I and type II diabetes are two distinct disorders with different aetiology and pathogenesis. The 'accelerator hypothesis' considers both types of diabetes to be the same disease of insulin resistance where a specific genetic inheritance and some environmental and behavioural factors determine the age of onset.[4]

The International Pancreas Transplant Registry (IPTR) began recording data on type II diabetes in the mid-1990s. Until 5 years ago, there had been a slow increase in the proportion of simultaneous pancreas–kidney (SPK) transplant recipients reported as having type II diabetes, reaching 7%. This proportion has remained stable over the last 5 years.[5,6] Most registry analyses confirmed that type II diabetics do as well as those with type I following pancreas transplantation.

> ✅ An analysis of 3858 type I versus 292 type II diabetes mellitus cases transplanted between 2004 and 2008 revealed for the first time that type II patients may do less well, having 80% 1-year pancreas graft survival compared with 85% in type I patients.[5]

Pancreas transplantation from living donors

The pancreas transplant database of all US transplants performed between 1967 and 2011 records 72 living-donor transplants out of approximately 25 000 pancreas transplants (0.3%).[6] Only three centres in the USA have performed this procedure, more than 80% of reported cases coming from the University of Minnesota. A recent review article[7] by the authors of the largest series quotes the worldwide experience as approximately 160 cases, with only two centres outside the USA contributing several cases each. One-year pancreas graft survival after living-donor pancreas transplantation in the Minneapolis series was inferior to graft survival after deceased donor transplantation. Long-term outcome was comparable. The experience regarding perioperative morbidity and the long-term risks

for the donor is inadequate to allow comment. It is of concern that only 67 of the first 115 live pancreas donors were traced to complete a follow-up survey. The survey revealed that three of these donors needed to start insulin some time after donation and 10 had elevated HbA1c levels.

The fact that it remains a small fringe activity confined to very few centres presumably indicates that living-donor pancreas transplantation is not endorsed by the transplantation community in general. This is certainly the view that prevails in the UK and the rest of Europe. The discussion in the remainder of this chapter is confined to allogeneic pancreas transplantation from deceased organ donors.

Patient selection for pancreas transplantation

Pancreas transplantation is performed in three distinct clinical settings, as presented below.

Simultaneous pancreas–kidney transplantation (SPK)

There is little debate that diabetic patients with renal failure should be offered kidney transplantation and there is good evidence that their prognosis is poor on dialysis.[8] Such patients will already be obligated to immunosuppression on account of kidney transplantation. Combined kidney and pancreas transplantation offers these patients the opportunity to become insulin independent as well as dialysis independent. The risks and potential benefits of SPK transplantation compared with kidney transplantation alone for diabetic patients are summarised in Box 9.1. The evidence for the risks and benefits alluded to in Box 9.1 is reviewed in the final part of the chapter.

Experience has taught us the crucial importance of recipient selection for success in pancreas transplantation. Cardiovascular comorbidity is the most important factor leading to patient death in the early postoperative period after transplantation in diabetic patients. Patient selection needs to include a comprehensive medical evaluation, ideally performed by a multidisciplinary team within each transplant unit. Asymptomatic ischaemic heart disease is not uncommon in diabetics. The cardiac

Box 9.1 • Potential risks and benefits of simultaneous pancreas–kidney (SPK) transplantation

Risks

Perioperative morbidity and mortality

Potential for pancreas transplant to adversely affect kidney transplant outcome

Consequences of higher immunosuppression

Benefits

Improved quality of life, insulin independence

Potential benefits on diabetic complications

Improved life expectancy

Box 9.2 • Contraindications and risk factors for pancreas transplantation

- Inability to give informed consent
- Active drug abuse
- Major psychiatric illness or non-compliant behaviour
- Recent history of malignancy
- Active infection
- Recent myocardial infarction
- Evidence of significant uncorrectable ischaemic heart disease
- Insufficient cardiac reserve with poor ejection fraction
- Any other illness that significantly restricts life expectancy
- Age greater than 60
- Significant obesity (BMI >30)
- Severe aortoiliac atherosclerosis

assessment should include as a minimum a 12-lead electrocardiogram (ECG), echocardiography, exercise tolerance test and a non-invasive test of myocardial perfusion (a radioisotope scan or dobutamine stress echocardiography). There is insufficient evidence to comment on the value of routine angiography.[9] Any patient with an abnormality detected in non-invasive tests or those with symptoms of ischaemic heart disease should be investigated further, including angiography. Any correctable coronary artery disease should be dealt with prior to transplantation.[10]

✅ Most pancreas transplant units will have an arbitrary and flexible upper age limit – around 50 years – in determining suitability for SPK transplantation. With increasing experience, criteria for suitability of individuals for SPK transplantation have become more liberal. In the USA 19% and 15% of patients receiving SPK transplantation were aged 50 or older in 2004 and 2005, respectively.[11]

Two per cent of SPK transplants between 2006 and 2010 were performed in recipients aged 60 or older. Strong evidence to differentiate between contraindications and relative contraindications does not exist (Box 9.2). Neither blindness nor previous amputation are regarded as contraindications. Hepatitis B, hepatitis C or human immunodeficiency virus (HIV) infection in the potential recipient are not contraindications to pancreas transplantation either. Box 9.2 is intended as a guide only. No attempt has been made to separate absolute and relative contraindications. The use of imprecise definitions such as 'significant', 'severe' or 'recent' is also intentional. Appropriate patient selection requires a balanced assessment by experienced clinicians of the risk factors versus potential benefits.

Pancreas after kidney transplantation (PAK)

Historically, the large majority of pancreas transplants performed have been SPKs. This was largely because of the relatively poor outcomes following solitary pancreas transplantation. Improved success of pancreas transplantation in the last 15 years[12,13] has encouraged many transplant units to offer pancreas transplantation for diabetic patients who have previously undergone successful kidney transplantation. Until the end of 2000, PAK transplants constituted 11% of all pancreas transplants performed in the USA and 5% of pancreas transplants performed outside the USA. Thereafter a rapid increase in PAK transplant rate was observed, reaching a peak of 400 (around a third of all pancreas transplants) in the USA in 2004.[6,11] There has since been a sharp decline in PAK numbers in the USA. More detailed analysis of activity and outcome in different forms of pancreas transplantation is given in the next section.

Contraindications to PAK transplantation are the same as those for SPK (Box 9.2). Within the confines of these contraindications, all diabetics who have previously undergone successful kidney transplantation are potentially suitable candidates for PAK. In practice the procedure is most useful for those diabetics who have a potential living donor for kidney transplantation. Since PAK outcomes are now approaching those of SPK, an elective and early living-donor kidney transplantation has obvious benefits to the potential recipient and has additional benefits to the overall pool of patients awaiting transplantation by releasing another deceased donor kidney. Clearly some time should elapse after kidney transplantation to allow for recovery from surgery and stabilisation of allograft function and immunosuppression. The optimal timing has not been determined. A study comparing early (within the first 4 months) with late (more than 4 months after kidney transplantation) PAK did not reveal any significant difference in the incidence of morbidity or outcome.[14] More recent data suggest that longer intervals (greater than 3 years) between kidney transplantation and subsequent PAK transplantation can be associated with increased risk to the kidney graft.[15]

There are also unique immunological considerations for patients who are being considered for PAK. Previous kidney transplantation may have influenced sensitisation profiles for such patients. In the presence of good renal allograft function and no history of acute rejection following kidney transplantation, shared human leucocyte antigens (HLAs) between the pancreas allograft and the previous renal allograft may have a favourable impact on the outcome, an assertion that remains untested. Whether acute rejection following previous kidney transplantation predisposes PAK recipients to acute rejection of the pancreatic allograft is not known.

An important consideration, in particular for patients who are being assessed some considerable time after kidney transplantation, is the adequacy of kidney function. The level of kidney function at the time of PAK transplantation, independent of the time interval between the two transplants, is a factor associated with mortality risk.[16] Criteria based on strong evidence do not exist but a creatinine clearance of greater than 40 mL/min is a useful guide as a minimum requirement.[17] For recipients of kidney transplants who are not receiving calcineurin inhibitors, a higher creatinine clearance of not less than 55 mL/min is recommended. A renal allograft biopsy prior to PAK is useful for documentation of the baseline renal reserve and for the monitoring of the progression of allograft nephropathy (diabetic or otherwise).

The discussion above relating to SPK and PAK highlights the difficult choice facing patients. The experience of the local pancreas transplant centre, long waiting times for SPK transplantation and individual risk factors (age, obesity, race, etc.) that may adversely affect pancreas transplant outcome may favour early live-donor kidney transplantation followed by PAK. On the other hand, most fit patients in experienced centres without unduly long waiting times are likely to fare better with SPK.[15]

Pancreas transplantation alone (PTA)

Universally agreed criteria that constitute indications for PTA are more difficult to find compared with those for SPK or PAK. The risk of transplantation for non-uraemic diabetics needs to take account of not only perioperative morbidity but also long-term risks associated with immunosuppression. At present the majority of patients developing type I diabetes will be better served by insulin injections at the onset of disease. Clear indications for PTA are life-threatening complications of diabetes in patients managed with insulin, namely intractable hypoglycaemic unawareness and cardiac autonomic neuropathy. In these two subpopulations of diabetic patients pancreas transplantation is truly life saving. Other indications for PTA are more controversial. The presence of two or more diabetic complications has been advocated as an indication.[18] In the absence of conclusive data on some of the diabetic complications, as reviewed in the final section of this chapter, it is difficult to defend the logic behind the assertion that two or more complications constitute an indication for PTA. Disabling and intractable symptoms of diabetic neuropathy or early nephropathy with preserved renal function may be considered as indications. In diabetics with overt nephropathy and impaired renal function, the nephrotoxicity of the immunosuppressive drugs will need to be considered. Available evidence does not permit precise guidelines but patients with creatinine clearance less than 40 mL/min may be better served by SPK transplantation.

Pancreas transplantation activity worldwide

At the beginning of 2011 the total number of pancreas transplants performed worldwide was close to 40 000.[6] Nearly two-thirds of these have been performed in the USA. The International Pancreas Transplantation Registry (IPTR) shares US transplant data with the United Network for Organ Sharing (UNOS). Reporting of data to the UNOS is compulsory, hence IPTR data regarding US pancreas transplantation activity are accurate and complete. Non-US pancreas transplants are reported to the IPTR on a voluntary basis. Some national organisations, such as Eurotransplant, share data with the international registry. The IPTR estimates that around 90% of non-US transplants are reported. Worldwide pancreas transplantation activity reported in a Council of Europe document suggests[19] that a much greater proportion of non-US transplants are missing from the IPTR database (**Fig. 9.1**). Despite this probable under-representation of non-US transplants, there seems to be a genuine difference in the utilisation of pancreas transplantation between the USA and the remainder of the world. **Figure 9.2** shows worldwide pancreas transplantation activity as recorded by the IPTR at the beginning of 2011.[6]

In the USA, SPK transplantation activity reached a peak of 972 transplants in 1998. Thereafter there has been a continuous slow decline in SPK activity, with just over 800 SPK transplants recorded in 2010. Solitary pancreas transplantation activity (PAK+PTA) continued to increase until 2004, reaching a peak of 520 transplants in 2004 (**Fig. 9.3**). Since then there has been a decline. The decline in the number of solitary pancreas transplants, in particular PAK transplants, has been sharper than the reduction in SPK numbers. In 2010 less than half as many PAK transplants were performed in the USA compared with 2004.

The total numbers of pancreas transplants performed in the UK and in the Eurotransplant zone are shown in Table 9.1 for comparison.[20,21] In Europe, within the Eurotransplant zone, pancreas transplantation activity has declined slowly since the peak of 2003. In the UK pancreas transplantation activity reached a peak in 2007 and some decline has occurred since. Pancreas transplant rate (the number of transplants per million population per annum) in the UK exceeded that of the Eurotransplant area in 2006 and has remained well above the Eurotransplant rate since then.

The age profile of pancreas transplant recipients has changed markedly over the last two decades. In the USA between 1987 and 1992, 9% of pancreas transplant recipients were older than 45. This proportion had risen to 34% in 2000–2004 and further to 41% in 2006–2010.[6,11]

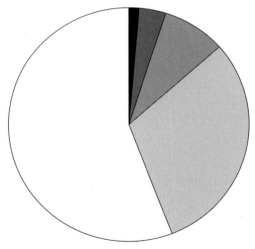

	Number of transplants	Population (millions)
☐ USA	1387	301
▥ Europe	762	488
▦ Latin America	214	470
▨ Canada	90	33
■ Australia/New Zealand	34	23

Figure 9.1 • Pancreas transplants performed worldwide in 2006. Data from International Figures on Organ Donation and Transplantation 2006. Transplant Newsletter 12(1), September 2007. Council of Europe.

✓ Management of exocrine secretions has also seen significant change (**Fig. 9.4**). Enteric drainage has been the predominant method in Europe but in the USA until the mid-1990s less than 10% of pancreas transplants were enterically drained. Enteric drainage has since surged in popularity in the USA also. Between 1996 and 2002 about half of US solitary pancreas transplants and two-thirds of US SPK transplants were enterically drained. In 2004 this proportion reached 81% for SPK transplants and exceeded 90% in 2010.[6,11]

✓✓ Enteric drainage has emerged as the preferred method of exocrine drainage worldwide in all but a small proportion of pancreas transplants.

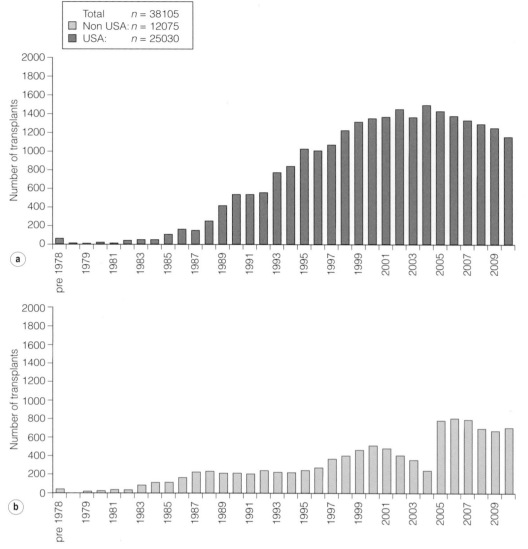

Figure 9.2 • Pancreas transplants reported to the International Pancreas Transplant Registry (1 January 2011). **(a)** USA. **(b)** Non-USA.

Portal venous drainage gained in popularity in the mid-1990s. In the USA between 1996 and 2002, 1091 of the 4394 (25%) enterically drained primary SPK cases have been performed with the portal venous drainage technique.[6] There has since been a decline in the utilisation of portal venous drainage, with recorded rates of 18% in SPK and PAK transplants and 10% in PTA transplants in 2010.[6]

Other demographic data for patients transplanted in the USA between 2004 and 2009 are summarised in Table 9.2.

The pancreas donor and the organ retrieval procedure

Criteria for eligibility for pancreas donors

Contraindications to organ donation are clinical HIV infection, diagnosis of Creutzfeldt–Jakob disease (CJD), history of malignancy (except non-melanoma skin cancer and certain primary central nervous system tumours) and active systemic sepsis.

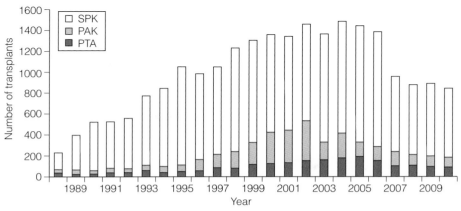

Figure 9.3 • Pancreas transplant activity by category of transplant in the USA.

Table 9.1 • Pancreas transplantation activity in the Eurotransplant area and in the United Kingdom

	Eurotransplant*		United Kingdom	
Year	**No. of transplants**	**pmp†**	**No. of transplants**	**pmp**
2000	309	2.58	33	0.56
2001	267	2.23	47	0.78
2002	337	2.81	60	1.0
2003	385	3.21	54	0.9
2004	334	2.78	79	1.31
2005	302	2.52	118	1.96
2006	245	2.04	162	2.69
2007	249	2.08	221	3.68
2008	257	2.14	214	3.57
2009	226	1.88	199	3.32
2010	273	2.28	188	3.18

*Eurotransplant zone includes Austria, Belgium, Croatia, Germany, Luxembourg, the Netherlands and Slovenia.
†pmp = per million population.

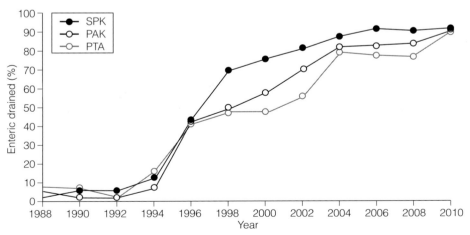

Figure 9.4 • Evolution of exocrine management technique in pancreas transplantation. US pancreas transplants 1 January 1988–31 December 2010. Data from the IPTR.

Table 9.2 • Patient characteristics for USA primary deceased donor pancreas transplants (January 2004 to January 2009)

	SPK	PAK	PTA
No. of transplants (%)	4320 (73%)	1148 (19%)	494 (8%)
Recipient age			
<15	3	–	–
15–29	312	60	75
30–44	2396	628	236
45–49	1556	447	168
>60	53	13	15
Gender			
Male	2728 (63%)	665 (58%)	
Female	1592 (37%)	483 (42%)	
Ethnicity			
Caucasian	3160 (77%)	971 (88%)	464 (95%)
All other ethnic groups	979 (23%)	133 (12%)	22 (5%)
Proportion with type II diabetes	7%	4%	3%
Exocrine management			
Enteric drainage	3656 (90%)	936 (85%)	383 (80%)
Bladder drainage	417 (10%)	172 (15%)	99 (20%)
Venous management			
Systemic	2871 (79%)	778 (83%)	324 (85%)
Portal	770 (21%)	157 (17%)	58 (15%)
Waiting time (months)			
0–5	1824	471	303
6–11	940	281	95
12–17	621	169	37
18–23	370	89	31
>24	565	138	28
Transplant centre volume			
Low-volume centre	2689 (62%)	744 (65%)	215 (44%)
High volume centre	1631 (38%)	404 (35%)	279 (66%)

Additional specific contraindications to pancreas donation are the presence of diabetes mellitus or gross pancreatic disease in the donor (including trauma, acute or chronic pancreatitis, excessive fatty infiltration). Neither hyperglycaemia nor hyperamylasaemia should preclude pancreas donation providing the pancreas appears normal on inspection. Increasing donor age, cerebrovascular/cardiovascular cause of death and donor obesity are associated with poorer pancreas transplant outcomes.[22–24] A precise upper age limit for pancreas donors is difficult to define because of many confounding variables, the retrospective nature of the studies and small sample sizes of individual reports. IPTR analyses use 45 as the age cut-off distinguishing 'young' and 'old' donors. Historically no more than 3% of US pancreas donors were older than 49 and this has remained largely unchanged.[6,11] In practice an upper age limit of around 55 is used by most transplant units worldwide. The general consensus is that the ideal pancreas donor will be younger than 45.

It is similarly difficult to quote an acceptable weight limit for donors. Body mass index (BMI) >30 should be regarded as a relative contraindication. Pancreas grafts from paediatric donors (age >4 years) and selected non-heart-beating donors can be used with excellent results.[25,26] The influence of donor related factors on pancreas transplant outcome is discussed on p. 168.

Pancreas retrieval operation

The pancreas is a close neighbour of the liver and shares important vascular structures with it. During multiorgan retrieval procedures priority clearly needs to be given to the liver. The key to successful retrieval of both the liver and the pancreas is good cooperation between the two retrieval teams. The optimum scenario is for both organs to be retrieved and transplanted by the same team. Specific anomalies in the arterial blood supply to the liver that preclude successful liver and successful pancreas transplantation are very rare.

It is not intended to give a detailed description of the surgical procedure for pancreas retrieval in this section, but several pertinent points about pancreatic retrieval from multiorgan donors are highlighted below.

University of Wisconsin (UW) solution was first developed as a pancreatic preservation solution[27] and remains the benchmark for pancreas preservation. Other preservation solutions have been used but experience with these is more limited.[28] Recent experience with histidine–tryptophan–ketoglutarate (HTK) solution and Celsior solution suggests that both these solutions perform equally well as UW solution with short (<12 h) ischaemia times. UW solution may perform better in longer cold ischaemia times exceeding 12 hours (for further details see Chapter 6).[29]

The cold ischaemia tolerance of the pancreas is somewhere between that of the liver and the kidney. In pancreas allografts perfused with UW solution, 20 hours was thought to be the limit for successful preservation, beyond which a time-dependent deterioration in outcome occurred.[30] Earlier data failed to demonstrate a clear benefit from a preservation time cut-off below 20 hours. Most surgeons intuitively aim for shorter preservation times. The mean (± SE) preservation time for the 2000–2004 cohort of pancreas transplants in the USA was 13.3 (± 5.9) hours for SPK, 15.3 (± 5.5) hours for PAK and 16.2 (± 5.8) hours for the PTA group.[31]

More recent data suggest that ischaemia time is of greater importance in recipients of suboptimal grafts and in such cases ischaemia times over 12 hours are likely to be associated with poorer outcomes. Registry data reveal that pancreas transplant surgeons have taken this message on board, resulting in a trend towards shorter preservation times. The median cold ischaemia time for all US pancreas transplants has been under 12 hours since 2006.[32,33]

The pressure gradient between mean arterial pressure and portal venous pressure that maintains blood flow through the pancreas can be significantly diminished during the perfusion of the abdominal organs in retrieval operations. Particular attention is required to maintain an adequate gradient if a cannula for perfusion is placed in the portal venous system as well as the aorta. Many transplant units perfuse abdominal organs with an aortic cannula only. Some evidence supports the view that additional portal perfusion is unnecessary.[34] For the interests of the pancreatic allograft, aortic perfusion alone is the most 'physiological' state that allows satisfactory perfusion and adequate drainage of the effluent.

It is common practice to flush the donor duodenum through a nasogastric tube with an antiseptic or antibiotic solution during the retrieval operation. No evidence exists to demonstrate the superiority of any solution used for duodenal decontamination.

Povidone–iodine during cold storage may be toxic to duodenal mucosa.[35] If povidone–iodine is used for flushing the allograft duodenal segment during organ retrieval, further flushing of the duodenal segment with preservation solution on the back table should be considered.

Donor duodenal contents should be submitted for bacterial and fungal culture. The results may be important in guiding the management of infection in pancreas transplant recipients.[36]

- Careful and minimal handling of the pancreas during retrieval is important. Removal of the spleen and the pancreatico-duodenal graft en bloc with the liver is the quickest and safest method for both organs. The organs are then easily and quickly separated on the back table at the retrieval centre.
- Further back-table preparation of the pancreas, which takes place in the recipient centre, is a crucial part of the procedure and takes a minimum of 2 hours. The short stumps of the gastroduodenal artery (GDA) and the splenic artery should be marked with fine polypropylene sutures at the time of retrieval. Demonstration of good collateral circulation within the pancreatico-duodenal arcade

(between the superior mesenteric artery (SMA) and the GDA) by flushing the arteries individually at the back table is reassuring. An iliac artery Y graft of donor origin anastomosed to the SMA and the splenic artery is the most common method of reconstruction for the graft arterial inflow (**Fig. 9.5**). Meticulous dissection and ligation of the lymphatic tissue and small vessels around the pancreas is important to prevent haemorrhage upon reperfusion of the graft in the recipient. Particular attention should be paid to secure the duodenal segment staple lines by inversion with further sutures.

Pancreaticoduodenal graft excised with an aortic patch

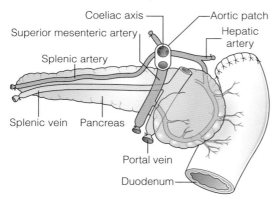

Reconstruction of arterial vessels

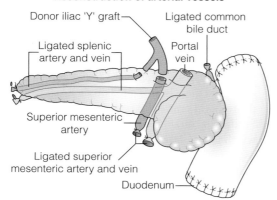

Figure 9.5 • In the absence of an aortic patch containing hepatic artery and the gastroduodenal artery, the pancreatic graft reconstruction requires a donor iliac 'Y' graft.

The pancreas transplant operation

General considerations

In SPK transplantation, pancreatic implantation is usually performed first because of the lower ischaemia tolerance of the pancreas. It is easier to implant the pancreatic graft on the right side. The renal allograft can also be placed intra-abdominally with anastomoses to the left iliac vessels. Alternatively, and perhaps more easily, an extraperitoneal renal transplant on the left side can be performed using the same incision or through a separate left iliac fossa incision. A further and equally satisfactory alternative is to implant the renal graft ipsilaterally, using more caudal segments of the recipient right iliac vessels.

In PAK transplantation, even in the presence of a right-sided renal allograft, the preferred site for the pancreas would be on the right-hand side cranial to the renal allograft. The arterial inflow to the pancreatic allograft usually comes from the right common iliac artery. Unless the lower aorta is clamped the renal graft does not suffer any ischaemia during pancreatic implantation.

Severely atherosclerotic and calcified vessels in some diabetic recipients can be a challenge during pancreatic implantation. Iliac Y grafts used for reconstruction offer greater flexibility in choosing a suitable arterial anastomotic site in the recipient vessels.

In the last 10 years the most common technique used for pancreas transplantation has been intra-abdominal implantation of the whole pancreas together with a donor duodenal segment. A list of previously employed techniques is given below (these are all associated with poorer outcomes and are rarely performed nowadays):

- segmental pancreas transplantation using only the tail and the body of the pancreas;
- pancreatic duct occlusion or ligation;
- free drainage of exocrine secretions into the peritoneal cavity;
- direct anastomosis of the transected pancreatic head into the bladder;
- utilisation of a small duodenal button.

Currently the choices available to the surgeon are related to the management of the exocrine secretions and the management of the venous drainage, as discussed below.

Management of exocrine secretions

Drainage of the exocrine secretions of pancreatic grafts into the recipient's bladder was the most common technique, accounting for 90% of US pancreas transplants during the 1980s and early 1990s. The popularity of this technique was due to its perceived safety, primarily less serious consequences of anastomotic leaks (compared with enteric drainage) in the days of higher corticosteroids and unrefined immunosuppression. The ability to monitor amylase levels in the urine has been considered an additional advantage of bladder drainage. The latter point is contentious. The evidence with respect to the usefulness of urinary amylase monitoring is reviewed later in this chapter. The unphysiological diversion of pancreatic exocrine secretions into the urinary bladder causes frequent complications, often leading to chronic and disabling symptoms. As a consequence, conversion of the urinary diversion to enteric drainage is required in many patients. Complications of pancreatic transplantation, including specific problems associated with bladder drainage, are discussed in detail later in the chapter.

As discussed earlier, enteric drainage has replaced bladder drainage as the method of choice for the management of exocrine secretions in the USA. Data regarding the prevalence of enteric versus bladder drainage for pancreas transplantation in Europe are not easy to find. Historically, enteric drainage has been the preferred method in Europe and it is likely that the majority of European pancreas transplant units employ this technique.

Any part of the recipient's small bowel can be used for anastomosis with the allograft duodenum. No data exist to demonstrate the superiority of one particular site over others. Roux-en-Y loops, which were commonly used, are becoming rare and a simple side-to-side entero-enterostomy is preferred.[31]

Delayed endocrine function from the transplanted graft is uncommon and insulin infusion should be discontinued at the time of reperfusion. Achieving insulin independence for the first time in many years in the recipient is a gratifying part of the operation for the surgeon. Patients can become hypoglycaemic at this stage. Blood sugar levels should be checked frequently and a low rate of dextrose infusion is often required.

Management of the venous drainage

Drainage of the venous outflow from pancreas grafts into the portal circulation was first described by Calne in 1984.[37] This complex surgical technique using a segmental graft and gastric exocrine diversion in a paratopic position has never gained popularity. Drainage of the venous outflow into the systemic circulation at the level of the lower inferior vena cava has been the norm in pancreatic transplantation. Since the mid-1990s there has been a resurgence of interest in portal venous (PV) drainage. The technique described by Shokouh-Amiri et al.[38] involves placement of the graft slightly more cranially in the abdominal cavity, with the utilisation of the superior mesenteric vein (SMV) for the venous drainage. Several studies, including prospective randomised comparisons, have shown that this offers at least equivalent outcome to that of systemic venous (SV) drainage, with no compromise in safety.[39–41] The impetus for PV drainage was to achieve a more physiological insulin delivery. A theoretical benefit was considered to be avoidance of hyperinsulinaemia, which has been linked with atherogenesis.[42] Systemic drainage does not always cause hyperinsulinaemia. Nor may it be the only factor, since hyperinsulinaemia occurs in non-diabetic recipients of kidney transplants receiving steroids.[43,44] None of the studies of metabolic function after PV drainage have shown a clear benefit in terms of glucose metabolism, lipid profiles or atherogenesis. There is some evidence suggestive of an immunological advantage to PV drainage in the form of a reduction in the incidence of acute rejection. The mode of antigen delivery is known to modulate the immune response, which has been proposed as the mechanism responsible for the observed reduction in acute rejection rates in portal venous drained grafts.[39–41]

Technically, PV drainage may be attractive for retransplants or for patients who have had previous lower abdominal surgery. It requires the use of a long donor iliac Y graft to reach a suitable arterial anastomotic site on the recipient vessels. Suturing the graft portal vein to the recipient SMV or its main feeding tributary requires delicate handling of these fragile vessels. In obese patients and in those with thickened or foreshortened bowel mesentery, the SMV may not be easily accessible and PV drainage may be difficult to perform.

Immunosuppression in pancreas transplantation

Historically there is ample evidence that the incidence of acute rejection is higher after pancreas transplantation compared with kidney transplantation.[18,30] The reasons for this difference are not clear. Nevertheless, there has been general acknowledgement of the higher immunological risk of pancreas transplantation. This has resulted in the evolution of strategies that employ more intense immunosuppressive protocols for pancreas transplantation compared with kidney transplantation.

In Europe immunosuppressive protocols in solid-organ transplantation in general have been less aggressive compared with the USA. In the evolution of immunosuppression for pancreas transplantation tacrolimus has largely replaced ciclosporin starting from the mid-1990s. Similarly, mycophenolate mofetil (MMF) has replaced azathioprine in most immunosuppressive protocols (**Fig. 9.6**). There is a sound evidence base for this evolution. This evidence, reviewed below, has been provided not only by single-centre reports or registry analyses but also by prospective randomised trials.

Two prospective controlled studies and many single-centre reports and registry analyses have demonstrated improved outcomes with tacrolimus in pancreas transplant recipients compared with

ciclosporin.[45–47] MMF has been shown to reduce the incidence of acute rejection compared with azathioprine in two large prospective randomised trials in the USA and Europe in kidney transplant recipients[48,49] and one prospective randomised trial in pancreas transplant recipients.[50]

Other studies have compared rapamycin versus MMF in tacrolimus-based protocols. A multicentre study of 167 patients found no significant differences in any of the outcome measures comparing the two agents.[51] A small single-centre prospective randomised trial of tacrolimus/MMF versus tacrolimus/rapamycin and steroid withdrawal at 6 months in PAK transplant recipients showed similar outcome for primary end-points (patient survival, graft survival, graft loss from rejection). Wound infections, intra-abdominal infections and the need for lipid-lowering agents at 1 year was higher with rapamycin.[52] Another small single-centre prospective randomised trial compared rapamycin with MMF, in the setting of antibody induction and tacrolimus/steroid maintenance. A significantly higher incidence of acute rejection was noted in the MMF group and the tolerability of MMF was poorer.[53]

Steroid withdrawal or avoidance has been a focus of study in the last decade. There is as yet no evidence demonstrating significant benefit from steroid avoidance or withdrawal but experience reveals that it is feasible without adversely affecting outcome in pancreas transplant patients.[52,54]

Figure 9.7 shows the use of antibody therapy as part of the induction immunosuppression in pancreas transplant recipients. Induction therapy with biological agents is used more often for pancreas transplant recipients compared with recipients of any other solid-organ transplant. In the early years of pancreas transplantation (1987–1993) 90% of pancreas transplant recipients were given antibody induction. This gradually decreased to 83% in 1994–1997 and to 76% for those transplanted in 2001. There has since been a gradual increase again in the use of antibodies for induction. In 2005, 88% of SPK and 85% of PAK transplant recipients were given antibodies as part of their induction immunosuppression. The most recent report of the IPTR shows that antibody induction remains part of the immunosuppressive protocol in nearly all pancreas transplants.[6]

Studies of induction therapy with antithymocyte globulin (ATG) or OKT3 were conducted in the

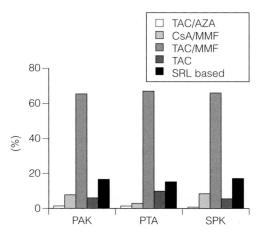

Figure 9.6 • Immunosuppressive protocols used for maintenance in pancreas transplant recipients in the USA. US primary deceased donor pancreas transplants 1 January 2000–6 June 2004. CsA, ciclosporin; MMF, mycophenolate mofetil; SRL, sirolimus; TAC, tacrolimus. Data from the IPTR.

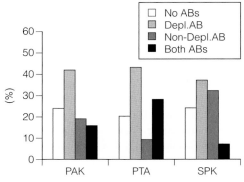

Figure 9.7 • The use of biological agents as part of induction in pancreas transplantation in the USA. US primary deceased donor pancreas transplants 1 January 2000–6 June 2004. Depl. AB, depleting antibodies; Non-Depl. AB, non-depleting antibodies. Data from the IPTR.

early 1990s, in the ciclosporin era. Two prospective multicentre randomised trials[55,56] show that these agents delay the onset and lessen the severity of rejection episodes at the expense of increased cytomegalovirus (CMV) disease but with no demonstrable influence on patient survival. Pancreas graft survival in the medium term, in this Sandimmune era, was better in patients given ATG or OKT3 for induction.

Two prospective randomised multicentre studies were published in 2003 investigating the role of induction therapy combined with tacrolimus- and MMF-based immunosuppression. Stratta et al. reported a significant reduction in the incidence of kidney and pancreas rejection with daclizumab induction.[57] Adverse events, including infectious complications, were not different with or without induction therapy. A modified two-dose daclizumab regime gave overall better results than the standard five-dose regime. Another prospective randomised trial at 18 US centres compared induction using any one of the biological agents (OKT3, ATG, basiliximab or daclizumab) with no induction.[58] A trend towards reduction in the incidence of acute rejection by induction therapy was seen. The 1-year incidence of acute rejection (kidney or pancreas) was 24.6% and 31.2% in induction therapy and control groups, respectively (P=0.28). The incidence of biopsy-confirmed acute kidney allograft rejection was 13.1% and 23% (P=0.08). No clear and consistent pattern emerges to demonstrate the superiority of any one of the biological agents discussed above, when used in conjunction with tacrolimus-based immunosuppression.

> ✔ More recent evidence from a single-centre randomised comparison suggests that alemtuzumab induction is associated with similar graft and patient survival rates compared with ATG induction, but results in lower incidence of acute rejection and better safety profile, with significantly lower incidence of CMV infection.[59]

Individualised immunosuppressive therapy is required for the greater immunological risk in young patients, black patients and recipients of re-transplants. SPK transplant recipients with delayed graft function can be maintained on antibodies for longer periods and commence calcineurin inhibitors late, after the kidney function starts to improve. Older recipients require less potent immunosuppression.

Acute rejection following pancreas transplantation

Diagnosis of acute rejection

One of the notable features about pancreas transplantation over the last 15 years has been the considerable reduction in the incidence of acute rejection. In 1992, 74% of SPK transplant recipients and 50% of solitary pancreas transplant recipients (this probably underestimates the true incidence) were reported to have received anti-rejection therapy.[18,30] This had reduced to 19% and 17%, respectively, by 2000.[31]

An important feature of pancreatic graft rejection, for the purposes of patient management, is the lack of a reliable early marker. In SPK transplants diagnosis of acute rejection almost completely relies on monitoring of the renal allograft function by serum creatinine levels and further assessment when indicated by renal biopsy. Discordant rejection of allografts is thought to occur rarely following SPK transplantation. Isolated rejection of the pancreas is said to represent no more than 5–10% of acute rejection episodes.[18] Direct evidence from series with simultaneous kidney and pancreas biopsies has been limited until recently. Experimental work in dogs by the Westmead team in Sydney showed isolated pancreas rejection to occur with an incidence of no more than 2% following combined kidney and pancreas transplantation.[60] The most convincing evidence for the security of the implied diagnosis of rejection in the pancreas by diagnosing kidney rejection comes from consistent clinical observations of higher pancreatic graft survival rates following SPK transplantation compared with solitary pancreas transplantation. Monitoring for acute rejection and patient management in the early postoperative period is therefore a particular challenge in solitary pancreas transplants.

Acute rejection of the pancreas affects the exocrine pancreas first. The inflammation may cause pain and a low-grade fever associated with a rise in serum amylase. These symptoms and signs are non-specific, can be subtle and do not distinguish between acute rejection and other causes of graft inflammation (such as ischaemia–reperfusion injury or allograft pancreatitis). Islets of Langerhans are scattered sparsely throughout the exocrine pancreas and beta cells have considerable functional reserve. Therefore, dysfunction of the majority of islets resulting in hyperglycaemia as a consequence of rejection occurs only very late in the course of pancreatic rejection. Imaging modalities such as computed tomography (CT) or magnetic resonance imaging (MRI) visualise the pancreas and are helpful to exclude other pathology (such as lack of perfusion, which may be segmental or intra-abdominal collections). There are no specific signs of acute rejection on any radiological investigation. Unlike the kidney, the pancreas lacks a firm capsule. Therefore, vascular resistance is not reliably altered as a consequence of inflammation and duplex scan monitoring is not useful. Detection of urinary amylase in bladder-drained grafts is a sensitive indicator of exocrine function. However, detection of hypoamylasuria lacks specificity. Factors other than acute rejection such as diuresis or fasting also cause hypoamylasuria.[61] Greater than 25% reduction in urinary amylase correlates with acute rejection in no more than half of the cases when assessed by biopsy.[62] A stable urinary amylase may therefore be helpful in excluding acute rejection but detection of hypoamylasuria is non-specific and unhelpful. Other tests have been shown to be better correlated with early endocrine dysfunction of pancreas grafts, such as glucose disappearance rate or insulin secretion dynamics following an intravenous glucose load.[63] Owing to their complexity and lack of availability, such tests are not practical for use as routine daily monitoring tools in patient management.

Pancreas allograft biopsy has recently become established as a reliable and safe technique and is the gold standard in the diagnosis of acute rejection in solitary pancreas transplants. Percutaneous biopsy under ultrasound or CT guidance is the most common method. Histological criteria for the diagnosis and grading of rejection have been standardised.[64]

Histological examinations of pancreas graft biopsies correlated with clinical and serological findings have revealed two distinct pathways of rejection (similar to the more widely recognised pattern in kidney transplantation): T-cell-mediated rejection and antibody-mediated rejection.

> ✅ A recent article by Papadimitriou and Drachenberg[65] provides an authoritative and up-to-date review of the histological criteria for these two subtypes of acute pancreas allograft rejection, as well as mechanisms leading to graft injury and differential diagnosis.

The recognition of antibody-mediated rejection as a distinct entity in pancreas transplantation explains conflicting results in published data from earlier years showing some cases of treatment-resistant acute pancreas allograft rejection thought to be cell-mediated rejection. It also partially explains the success rate of clinical programmes with much improved success in solitary pancreas transplantation as a consequence of liberal use of surveillance biopsies.[59] Finally, the increasing utilisation of pancreas allograft biopsies has cast doubt on the validity of the assumption that isolated rejection of the kidney or the pancreas graft in SPK recipients is uncommon.

Management of acute rejection

Recipients of pancreas transplants have more to lose than recipients of other organ transplants from unnecessary treatment for presumed acute rejection. Diagnosis of acute rejection of the pancreas should always be confirmed histologically prior to the institution of treatment. The recent evidence allowing the distinction between cell-mediated and antibody-mediated acute rejection[63,65] provides a further rationale for pancreas allograft biopsies.

Early or mild cell-mediated acute rejection of the pancreas allograft concurrent with kidney rejection can be successfully treated with high-dose corticosteroids. Recurrent acute rejection or moderate to severe rejection episodes require treatment with anti-T-cell agents. IPTR data show that steroids were used in 85% of SPK and 80% of solitary pancreas transplant recipients diagnosed as having acute rejection.[31] However, 48% of SPK recipients and 80% of solitary pancreas recipients with acute rejection were given anti-T-cell agents also, suggesting that many patients were treated with both. There are not enough data to make evidence-based recommendations on the optimum treatment for acute antibody-mediated rejection. Experience with the management of antibody-mediated rejection in kidney transplantation would suggest a potential role for plasma exchange with or without intravenous immunoglobulin and/or rituximab.

Acute rejection in pancreas allografts is not life threatening and caution is advised against overimmunosuppression. If diagnosed before the onset of hyperglycaemia most rejection episodes are reversible.

Impact of acute rejection on outcome

The UNOS data for 4251 patients who received SPK transplants between 1988 and 1997 were analysed by Reddy et al. in order to determine the influence of acute rejection on long-term outcome.[66] Acute rejection of either graft increased the relative risk of pancreas and kidney graft failure at 5 years. The relative risks, adjusted for other risk factors, were 1.32 and 1.53 for pancreas and kidney, respectively, if acute rejection occurred. In this analysis 45% of the cohort had no acute rejection. The worst outcome was in patients who had both kidney and pancreas rejection.

Complications of pancreas transplantation

Introduction

Pancreas transplantation is associated with a higher incidence and a greater range of complications than kidney transplantation, and the postoperative patient management constitutes a greater challenge (Box 9.3). Between a quarter and a third of patients require re-laparotomy following pancreas transplantation to deal with complications. Part of the reason for the increased incidence of complications is the higher level of immunosuppression in a high-risk diabetic population who already exhibit impaired infection resistance, poor healing and a

---

Box 9.3 • Complications of pancreas transplantation

Vascular complications
- Thrombosis: allograft venous or arterial thrombosis
- Haemorrhage: early haemorrhage from allograft vessels and late haemorrhage (rupture of pseudoaneurysms)

Infective complications
- Systemic infection: opportunistic infections associated with immunosuppression
- Local infections: peritonitis, localised collections, enteric or pancreatic fistulas

Allograft pancreatitis
- Ischaemia–reperfusion injury or reflux pancreatitis (especially after bladder drainage)

Complications specific to bladder drainage
- Chronic dehydration, acidosis, recurrent urinary tract infections, haematuria, chemical cystitis, urethral strictures or urethral disruption

---

high prevalence of comorbidity. Other factors relate to the allograft, which unlike kidney or liver allografts is not sterile and uniquely possesses rich proteolytic enzymes, making it susceptible to specific complications such as secondary haemorrhage, pancreatitis, leaks and fistula formation. The blood flow to the pancreas is much lower compared with the kidney. This is a further risk factor specifically for thrombotic complications. Finally, bladder drainage of the exocrine secretions is associated with a high incidence of complications unique to this unphysiological diversion.

Increasing donor age, prolonged preservation time, recipient obesity and donor obesity are factors associated with increased probability of complications and early graft loss.

Vascular complications

Thrombosis

Allograft venous or arterial thrombosis occurs more commonly following pancreatic transplantation compared with kidney transplantation. Venous thrombosis is more common than arterial thrombosis by a factor of 2:1.[67] Graft thrombosis is by far the most common cause of early graft loss following pancreas transplantation. An analysis of US pancreas transplants performed until the end of 2008 reveals that 5% of SPK transplants and 7%

Table 9.3 • Causes of early graft loss after pancreas transplantation in USA primary deceased donor pancreas transplants (January 2004 to January 2009)

Causes of early graft loss	SPK n=4320	PAK n=1148	PTA n=494
Thrombosis	5.1%	7.4%	6.6%
Infection	0.6%	0.8%	0.4%
Pancreatitis	0.6%	0.4%	0.4%
Anastomotic leak	0.4%	0.2%	0.3%
Bleeding	0.2%	0.3%	0.3%
Total graft loss	6.9%	9.1%	7.9%

SPK, simultaneous pancreas–kidney transplants; PAK, pancreas after kidney transplants; PTA, pancreas transplantation alone.

of solitary pancreas transplants fail as a result of thrombosis[66] (Table 9.3). Among the recognised risk factors for thrombosis, donor-related factors have the greatest impact. These include donor age, donor BMI, cardiovascular and cerebrovascular cause of donor death, prolonged preservation time, excessive flush volumes and pressure, and the type of preservation solution. As discussed before,[29] the use of HTK solution may be associated with inferior outcome compared with UW solution. The effect of HTK may partly be because of the lower viscosity, hence the larger volumes traditionally used. It is also dependent on preservation time. HTK appears to be a risk factor only when cold ischaemia time exceeds 12 hours.[29,67,68]

IPTR data suggest that solitary pancreas transplantation and enteric drainage in some categories of pancreas transplantation may be associated with a marginally higher risk of thrombosis.[6] This may reflect the higher probability of rejection-related graft thrombosis, in particular in enteric-drained solitary transplants, rather than being a function of the exocrine drainage method per se.[68] Ciclosporin compared with tacrolimus has been shown to be a risk factor for thrombosis in a randomised controlled trial.[69] Intravenous administration of tacrolimus, now virtually abandoned, may be associated with increased risk of thrombosis. Of greater clinical relevance is a recent publication reporting pancreas graft thrombosis associated with the administration of intravenous immunoglobulin.[70] A technical factor predisposing to thrombosis could be the use of venous extension grafts for the portal vein anastomosis, which should be only very rarely required. Concern about a potentially higher incidence of thrombosis following portal venous drainage has not been borne out by clinical experience. There is no difference in the incidence of technical failure

rate with portal venous drainage compared with systemic venous drainage.

Graft thrombosis, once diagnosed, requires prompt laparotomy and graft pancreatectomy. There are reports of surgical, radiological and pharmacological interventions in small numbers of cases.[71–73] Virtually all of these refer to highly selected cases of segmental, incomplete thrombosis.

Routine use of heparin for prophylaxis against allograft vascular thrombosis is used by some but is not standard practice in many units and will be associated with increased haemorrhage risk. Published evidence does not permit recommendations for a universal or selective anticoagulation policy. The authors from the University of Minnesota have reported a small reduction in the incidence of graft thrombosis with heparin.[30]

Table 9.3 illustrates the relative prevalence of early complications of pancreas transplantation leading to graft loss from the IPTR database.

Haemorrhage

Release of the vascular clamps and reperfusion of the pancreatic allograft during the recipient operation can be tricky, with potential for bleeding from multiple points on the allograft. The key to avoiding this is meticulous preparation of the allograft on the back table prior to implantation.

Haemorrhage in the early postoperative hours is often a result of the proteolytic and fibrinolytic activity of the pancreatic exocrine secretions leaking from the surface of the pancreas and coming into contact with thrombus-sealing small vessels or with vascular anastomoses. This is a complication unique to pancreas transplantation. Early postoperative bleeding is the most common indication for re-laparotomy after pancreas transplantation. Unlike graft thrombosis however, bleeding has little impact on ultimate outcome. Less than 1% of pancreas grafts are lost to bleeding[69] (Table 9.3).

Late haemorrhage following pancreas transplantation is an uncommon but catastrophic complication, often due to the rupture of a pseudoaneurysm or direct erosion of one of the anastomoses secondary to a leak. Any unexplained fever, tachycardia, leucocytosis or abdominal pain in recipients of pancreas transplants should lead to investigations to look for a leak or an intra-abdominal collection.

Infective complications

Pancreas transplantation, in common with all transplant procedures that require immunosuppression, is associated with an increased risk of mostly opportunistic infections. CMV disease is more common after pancreas transplantation compared with kidney or liver transplantation. Antiviral prophylaxis in CMV-mismatched donor/recipient pairs is mandatory. Unique to pancreatic transplantation are intra-abdominal septic complications, which occur as a consequence of bacteria or fungi transmitted from the donor via the allograft or as a consequence of anastomotic leaks. Patients on peritoneal dialysis at the time of transplantation have a higher rate of intra-abdominal infection compared with those on haemodialysis.[30]

Intra-abdominal infections can be localised or diffuse and often occur within the first 4–6 weeks after transplantation. In contrast with graft thrombosis, which leads to graft loss but not mortality, intra-abdominal infections can lead to both graft loss and patient death. Most localised intra-abdominal collections can be treated with percutaneous drainage when patients are not unwell. However, any clinical deterioration mandates laparotomy and in severe infections the treatment should be focused on saving the patient's life rather than saving the graft.

It is not known whether duodenal decontamination during organ retrieval has any influence on recipient intra-abdominal or wound infections. A bacteriology specimen of the donor duodenal contents should be routinely taken and results used to guide antimicrobial therapy in the event of intra-abdominal sepsis. Abdominal lavage with warm saline or antibiotic/antifungal solutions is also common practice after implantation of pancreatic allografts. This practice, intuitively useful, is supported by indirect evidence from other clinical settings but there are no controlled trials demonstrating its efficacy for pancreas transplantation.

Allograft pancreatitis

Cold storage and ischaemia–reperfusion injury inevitably result in a degree of oedema of the pancreatic allograft. This is a commonly encountered finding if a re-laparotomy becomes necessary in the first few postoperative days and it is not always associated with an elevation in serum amylase. There is no universally agreed definition of allograft pancreatitis. The condition has a different clinical course to native pancreatitis. It is rarely severe or life threatening. Ischaemia–reperfusion injury may be the cause or a predisposing factor. It is not known whether drugs associated with native pancreatitis can also cause allograft pancreatitis. Bladder drainage (especially in the presence of autonomic neuropathy affecting bladder function and causing high intravesical pressures) can be associated with recurrent episodes of allograft pancreatitis due to reflux. Catheter drainage of the bladder for at least 7–10 days is usually adequate for the management of the acute episode but ultimately enteric conversion may be required.

During the pancreas transplant operation, the allograft exocrine function starts very promptly upon revascularisation and the duodenal segment quickly fills with pancreatic juice. Excessive distension of the stapled duodenal segment and the consequent reflux could cause postoperative pancreatitis. Even if the exocrine diversion is not going to be performed straight away, the duodenal segment should be decompressed and excessive distension of the graft duodenum should be avoided during the recipient operation. Donor age, donor obesity and prolonged preservation times are other factors associated with allograft pancreatitis.

The distinction between allograft pancreatitis and acute rejection in the presence of an oedematous pancreas, abdominal pain and a slightly raised serum amylase is a difficult clinical diagnosis.

Complications specific to bladder drainage

The most common consequence of the diversion of the exocrine pancreatic secretions into the bladder is a chemical cystitis, which predisposes patients to infection, persistent haematuria and troublesome dysuria. Dysuria is more troublesome in men, with urethritis that can progress to urethral disruption. Failure of reabsorption of the exocrine secretions results in chronic dehydration and acidosis. Urinary tract infections are much more common compared with intestinal drainage. Persistent haematuria can require repeated blood transfusions. In the presence of autonomic neuropathy affecting the bladder, repeated episodes of reflux allograft pancreatitis are another potential complication. As a consequence of one or more of these complications enteric conversion of the exocrine drainage may become necessary. The enteric conversion rate in bladder-drained pancreas transplants increases with increasing follow-up and could be as high as 40% at 5 years.[18]

Outcome following pancreas transplantation

Introduction

There is little doubt that patient and graft survival rates following pancreas transplantation continued to improve throughout the 1990s. Detailed analyses of outcomes reported to the IPTR have been available as annual reports from the registry. They remain as valuable sources of data attesting to this improvement. The IPTR reports, however, refer to short- or medium-term outcome and should be interpreted within the context of their limitations. For instance, the analysis of 1996–2000 US pancreas transplants refers to 5276 transplants performed in this period. The outcome figures were based on data from 4073 of these patients for whom complete information was available. It is not mentioned what information was missing in the remaining 1203 patients. Table 9.4 summarises the improvements observed in the success rate of pancreatic transplantation in the USA between 1987 and 2010. The most recent analysis of the IPTR data reveals that short- and medium-term results have remained excellent, with 95% and 92% 1-year and 3-year patient survival in all three pancreas transplant categories for patients transplanted in 2009[5] (Table 9.5).

Table 9.4 • One-year patient and graft survival rate after pancreas transplantation in the USA in three different eras

	1987–1990	1998–2000	2004–2009
SPK transplants			
Patient survival	89%	95%	95%
Kidney graft survival	84%	92%	92%
Pancreas graft survival	72%	82%	85%
PAK transplants			
Patient survival	91%	94%	97%
Pancreas graft survival	52%	74%	79%
PTA transplants			
Patient survival	93%	100%	97%
Graft survival	47%	76%	79%

SPK, simultaneous pancreas–kidney transplants; PAK, pancreas after kidney transplants; PTA, pancreas transplantation alone.

Table 9.5 • Patient survival and pancreas graft survival rates after primary deceased donor pancreas transplantation in the USA (January 2004 to January 2009)

	Patient survival		Graft survival	
	1-year	3-year	1-year	3-year
SPK transplants (n=4206)	95.2%	91.9%	84.9%	77.9%
PAK transplants (n=1130)	96.6%	90.2%	78.6%	78.9%
PTA transplants (n=491)	96.5%	91.9%	65.1%	57.2%

SPK, simultaneous pancreas–kidney transplants; PAK, pancreas after kidney transplants; PTA, pancreas transplantation alone.

Short-term patient survival and graft survival rates remain as the standard primary outcome measures in organ transplantation. As illustrated in Table 9.5, these rates have improved considerably in pancreas transplantation, to the extent that demonstration of any further significant improvement as a consequence of any intervention requires prospective studies with very large patient groups. In order to circumvent this difficulty in kidney transplantation, surrogate end-points (or secondary outcome measures) such as the incidence of acute rejection or the quality of graft function have been used. Similar surrogate outcome measures applicable to pancreas transplantation are more difficult to define. Data referring to the immunological benefits of portal venous drainage are an example illustrating the point. The fact that portal drainage is not associated with improved graft survival rates may indeed be a genuine finding. However, it could also be that a small benefit is not evident because of the already excellent graft survival rates with systemic venous drainage and the relatively infrequent application of portal venous drainage in selected patients. Distorted reporting with more complete data in the registry from the portal-drained subgroup of patients may also be a confounding factor.

Any enquiry into the outcome of pancreas transplantation worldwide suffers from the lack of a truly representative and complete international database. The IPTR and the UNOS/SRTR databases have given a remarkably useful insight into the picture in the USA. Information with respect to the outcome of pancreas transplantation outside the USA is more sketchy. The responsible attitude for the pancreas transplantation community worldwide should be to regard complete and accurate reporting of pancreas transplantation activity and outcome as an indispensable priority.

Factors influencing pancreas transplantation outcome

Recipient age

Increasing recipient age is a small but significant risk factor in the outcome of pancreas transplantation. Historically patient and graft survival rates have been higher in younger recipients. In recent years more careful patient selection has influenced the outcome in older recipients favourably, to the extent that the short-term outcome following pancreas transplantation is no different for patients older than 45 at the time of transplant compared with those who are younger than 45.[11] The number of patients in solitary pancreas transplant categories is smaller and most patients receiving solitary transplants tend to be in the younger age group. As a consequence the influence of recipient age is more readily demonstrable in SPK transplantation and becomes more pronounced with longer follow-up. Five years after SPK transplantation patient survival is 86.0% for recipients aged 35–49 at the time of transplantation compared with 81.7% for those aged 50–64.[11]

Re-transplantation

Re-transplantation appears as a consistent and significant risk factor for graft survival in all categories. One-year pancreas graft survival rate after re-transplantation in the SPK category is 70.8% (± 9.3%) compared with 85.4% (± 0.9%) in primary SPK transplants (**Fig. 9.8**).[11]

HLA matching

Analyses of US registry data over the years have inconsistently revealed some evidence for the influence of HLA matching on pancreas transplant outcome on some categories.[17] The effect of HLA matching, when present, has been small and seemed to affect different categories in different eras or was confined to different classes of HLA mismatches. The likely explanation is that HLA matching has a negligible influence or no influence on the outcome of pancreas transplantation. This is indeed what the most recent analysis of the IPTR database reveals.[5]

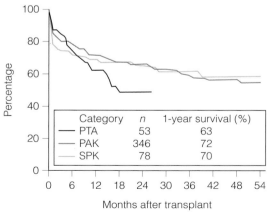

Figure 9.8 • Pancreas *re-transplant* graft function. These are US deceased donor re-transplants from January 1996 to July 2003.

Management of exocrine secretions: management of venous drainage

The surgical technique employed for the exocrine diversion has no influence on outcome in pancreas transplantation. Pancreas graft survival rates at 1 year following SPK transplantation for the 2000–2004 cohort in the USA were 87% and 85% for bladder-drained and enteric-drained grafts, respectively. More recent analyses confirm that method of exocrine diversion has no influence on patient or graft survival rates.[6]

Similarly, systemic versus portal venous drainage has not been found to be associated with pancreas transplantation outcome.[11]

Immunosuppression

Immunosuppressive therapy has a major influence on the outcome of pancreas transplantation. In the last decade, tacrolimus and MMF have been the basis of maintenance immunosuppression in the large majority of patients (Fig. 9.6). Multivariate analyses reveal the tacrolimus/MMF combination to be associated with significant reductions in pancreas graft loss (relative risk (RR)=0.74, P=0.08 for SPK; RR=0.51, P=0.001 for PAK; and RR=0.46, P=0.014 for PTA) categories. In multivariate analyses, sirolimus use considered as a variable is also associated with a significant reduction in pancreas graft loss (RR=0.81, P=0.17 for SPK; RR=0.54, P=0.01 for PAK; and RR=0.16, P=0.001 for PTA categories).[31] In a cohort of 2006–2010 transplants, antibody induction was associated with lower risk of pancreas graft failure in SPK but not in PAK or PTA and only when depleting antibodies were used.[6]

Donor factors

Donor age, donor obesity and donor cause of death have been linked with the outcome of pancreas transplantation. Whilst all of these variables may be independently associated with outcome, they are likely to be inter-related; for instance, younger donors are more likely to have died of trauma whilst older and obese donors are more likely to have died of a cerebrovascular cause.

An analysis of all SPK transplants performed in the USA during a 12-year period between 1994 and 2005 (n = 8850) has conclusively shown increasing donor age to be a risk factor in pancreas transplantation.[22] During this period 776 transplants (8.8%) were performed using organs from deceased donors aged 45 or older (mean age ± SD = 49.2 ± 3.7). A large majority of patients (8074, 91.2%) received organs from donors younger than 45 (mean age ± SD = 24.6 ± 9.1). Pancreas and kidney graft survival and patient survival were significantly inferior in the 'old donor' group (77% vs. 85%, 89% vs. 92% and 95% vs. 93%, respectively, at 1 year). A larger decrement in early graft survival after old versus young donor transplants was observed for pancreas compared to kidney transplants. Graft survival for young and old donor transplants continued to diverge over time for both grafts. Five-year pancreas graft survival was 72% versus 60% for young versus old donor transplants, respectively.

Humar et al.[23] reported the outcome of 711 deceased donor pancreas transplants in Minneapolis performed between 1994 and 2001. The outcomes were analysed for three groups based on donor BMI (BMI <25; n=434; BMI 25–30, n=196; BMI >30, n=81). Patients who received grafts from obese donors (BMI >30) had a higher incidence of complications and inferior graft survival. The incidence of technical failure was 9.7% in the BMI <25 group, 16.3% in the BMI 25–30 group and 21% in the BMI >30 group (P=0.04). More recently the same group of authors published an analysis in a slightly larger cohort of pancreas transplant patients from Minneapolis[24] in order to determine risk factors for technical failure following pancreas transplantation. Technical failure, defined as thrombosis, bleeding, leaks, infections or pancreatitis, was responsible for the loss of 13.1% of transplants (131 of 973). By multivariate analysis the following were significant risk factors: recipient BMI >30 (RR=2.42, P=0.0003), preservation time >24 hours (RR=1.87, P=0.04) and cause of donor death other than trauma (RR=1.58, P=0.04). Donor obesity had borderline significance.

Pancreas grafts from paediatric donors (aged >4 years) can be used with excellent results, not inferior to those obtained from optimum deceased donor grafts.[25] Organs from DCD (donation after circulatory death or donation after cardiac death) donors constitute an increasing proportion of the deceased donor pool. University of Wisconsin experience and the pooled US data suggest that the outcome of pancreas transplantation using DCD grafts is equivalent to that achieved with DBD (donation after brain death) donor organs.[25,26] More recent data from Oxford in the UK, where one of the world's largest pancreas transplant programmes is based, reveal a higher risk of pancreas graft failure with DCD grafts. The poorer outcome was confined to solitary pancreas transplant recipients with prolonged preservation times.[32,33]

It is evident that donor selection has a major influence on the outcome of pancreas transplantation. Therefore, other risk factors such as preservation time, recipient BMI and comorbidity need to be considered when using suboptimal grafts for pancreas transplantation.

Long-term outlook following pancreas transplantation

Pancreas transplantation and life expectancy

Clearly, one of the most important issues for patients considering pancreas transplantation is whether their life expectancy will be influenced by the transplant. Numerous studies and analyses of databases have consistently shown that successful pancreas transplantation is associated with improved survival prospects in diabetic patients. No prospective controlled study has ever been carried out that compares pancreas transplantation with insulin therapy. Hence all available evidence is subject to selection bias. It would be reasonable to expect that in clinical practice younger fitter patients with lower risk would have been chosen for pancreas transplantation, creating bias in favour of this group. Nevertheless, a strong body of indirect evidence suggests that successful pancreas transplantation may truly increase life expectancy as well as improving quality of life.

Several studies have addressed the question of the impact of pancreas transplantation on long-term mortality in a number of different ways. The University of Wisconsin experience in 500 SPK transplant recipients published in 1998[74] simply quotes a 10-year patient survival rate of 70%. This is matched in their experience only by recipients of living-donor kidney transplants. Unsurpassed as they are, these results were obtained in a highly selective group of young patients with a relatively short duration of diabetes and kidney failure and strict eligibility criteria excluding those with ischaemic heart disease.

A large registry analysis from the USA published in 2001 by Ojo et al. looked at the outcome in 13 467 adults with type I diabetes registered in kidney and SPK transplant waiting lists between 1988 and 1997.[75] Adjusted 10-year patient survival was 67% for SPK transplant recipients, 65% for living-donor kidney (LKD) transplant recipients and 46% for cadaveric kidney (CAD) transplant recipients. Taking the mortality of patients who remained on dialysis as reference, the adjusted relative risk of 5-year mortality was 0.40, 0.45 and 0.74 for SPK, LKD and CAD recipients. Another large review of the UNOS database published by Reddy et al.[76] in 2003 analysed long-term survival in 18 549 type I diabetic patients transplanted between 1987 and 1996. There was a long-term survival advantage in favour of pancreas transplant recipients (8-year crude survival rates: 72% for SPK, 72% for LKD and 55% for CAD). This diminished but persisted after adjusting for donor and recipient variables and kidney graft function. Tyden et al. from Sweden demonstrated a striking difference in long-term survival in a small group of diabetic patients transplanted between 1982 and 1986 and followed up for at least 10 years.[77] Fourteen patients received successful SPK transplants. The control group consisted of 15 patients who had undergone the same assessment, had been accepted for SPK transplants but either declined pancreas transplantation or received SPK but lost the pancreas graft within the first year because of a technical complication. Ten years later three of the SPK transplant recipients had died (20%), compared with 12 of the 15 kidney transplant recipients (80%). Another interesting study addressing the long-term survival after transplantation in type I diabetics came from the Netherlands. Smets et al. studied all 415 adults with type I diabetes who started renal replacement therapy in the Netherlands between 1985 and 1996. Patients were divided into two groups depending on where they lived. The basis for this was the fact that in the Leiden area the treatment of choice for such patients was SPK transplantation (73% of transplants), whereas in the remainder of the country kidney transplantation alone was the predominant type of therapy and SPK was performed uncommonly (37%). The relative risk for death for patients who lived outside the Leiden area was 1.9. When the transplanted patients only were analysed the relative risk for death was 2.5 for those outside the Leiden area.[78]

Influence of pancreas transplantation on diabetic complications

Nephropathy

There is convincing evidence that successful pancreas transplantation can stop the progression of diabetic nephropathy and reverse associated histological changes. This evidence largely comes from studies that have assessed the course of diabetic nephropathy in kidney allografts in SPK or PAK transplant recipients.[79,80] Fioretto et al. have shown that established lesions of diabetic nephropathy in native kidneys can be reversed with successful pancreas transplantation (PTA).[81] In the setting of clinical transplantation the beneficial effect of the pancreas graft is counterbalanced by the nephrotoxicity of the immunosuppressive drugs.

Retinopathy

✓✓ Patients with type I diabetes often quote preservation of eyesight as one of the main reasons for considering pancreas transplantation. There is good evidence that better blood glucose control reduces the risk of progression of retinopathy.[82] However, in practice the large majority of patients undergoing pancreas transplantation will have advanced proliferative retinopathy. Hence prevention of retinopathy is seldom a major factor in the consideration of the risks and benefits of pancreas transplantation.[83]

Retinopathy needs to be treated prior to transplantation with laser photocoagulation, which is an effective treatment. For the minority of patients who present with non-proliferative retinopathy or those who recently underwent treatment for proliferative retinopathy there is a risk of rapid progression of the retinopathy following transplantation. Such patients require close ophthalmic follow-up within the first 3 years of transplantation. Stabilisation of retinopathy after pancreas transplantation takes 3 years.[83–85] During this time any patient who has an indication or develops an indication for laser treatment should undergo treatment.

Patients often report improved vision soon after pancreas transplantation. Improvement in macular oedema is demonstrable soon after transplantation and can result in early improvement of vision. It is unclear whether this is a consequence of euglycaemia or a consequence of the kidney transplant resulting in improved fluid balance. It is probable that euglycaemia offered by pancreas transplantation, over and above the benefits of the non-uraemic environment, results in better elimination of osmotic swelling of the lens, hence improving fluctuations in vision that diabetic patients experience.[83]

Neuropathy

Patients with end-stage renal failure and type I diabetes almost universally exhibit an autonomic and peripheral (somatic) diabetic polyneuropathy as well as uraemic neuropathy. Improvement in neuropathy following SPK transplantation using objective measures of nerve function has been demonstrated by several transplant centres.[86,87] For individuals with intractable and distressing symptoms of neuropathy the clinical benefit may be considerable. Reversal of neuropathic symptoms takes many months and clinically relevant benefit may not be evident earlier than 6–12 months after transplantation. Obesity, smoking, presence of advanced neuropathy and poor renal allograft function are predictors of poor recovery in nerve function after SPK transplantation.[88]

Cardiovascular disease

Pancreas transplantation has demonstrable benefits on microangiopathy in diabetics.[89] Some of its effects on retinopathy, nephropathy and neuropathy may be mediated through this mechanism. It has been more difficult to demonstrate any improvement in macroangiopathy. The enhanced survival prospects after pancreas transplantation ought to be, at least in part, due to the improvement in the cardiovascular risk profile. Evidence to support this is accumulating. Fiorina et al. in Milan demonstrated favourable influences of pancreas[90] and islet[91] transplantation on atherosclerotic risk factors, including plasma lipid profile, blood pressure, left ventricular function and endothelial function. This translates into reduced cardiovascular death rate.[92,93] Similar improvements occur in early non-uraemic diabetics after PTA.[94]

Key points

- By the end of 2010, over 35 000 pancreas transplants have been performed worldwide. In the USA alone there are more than 100 000 patients with functioning transplants; around 10 000 of these are pancreas allografts.
- The outcome following pancreas transplantation has improved considerably in the last 10–15 years. It is now comparable to the outcome for other solid-organ transplants.
- The number of pancreas transplants reached a peak in 2004. Activity has been declining in the USA since then in all three categories. An overall decrease of 20% was observed in 2010, compared with 2004. The largest decrease was observed in the PAK category (55%), followed by PTA (30%) and SPK (8%).
- Pancreas transplantation activity in the UK has followed a different pattern, with a much sharper increase in activity between 2000 and 2007, followed by a more modest decline since then.
- Despite the reduction in activity, pancreas transplant outcomes have remained at least as good in the last decade.
- Induction immunosuppression with biological agents is used in pancreas transplantation more often than any other solid-organ transplant. Tacrolimus/MMF combination is the basis of the most commonly used maintenance immunosuppression protocols. Steroid minimisation or avoidance is gaining momentum.
- Over the last 15 years enteric drainage has gradually replaced bladder drainage as the preferred technique for the management of exocrine secretions in pancreas transplantation.
- Portal venous drainage, introduced in the mid-1990s, has not gained increasing popularity. It is used in just under a fifth of SPK and PAK and in 10% of PTA transplants.
- Evidence regarding the influence of pancreas transplantation on diabetic complications and life expectancy is not available from prospective controlled trials. Nevertheless, accumulating evidence from many studies strongly suggests that successful pancreas transplantation has a favourable influence on diabetic complications and survival prospects for patients.

References

1. Kelly KD, Lillehei KC, Merkle FK, et al. Allotransplantation of pancreas and duodenum along with kidney in diabetic nephropathy. Surgery 1967;61:827–37.

2. Sasaki TM, Gray RS, Ratner RE, et al. Successful long term kidney–pancreas transplants in diabetic patients with high C-peptide levels. Transplantation 1998;65:1510–2.

3. Orlando G, Stratta RJ, Light J. Pancreas transplantation for type 2 diabetes mellitus. Curr Opin Organ Transplant 2011;16:110–5.

4. Wilkin TJ. The accelerator hypothesis: a review of the evidence for insulin resistance as the basis for Type I as well as Type II diabetes. Int J Obes (Lond) 2009;33:716–26.

5. Gruessner AC, Sutherland DER, Gruessner RWG. Pancreas transplantation in the United States: a review. Curr Opin Organ Transplant 2010;15:93–101.

6. Gruessner AC. 2011 update on pancreas transplantation: comprehensive trend analysis of 25,000 cases followed up over the course of 24 years at the IPTR. Rev Diabet Stud 2011;8:6–16.

7. Sutherland DER, Radosevich D, Gruessner R, et al. Pushing the envelope: living donor pancreas transplantation. Curr Opin Organ Transplant 2012;17:106–15.

8. McMillan MA, Briggs JD, Junor BJ. Outcome of renal replacement treatment in patients with diabetes mellitus. Br Med J 1990;301:540–4.

9. Rabbat CG, Treleaven DR, Russell DJ, et al. Prognostic value of myocardial perfusion studies in patients with end-stage renal disease assessed for kidney or kidney–pancreas transplantation: a meta-analysis. J Am Soc Nephrol 2003;14:431–9.

10. Kumar N, Baker CSR, Chan K, et al. Cardiac survival after pre-emptive coronary angiography in transplant patients and those awaiting transplantation. Clin J Am Soc Nephrol 2011;6:1912–9.

11. 2006 Annual Report of the US Organ Procurement and Transplantation Network and the Scientific Registry of Transplant Recipients: Transplant Data 1996–2005. Rockville, MD: Health Resources and Services Administration, Healthcare Systems

Bureau, Division of Transplantation (2006 OPTN/ SRTR Annual Report 1996–2005. HHS/HRSA/ HSB/DOT); http://www.transplant.hrsa.gov/.

12. Kleinclauss F, Fauda M, Sutherland DER, et al. Pancreas after living donor kidney transplants in diabetic patients: impact on long-term kidney graft function. Clin Transplant 2009;23:437–46.

13. Poommipanit N, Sampaio MC, Cho Y, et al. Pancreas after living donor kidney versus simultaneous pancreas–kidney transplant: an analysis of the Organ Procurement Transplant Network/ United Network of Organ Sharing database. Transplantation 2010;89:1496–503.

14. Humar A, Sutherland DE, Ramcharan T, et al. Optimal timing for a pancreas transplant after successful kidney transplant. Transplantation 2000;70:1247–50.

15. Wiseman AC. Pancreas transplant options for patients with type 1 diabetes mellitus and chronic kidney disease: simultaneous pancreas kidney or pancreas after kidney? Curr Opin Organ Transplant 2012;17:80–6.

16. Luan FL, Kommareddi M, Cibrik DM, et al. The time interval between kidney and pancreas transplantation and the clinical outcomes of pancreas after kidney transplantation. Clin Transplant 2012;26(3):403–10.

17. Hariharan S, Pirsch JD, Lu CY, et al. Pancreas after kidney transplantation. J Am Soc Nephrol 2002;13:1109–18.

18. Odorico JS, Sollinger HW. Technical and immunological advances in transplantation for insulin dependent diabetes mellitus. World J Surg 2002;26:194–211.

19. International Figures on Organ Donation and Transplantation 2006. Transplant Newsletter September 2007;12(1). Council of Europe.

20. http://www.organdonation.nhs.uk.

21. http://www.eurotransplant.org/cms/; [accessed 13.10.12].

22. Salvalaggio PR, Schnitzler MA, Abbott KC, et al. Patient and graft survival implications of simultaneous pancreas kidney transplantation from old donors. Am J Transplant 2007;7:1561–71.

23. Humar A, Thigarajan R, Kandaswamy R, et al. The impact of donor obesity on outcomes after cadaver pancreas transplants. Am J Transplant 2004;4:605–10.

24. Humar A, Thigarajan R, Kandaswamy R, et al. Technical failures after pancreas transplants: why grafts fail and the risk factors – a multivariate analysis. Transplantation 2004;78(8):1188–92.

25. Krieger NR, Odorico JS, Heisey DM, et al. Underutilization of pancreas donors. Transplantation 2003;75:1271–6.

26. Salvalaggio PR, Davies DB, Fernandez LA, et al. Outcomes of pancreas transplantation in the United States using cardiac death donors. Am J Transplant 2006;6:1059–65.

27. D'Allessandro AM, Stratta JR, Sollinger HW, et al. Use of UW solution in pancreas transplantation. Diabetes 1989;38(Suppl. 1):7–9.

28. Potdor S, Eghtesad B, Jain A, et al. Comparison of early graft function and complications of pancreas transplant recipients in Histidine–Tryptophan–Ketoglutarate (HTK) solution and University of Wisconsin (UW) solutions. Transplantation 2003;76:S288.

29. Fridell JA, Mangus RS, Powelson JA. Organ preservation solutions for whole organ pancreas transplantation. Curr Opin Organ Transplant 2011;16:116–22.

30. Sutherland DER, Gruessner RW, Dunn DL, et al. Lessons learned from more than 1000 pancreas transplants at a single institution. Ann Surg 2001;233:463–501.

31. International Pancreas Transplant Registry. 2004 Annual Report, http://www.iptr.umn.edu/IPTR/annual_reports/2004_annual_report/home.html; August 2006.

32. Muthusamy AS, Mumford L, Hudson A. NHBD pancreas transplantation in the UK: should we go on? Transplant Int 2010;23(Suppl. s1):6.

33. Muthusamy AS, Vaidya A. Expanding the donor pool in pancreas transplantation. Curr Opin Organ Transplant 2010;15:123–7.

34. de Ville de Goyet J, Hausleithner V, Malaise J, et al. Liver procurement without in situ portal perfusion. A safe procedure for more flexible multiple organ harvesting. Transplantation 1994;57:1328–32.

35. Olson DW, Kadota S, Cornish A, et al. Intestinal decontamination using povidone iodine compromises small bowel storage quality. Transplantation 2003;75:1460–2.

36. Woeste G, Wallstein C, Vogt J, et al. Value of donor swabs for intra-abdominal infection in simultaneous pancreas kidney transplantation. Transplantation 2003;76:1073–8.

37. Calne RY. Para-topic segmental pancreas grafting: a technique with portal venous drainage. Lancet 1984;1:595–7.

38. Shokouh-Amiri MH, Gaber AO, Gaber LW, et al. Pancreas transplantation with portal venous drainage and enteric exocrine diversion: a new technique. Transplant Proc 1992;24:776–7.

39. Petruzzo PA, Palmina A, DaSilva MA, et al. Simultaneous pancreas–kidney transplantation: portal versus systemic venous drainage of the pancreas allografts. Clin Transplant 2000;14:287–91.

40. Stratta RJ, Shokouh-Amiri MH, Egidi MF, et al. A prospective comparison of simultaneous kidney–pancreas transplantation with systemic-enteric versus portal-enteric drainage. Ann Surg 2001;233:740–51.

41. Stratta RJ, Lo A, Shokouh-Amiri MH, et al. Improving results in solitary pancreas transplantation with portal enteric drainage, thymoglobulin induction and tacrolimus/mycophenolate mofetil based immunosuppression. Transplant Int 2003;16:154–60.

42. Despres JP, Lamarche B, Mauriege P, et al. Hyperinsulinemia as an independent risk factor for ischaemic heart disease. N Engl J Med 1996;334:952–7.

43. Ost LD, Tyden G, Fehrman I. Impaired glucose tolerance in Ciclosporine–prednisolone treated renal allograft recipients. Transplantation 1988;46:370–2.

44. Christiansen E, Vestergaard H, Tibell A, et al. Impaired insulin-stimulated non-oxidative glucose metabolism in pancreas–kidney transplant recipients: dose–response effects of insulin on glucose turnover. Diabetes 1996;45:1267–75.

45. Stratta RJ. Review of immunosuppressive usage in pancreas transplantation. Clin Transplant 1999;13:1–12.

46. Gruessner RWG. Tacrolimus in pancreas transplantation: a multi-center analysis. Clin Transplant 1997;11:299–312.

47. Bartlett ST, Schweitzer EJ, Johnson LB, et al. Equivalent success of simultaneous pancreas–kidney and solitary pancreas transplantation. A prospective trial of tacrolimus immunosuppression with percutaneous biopsy. Ann Surg 1996;224:440–9.

48. European Mycophenolate Mofetil Co-operative Study Group. Placebo controlled study of mycophenolate mofetil combined with ciclosporine and corticosteroids for prevention of acute rejection. Lancet 1995;345:1321–5.

49. Sollinger HW, for the US Renal Transplant Mycophenolate Mofetil Study Group. Mycophenolate mofetil for the prevention of acute rejection in primary cadaveric renal allograft recipients. Transplantation 1995;60:225–32.

50. Merion RM, Henry ML, Melzer JS, et al. Randomized prospective trial of mycophenolate mofetil versus azathioprine for prevention of acute renal allograft rejection after simultaneous kidney–pancreas transplantation. Transplantation 2000;70:105–11.

51. Garcia VD, Keitel E, Santos AF, et al. Immunosuppression in pancreas transplantation: mycophenolate mofetil versus sirolimus. Transplant Proc 2004;36(4):975–7.

52. Kandaswamy R, Khwaja K, Gruessner A, et al. A prospective randomized trial of steroid withdrawal with mycophenolate mofetil (MMF) versus sirolimus (SRL) in pancreas after kidney transplants. Am J Transplant 2003;3(Suppl. 5):292.

53. Burke GW, Ciancio G, Mattiazzi A, et al. Lower rate of acute rejection with rapamycin than with mycophenolate mofetil in kidney pancreas transplantation. A randomized prospective study with Thymoglobulin/Zenapax induction, tacrolimus and steroid maintenance: comparing rapamycin with mycophenolate mofetil. Am J Transplant 2003; 3(Suppl. 5):322.

54. Gruessner RWG, Kandaswamy R, Humar A, et al. Calcineurin inhibitor and steroid free immunosuppression in pancreas kidney and solitary pancreas transplantation. Transplantation 2005;79(9):1184–9.

55. Wadstrom J, Brekke B, Wrammer L, et al. Triple versus quadruple induction immunosuppression in pancreas transplantation. Transplant Proc 1995;27:1317–8.

56. Cantarovich D, Karam G, Giral-Classe M, et al. Randomized comparison of triple therapy and antithymocyte globulin induction treatment after simultaneous pancreas kidney transplantation. Kidney Int 1998;54:1351–6.

57. Stratta RJ, Alloway RR, Lo A, et al. Two dose daclizumab regimen in simultaneous kidney pancreas transplant recipients: primary endpoint analysis of a multi-center randomised study. Transplantation 2003;75:1260–6.

58. Kaufman DB, Burke GW, Bruce DS, et al. Prospective randomised multi-center trial of antibody induction therapy in simultaneous kidney–pancreas transplantation. Am J Transplant 2003;3:855–64.

59. Rogers J, Farney AC, Al-Geizawi S, et al. Pancreas transplantation: lessons learned from a decade of experience at Wake Forest Baptist Medical Center. Rev Diabet Stud 2011;8:17–27.

60. Hawthorne WJ, Allen RDM, Greenberg ML, et al. Simultaneous pancreas and kidney transplant rejection: separate or synchronous events. Transplantation 1997;63:352–8.

61. Munn SR, Engen DE, Barr D, et al. Differential diagnosis of hypoamylasuria in pancreas allograft recipients with urinary exocrine drainage. Transplantation 1990;49:359–62.

62. Benedetti E, Najarian JS, Gruessner A, et al. Correlation between cystoscopic biopsy results and hypoamylasuria in bladder drained pancreas transplants. Surgery 1995;118:864–72.

63. Elmer DS, Hathaway DK, Bashar AA, et al. Use of glucose disappearance rates (kG) to monitor endocrine function of pancreas allografts. Clin Transplant 1998;12:56–64.

64. Drachenberg G, Klassen D, Bartlett S, et al. Histologic grading of pancreas acute allograft rejection in percutaneous needle biopsies. Transplant Proc 1996;28:512–3.

65. Papadimitriou JC, Drachenberg CB. Distinctive morphological features of antibody mediated and T-cell mediated acute rejection in pancreas allograft biopsies. Curr Opin Organ Transplant 2012;17:93–9.

66. Reddy KS, Davies D, Ormond D, et al. Impact of acute rejection episodes on long term graft survival following simultaneous kidney pancreas transplantation. Am J Transplant 2003;3:439–44.

67. Farney AC, Rogers J, Stratta RJ. Pancreas graft thrombosis: causes, prevention, diagnosis and intervention. Curr Opin Organ Transplant 2012;17:87–92.

68. Troppmann C. Complications after pancreas transplantation. Curr Opin Organ Transplant 2010;15:112–8.

69. Steurer W, Malaise J, Mark W, et al. Spectrum of surgical complications after SPK transplantation in a propectively randomized study of two immunosuppressive protocols. Nephrol Dial Transplant 2005;20:54–61.

70. Muthusamy AS, Vaidya AC, Sinha S, et al. Pancreas allograft thrombosis following intravenous immunoglobulin administration to treat parvovirus B19 infection. Transpl Infect Dis 2009;11:463–6.

71. Stockland AH, Willingham DL, Paz-Fumagalli R, et al. Pancreas transplant venous thrombosis: role of endovascular interventions for graft salvage. Cardiovasc Intervent Radiol 2009;32:279–83.

72. Gilabert R, Fernandez-Cruz L, Real MI, et al. Treatment and outcome of pancreas graft thrombosis after kidney–pancreas transplantation. Br J Surg 2002;89:355–60.

73. Kuo PC, Wong J, Schweizer EJ, et al. Outcome after splenic vein thrombosis in the pancreas allograft. Transplantation 1997;64:933–5.

74. Sollinger HW, Odorico JS, Knechtle SJ, et al. Experience with 500 simultaneous pancreas–kidney transplants. Ann Surg 1998;228:284–96.

75. Ojo AO, Meier-Kriesche H, Hanson J, et al. The impact of simultaneous pancreas kidney transplantation on long-term patient survival. Transplantation 2001;71:82–9.

76. Reddy KS, Stablein D, Taranto S, et al. Long-term survival following simultaneous kidney–pancreas transplantation versus kidney transplantation alone in patients with type 1 diabetes mellitus and renal failure. Am J Kidney Dis 2003;41:464–70.

77. Tyden G, Bolinder J, Solders G, et al. Improved survival in patients with insulin-dependent diabetes mellitus and end-stage diabetic nephropathy 10 years after combined pancreas and kidney transplantation. Transplantation 1999;67:645–8.

78. Smets YFC, Westendorp RGJ, Van der Pijl JW, et al. Effect of simultaneous pancreas–kidney transplantation on mortality of patients with Type 1 diabetes and end stage renal failure. Lancet 1999;353:1915–20.

79. Wilczek HE, Jaremko G, Tyden G, et al. Evolution of diabetic nephropathy in kidney grafts. Transplantation 1995;59:51–7.

80. El-Gebely S, Hathaway DK, Elmer DS, et al. An analysis of renal function in pancreas kidney and diabetic kidney alone recipients at two years following transplantation. Transplantation 1995;59:1410–5.

81. Fioretto P, Steffes MW, Sutherland DER, et al. Reversal of lesions of diabetic nephropathy after pancreas transplantation. N Engl J Med 1998;339:69–75.

82. The Diabetes Control and Complications Trial Research Group. The effect of intensive treatment of diabetes on the development and progression of long-term complications in insulin dependent diabetes mellitus. N Engl J Med 1993;329:977–86.

83. Walsh AW. Effects of pancreas transplantation on seconday complications of diabetes – retinopathy. In: Gruessner RWG, Sutherland DER, editors. Transplantation of the pancreas. New York: Springer; 2004. p. 462–71.

84. Chow VCC, Pai RP, Chapman JR, et al. Diabetic retinopathy after combined kidney–pancreas transplantation. Clin Transplant 1999;13:356–62.

85. Pearce IA, Ilango B, Sells RA, et al. Stabilisation of diabetic retinopathy following simultaneous pancreas and kidney transplant. Br J Ophthalmol 2000;84:736–40.

86. Cashion AK, Hathaway DK, Milstead EJ, et al. Changes in patterns of 24 hour heart rate variability after kidney and kidney–pancreas transplant. Transplantation 1999;68:1426–30.

87. Hathaway DK, Abell T, Cardoso S, et al. Improvement in autonomic and gastric function following pancreas–kidney versus kidney alone transplantation and the correlation with quality of life. Transplantation 1994;57:816–22.

88. Allen RDM, Al-Harbi IS, Morris JG, et al. Diabetic neuropathy after pancreas transplantation: determinants of recovery. Transplantation 1997;63:830–8.

89. Abendroth D, Schmand J, Landgraf R, et al. Diabetic microangiopathy in Type 1 (insulin dependent) diabetic patients after successful pancreatic and kidney or solitary kidney transplantation. Diabetology 1991;34:131–4.

90. Fiorina P, LaRocca E, Venturini M, et al. Effects of kidney–pancreas transplantation on atherosclerotic risk factors and endothelial function in patients with uraemia and Type 1 diabetes. Diabetes 2001;50:496–501.

91. Fiorina P, Folli F, Maffi P, et al. Islet transplantation improves vascular diabetic complications in patients with diabetes who underwent kidney transplantation: a comparison between kidney–pancreas and kidney alone transplantation. Transplantation 2003;75:1296–301.

92. LaRocca E, Fiorina P, DiCarlo V, et al. Cardiovascular outcomes after kidney–pancreas and kidney alone transplantation. Kidney Int 2001;60:1964–71.

93. Jukema JW, Smets YF, van der Pijl JW, et al. Impact of simultaneous pancreas and kidney transplantation on progression of coronary atherosclerosis in patients with end-stage renal failure due to type 1 diabetes. Diabetes Care 2002;25:906–11.

94. Copelli A, Giannarelli R, Mariotti R, et al. Pancreas transplant alone determines early improvement of cardiovascular risk factors and cardiac function in type 1 diabetic patients. Transplantation 2003;76:974–6.

10

Islet transplantation

John J. Casey

Introduction

The discovery of insulin by Banting and Best in the early part of the 20th century saw type I diabetes become a treatable chronic illness rather than a rapidly fatal diagnosis. Since then, patients with diabetes have been able to lead relatively normal lives thanks to ongoing refinements in insulin therapy. Despite this, many patients will suffer from the secondary side-effects of diabetes including retinopathy, neuropathy, nephropathy and premature cardiovascular disease. The Diabetes Control and Complications Study Group Trial demonstrated that the incidence of these complications can be reduced by tight glycaemic control but the risk of severe hypoglycaemic reactions is increased.[1] Follow-up of this cohort of patients confirmed that these benefits were long lasting even if patients were unable to maintain tight control in the long term.[2]

Patients with type I diabetes and end-stage diabetic nephropathy may benefit from simultaneous pancreas and kidney transplantation (SPK). This not only removes the need for dialysis in these patients, but also results in normoglycaemia without the need for insulin in over 85% of patients.[3] Unfortunately, the morbidity and mortality associated with SPK transplantation mean that only a small number of patients are fit enough to undergo SPK transplantation and in addition many more patients have labile diabetes without concurrent renal failure.[4]

Many of the complications of whole pancreas transplantation are associated with the exocrine portion of the pancreas (pancreatitis, pancreatic fistula). The islets of Langerhans account for only 1% of the mass of the pancreas but contain the beta and alpha cells responsible for insulin and glucagon production necessary for glycaemic control. The concept of extracting and transplanting islets is not new and was initially attempted in 1893 by P. Williams in Bristol. He transplanted a fragmented sheep's pancreas subcutaneously into a 15-year-old boy dying of ketoacidosis.[5] This early xenograft was, not surprisingly, unsuccessful but predated the discovery of insulin by nearly 30 years. The era of experimental islet research began in 1911, when Bensley stained islets within the guinea-pig pancreas using a number of dyes, and was able to pick free the occasional islet for morphological study.[6] Mass isolation of large numbers of viable islets from the human pancreas has proven to be a challenge ever since. The average adult human pancreas weighs 70 g, contains an average of 1–2 million islets of average diameter 157 μm, constituting between 0.8% and 3.8% of the total mass of the gland.[7] It was almost 100 years after the work of Bensley that Scharp et al. reported insulin independence after islet transplantation; however, even this was short lived and difficult to reproduce.[8,9]

✓✓ In 2000 the Edmonton group reported a series of seven consecutive patients in whom insulin independence was achieved after islet transplantation.[10]

This remarkable outcome was achieved by transplanting at least two islet preparations from different donors and using a novel steroid-free immunosuppression regimen of tacrolimus, sirolimus and induction with daclizumab. This regimen has been termed 'the Edmonton protocol' and many units worldwide have attempted to replicate these outcomes, with variable success.[11,12] In the aftermath of the Edmonton protocol, islet transplantation is considered in many countries as 'standard of care' for a select group of patients with type I diabetes and is funded through the healthcare system in Canada and the NHS in the UK. The results of combined islet and kidney transplantation now match those of islet alone,[13,14] and recent data suggest that islets transplanted with a kidney may prolong the patient and kidney graft survival and protect against diabetic vascular complications.[15,16]

Patient selection and assessment

There are two principal indications for islet transplantation:

1. **Severely impaired awareness of hypoglycaemia (IAH) despite optimum insulin therapy.** IAH occurs in 20–25% of patients with type I diabetes and is potentially life threatening. These patients have a defective counter-regulatory hormonal response to hypoglycaemia, are unable to identify low blood sugars and therefore institute corrective measures.[4] Defective recognition

of hypoglycaemia increases the risk of severe hypoglycaemic episodes that can result in coma and death. The impact on quality of life for these patients is substantial, and social activities and employment can be severely restricted; indeed, in the UK, patents with IAH cannot hold a UK driving licence.

2. **Patients with type I diabetes and a functioning kidney allograft who are unable to maintain their HbA1c below 7%.** In this patient group it is not necessary to demonstrate IAH as they are already taking immunosuppression and it has been shown that the improved glycaemic control after islet transplantation in this setting is associated with a reduction in long-term diabetic complications.

Impaired awareness of hypoglycaemia can be assessed by patient history and by asking the patient to keep a diary of insulin usage, dietary intake and hypoglycaemic events, in particular those events requiring assistance from relatives or those requiring hospitalisation. The use of a continuous glucose monitoring sensor (CGMS) can be very useful in assessing daily glucose profiles pre- and post-islet transplantation (**Fig. 10.1**).[17] Scoring systems such as the Gold or Clark scores allow numerical documentation of the degree of IAH. The Gold score asks the question 'do you know when your hypos are commencing?' and the patient completes a linear scale from 1 to 7 (always aware to never aware). A score of 4 or above suggests IAH. The Clark method asks eight questions to document the patient's exposure and responses to moderate and severe hypoglycaemia, and

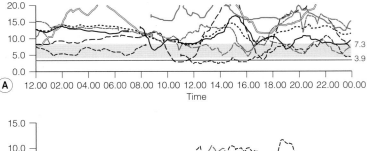

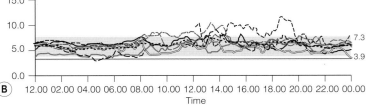

Figure 10.1 • CGMS profiles before **(a)** and after **(b)** islet transplantation.

again a score of 4 or more suggests IAH.[4] Ryan et al. have described a composite HYPO score based on 4 weeks of glucose values.[18] They suggest that this provides a more objective assessment of the metabolic instability of an individual patient and allows pre- and post-transplant comparison. Patients should be assessed by a multidisciplinary team consisting of a diabetologist, transplant surgeon, dietician and a diabetes nurse specialist. This will ensure that their current insulin regimen and dietary compliance are optimum and that the patient is fully informed about the likely outcome of islet transplantation and the risks involved, principally post-transplant immunosuppression.

Islet isolation

Donor factors contributing to successful islet isolation have been documented by Lakey et al. (Table 10.1).[19] This paper suggests that pancreata from older donors with a higher body mass index (BMI) should result in a significantly higher islet yield. O'Gorman et al. have suggested a scoring system from 1 to 100 to give a numerical assessment of the likelihood of successful isolation from a specific donor pancreas.[20] These studies, however, only predict successful isolation and do not take into consideration data that suggest that islets isolated from younger donors are functionally better.[21] In the UK a sharing scheme was introduced in December 2010 where patients for SPK transplantation and islet transplantation are placed on a common waiting list and pancreata offered on a named patient basis. Multiple donor and recipient factors are taken into consideration, allowing islet and whole pancreas recipients equal access to suitable organs.

Most of the outcome data on islet transplantation are based on organs from brain dead donors (DBD); however, there is growing evidence that pancreata from donation after circulatory death (DCD) can produce transplantable preps and good outcomes. Most of the data on DCD islet transplantation are from the Kyoto group and although long-term graft survival is obtained, insulin independence is less common.[22–26]

It is critical that the pancreas for islet isolation is retrieved with the same care as that for whole pancreas transplantation and that the cold ischaemic time is minimised, ideally to under 8 hours.[27] Pancreata should be transported rapidly and the staff in the isolation laboratory should be ready to begin the isolation immediately. It has been demonstrated that suspending the explanted pancreas in a bilayer of oxygenated perfluorocarbon (PFC) and University of Wisconsin (UW) solution during or after transport allows satisfactory islet preparations to be obtained from suboptimal pancreases and may even increase yields from pancreases with long ischaemia times.[28,29] PFC-based preservation may also help expand the donor pool by improving islet isolation from DCD pancreases and older donors.[30]

The semi-automated process for islet isolation that is used in most labs was described by Ricordi et al. in 1989.[31] This involves digestion of the pancreas using a combination of collagenase enzyme and mechanical dissociation of the pancreas in the Ricordi chamber (**Fig. 10.2**). A number of new enzyme blends have been developed for human isolation,

Table 10.1 • Donor-related variables predicting isolation success

Variable	P value	R value	Odds ratio
Donor age (years)	<0.05	0.18	1.10
Body mass index	<0.01	0.19	1.30
Local vs. distant procurement team	<0.01	0.21	7.04
Min. blood glucose	<0.01	−0.24	0.68
Duration of cardiac arrest	<0.01	−0.17	0.81
Duration of cold storage	<0.05	−0.13	0.86

Reproduced from Lakey JR, Warnock GL, Rajotte RV et al. Variables in organ donors that affect the recovery of human islets of Langerhans. Transplantation 1996; 61(7):1047–53. With permission from Lippincott, Williams & Wilkins.

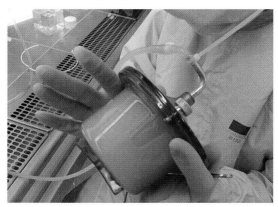

Figure 10.2 • Ricordi chamber.

including collagenase NB1 (Serva), Liberase MTF (Roche) and C1 collagenase HA (Vitacyte). Each of these differs slightly in the enzyme blend and manufacturing process but promises to deliver more consistent, better quality islet yields. The prep is then purified on a continuous density gradient using a COBE 2991 cell separator, resulting in a packed cell volume of only 1–2 mL (**Fig. 10.3**).[32] Although unpurified preps can be used (particularly in autotransplants), the risk of portal vein thrombosis, portal hypertension and disseminated intravascular coagulation (DIC) is increased.[33–36]

After isolation and purification, it is now standard practice to place the islet prep in culture for 12–48 hours. There are compelling data that this does not adversely affect islet graft function and does in fact increase purity of the prep.[37] Extended culture up to 48 hours can also be used to assess the viability of an islet graft, particularly after DCD isolation.

The number of islets in the prep is documented in terms of islet equivalents (IEQ). This counting method adjusts for the fact that islets vary greatly in size and cell viability stains such as fluorescenediacetate/propidium iodide and SytoGreen/ethidium bromide are used to determine the viable beta-cell mass.[38]

The minimum release criteria in the UK for an islet preparation are:

- >200 000 islet equivalents
- >70% viability
- >30% purity
- Gram stain negative
- endotoxin negative.

It is accepted that these criteria are subjective and open to observer variation and error. Some assessment of the 'quality' of the prep should also be made. Experienced islet lab staff can comment on the morphology of the cells, the integrity of the islets and whether or not there is evidence of central necrosis within the islets. Islet oxygen consumption rate and beta-cell ATP content show good correlation between product testing and in vivo islet function in animal studies, and may be useful in the future but are time consuming and expensive. The Minnesota group has demonstrated good correlation between marginal mass islet transplants in diabetic nude mice and outcome of human islet transplants from the same donor.[39]

Modern islet isolation facilities must comply with current good manufacturing practice (cGMP). The facility must be purpose built to comply with regulatory authorities, which in the UK comprise the Human Tissue Authority (HTA) and the Medicines and Healthcare products Regulatory Authority (MHRA). These regulations are designed to ensure that each lab produces a safe, consistent and traceable product, and influence the structural design of the laboratory, the documentation of standard operating procedures and of individual isolations and the training of members of the isolation team. Modern islet isolation is therefore expensive and requires a large number of staff to cover a 24/7 on-call rota. In the UK a hub and spoke model exists, whereby three isolation facilities provide islets for transplantation in seven centres.

The islet transplant

In the original Edmonton protocol, >11 000 IEQ/kg were required to achieve insulin independence and therefore at least two islet infusions are normally

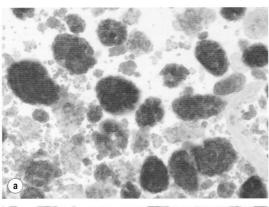

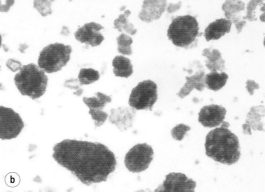

Figure 10.3 • Islets stained red with dithizone before **(a)** and after **(b)** purification.

required.[10] Islet preps are blood group matched with the potential recipient but the need for close tissue matching is not clear. There is no evidence that closely matched preps have a better outcome; however, it is likely to be beneficial to avoid repeated common mismatches as recipients may, in the event of graft rejection, become sensitised to multiple common alloantigens.

The islets are normally infused into the portal vein of the recipient under local anaesthetic and sedation in the radiology suite.[40] A 4F cannula is introduced under ultrasound and videofluoroscopy into the main portal vein and the islet prep infused under gravity feed over a period of 15–20 minutes (**Fig. 10.4**). Portal venous pressures are measured during the infusion process and if there is a significant rise, the infusion should be stopped until the portal pressure falls. The islet prep is heparinised (35 U/kg patient body weight) to reduce the risk of portal vein thrombosis. This should ideally be done by experienced interventional radiologists and the track of the cannula occluded on withdrawal to reduce the risk of bleeding. The infusion into the portal vein can also be carried out by surgical cannulation of an omental vessel or the umbilical vein. The intraportal site for islet embolisation was recognised to be the most efficient location for islet implantation in the rodent, with the benefit of high vascularity, proximity to islet-specific nutrient factors and physiological first-pass insulin delivery to the liver.[41] While many different sites have been tried for islet implantation, the optimal site appears to be through portal venous embolisation. Attempts to embolise the spleen have led to significant life-threatening complications of splenic infarction, rupture and even gastric perforation.[42,43] More recently, reports of experimental implantation of islets into the gastric submucosa have shown improved vascularisation of the graft.[44] Recent developments in encapsulation technology have stimulated interest in using alternative sites. Encapsulation devices protect the islets from immunological attack while allowing insulin to be secreted.[45] Such devices have been implanted subcutaneously, intramuscularly and into the omentum, but with limited clinical application so far.

After infusion into the liver, the islets undergo a process of angiogenesis, which takes 14–21 days. Interestingly, this is often reflected in the reduced need for insulin in islet graft recipients around 3–4 weeks post-transplant.

Immunosuppression and outcomes

All seven patients in the original Edmonton experience were insulin independent at 1 year post-transplant; however, follow-up of this cohort revealed that only 10% remained free of insulin at 5 years.[46] Alternative immunosuppression strategies have been reported in an attempt to improve these long-term outcomes. T-cell-depleting agents

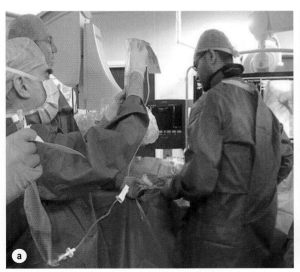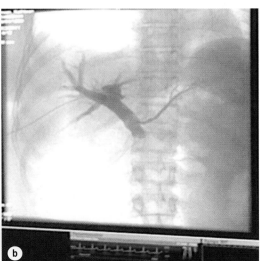

Figure 10.4 • Islet infusion into the portal vein.

such as antithymocyte globulin (ATG), anti-CD3 and alemtuzumab (campath/anti-CD52) have been used as alternative induction therapy and combined with agents such as etanercept/tumour necrosis factor (TNF)-α or mycophenolate mofetil/tacrolimus as maintenance therapy.[47] Barton et al. have published data from the Collaborative Islet Transplant Registry on 677 patients receiving 1375 islet infusions between 1999 and 2010.[48] These data demonstrate a significant improvement in long-term insulin independence in the 2007–2010 era compared to earlier years (**Fig. 10.5**), with 3-year insulin independence now approaching 50%. This report also demonstrates that patients who receive T-cell-depleting agents combined with TNF-α inhibition have better 3- to 5-year insulin independence rates (62% vs. 43%).

Serious adverse events after islet transplantation are either related to the infusion procedure or the immunosuppression. The more serious procedure-related complications of segmental portal vein thrombosis and bleeding have been reported in 4% and 10%, respectively.[49,50] The risk of portal vein thrombosis can be minimised by heparinisation of the recipient and by using only low-volume, high-purity preps. Bleeding from the liver puncture can be avoided by using a fine-bore (4 French) cannula and by ablating the track in the liver using coils, thrombostatic agents or a coagulative laser.[40] Leucopenia, neutropenia and sepsis have all been described after islet transplantation.[51] A reduction in estimated glomerular filtration rate has been described in islet transplant recipients in the long term post-transplant, but reports of clinically significant renal impairment are rare.[48]

One of the biggest challenges in islet transplantation is monitoring the graft. No reliable investigations exist to monitor graft function or detect acute rejection. Experimental studies in rats suggest that islets labelled with superparamagnetic iron oxide (SPIO) nanoparticles can be monitored using magnetic resonance imaging (MRI) scanning and that loss of the islet-related MRI spots correlates with rejection.[52] Metabolic studies such as the C-peptide response to a glucose challenge may give an indirect indication of ongoing graft mass but as yet cannot aid in predicting acute rejection.[53]

Barriers to long-term function

Figure 10.6 illustrates the multiple factors that contribute to islet death and subsequent graft failure. The organ retrieval process and subsequent cold ischaemic time (CIT) have a significant negative impact on the outcome of islet isolation. The increasing use of pancreata from DCD donors where there have not been the physiological changes associated with brain death may be beneficial for islet isolation, and techniques such as using extracorporeal membrane oxygenation (ECMO) circuits in the donor may result in islets that are protected from ischaemic change. There is no doubt that minimising the time between cross-clamp in the donor and beginning the isolation process in the lab improves the islet yield and long-term graft function, with the lesson that pancreata must be transported rapidly to the laboratory and the isolation process started immediately. Improvements in isolation techniques have seen an increase in the average number of islets that can be produced per isolation and ultimately improvements in graft survival.

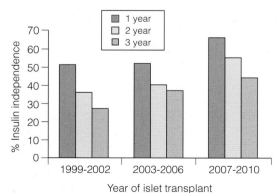

Figure 10.5 • Improvement in long-term insulin independence after islet transplantation from 1999 to 2010.[48]

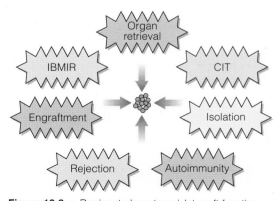

Figure 10.6 • Barriers to long-term islet graft function.

There is an immediate blood-mediated inflammatory reaction (IBMIR) to the islet graft as soon as the islets are infused into the portal vein. Platelets bind to the surface of the islets and leucocytes infiltrate the graft. This contributes largely to the early loss of islets post-transplant, which can be as high as 60% of the graft.[54] Strategies such as heparinisation of the recipient and ongoing insulin therapy may help to abrogate this process.[55] Little is known about the engraftment process of human islets within the liver. Transient elevation of liver enzymes is very common post-islet transplantation and it is interesting that the use of anti-inflammatory agents such as TNF-α blockers appears to improve graft survival.

Islets as a cell therapy

The shortage of organ donors coupled with the increased demand for islets has led to much research into alternative sources of insulin-producing cells that would be renewable and not depend solely on the availability of human cadaveric donors. The use of foetal or adult porcine islets for human xenotransplants has been explored; however, the high levels of immunosuppression required and the risk of transmission of porcine endogenous infections means that xenotransplantation is still some way in the future.

Stem cells are capable of both self-renewal and multilineage differentiation. They have the potential to proliferate and differentiate into any type of cell and to be genetically modified in vitro, thus providing a renewable source of cells for transplantation. Several potential strategies exist for developing a replenishable supply of beta cells. One of these is through directed differentiation of human embryonic stem cells (hESCs).[56] Functioning beta cells have been produced using this technology but concerns have been raised around the reproducibility of these processes and around the potential for these cells to develop into teratomas. In 2006, Takahashi and Yamanaka[57] described a technique whereby adult somatic cells could be de-differentiated and then induced to develop into different cell types. They used a cocktail of four transcription factors to produce these induced pluripotent stem cells (iPS cells), and many groups have reproduced this work and developed cells of multiple lineages using this technology. The Melton group from Cambridge demonstrated that, in vivo, three transcription factors are required for beta-cell development, namely Ngn3, Pdx1 and MafA.[58] These are encouraging steps forward in the development of stem-cell-derived islets but there are still issues around upscaling of cell numbers and the potential for residual de-differentiated cells to produce tumours in the recipient. One exciting prospect is the potential existence of stem cells within the pancreas that could develop into new beta cells or with the potential to transdifferentiate non-endocrine tissue into functioning islets.[59]

Key points

- Islet transplantation is now considered as 'standard of care' for patients with type I diabetes and severely impaired awareness of hypoglycaemia.
- The long-term outcomes of islet transplantation have improved significantly over the last 10 years, with insulin independence at 3 years approaching that of whole pancreas transplanation.
- Immunosuppression with T-cell-depleting agents appears to give the best long-term graft survival.

References

1. The Diabetes Control and Complications Trial Research Group. The effect of intensive treatment of diabetes on the development and progression of long-term complications in insulin dependent diabetes mellitus. N Engl J Med 1993;329:977–86.

2. DCCT/EDIC Research Group. Intensive diabetes therapy and glomerular filtration rate in type 1 diabetes. N Engl J Med 2011;365(25):2366–76.

3. Sutherland DER, Gruessener RWG, Gruessener AC. Pancreas transplantation for the treatment of diabetes mellitus. World J Surg 2001;25:487–96.

4. Graveling AJ, Frier BM. Impaired awareness of hypoglycaemia: a review. Diabetes Metab 2010;36(Suppl. 3):S64–74.

5. Williams P. Notes on diabetes treated with extract and by grafts of sheep's pancreas. Br Med J 1894;2:1303–4.

6. Bensley RR. Studies on the pancreas of the guinea pig. Am J Anat 1911;12:297–388.

7. Robertson GS, Dennison AR, Johnson PR, et al. A review of pancreatic islet autotransplantation. Hepatogastroenterology 1998;45(19):226–35.

8. Scharp DW, Lacy PE, Santiago JV, et al. Insulin independence after islet transplantation into type I diabetic patient. Diabetes 1990;39(4):515–8.

9. Brendel M, Hering B, Schulz A, et al. International Islet Transplant Registry Report. Germany: University of Giessen; 2001.

10. Shapiro AM, Lakey JR, Ryan EA, et al. Islet transplantation in seven patients with type 1 diabetes mellitus using a glucocorticoid-free immunosuppressive regimen. N Engl J Med 2000; 343(4):230–8.

11. Shapiro AM, Ricordi C, Hering B, et al. Edmonton's islet success has indeed been replicated elsewhere. Lancet 2003;362(9391):1242.

12. Shapiro AM, Ricordi C, Hering BJ, et al. International trial of the Edmonton protocol for islet transplantation. N Engl J Med 2006;355(13):1318–30.

13. Kaufman DB, Baker MS, Chen X, et al. Sequential kidney/islet transplantation using prednisolone free immunosuppression. Am J Transplant 2002;2:674–7.

14. Toso C, Morel P, Bucher P, et al. Insulin independence after conversion to tacrolimus and sirolimus based immunosuppression in islet-kidney recipients. Transplantation 2003;76:1133–4.

15. Fiorina P, Folli F, Zerbini G, et al. Islet transplantation is associated with improvement of renal function among uraemic patients with type I diabetes mellitus and kidney transplants. J Am Soc Nephrol 2003;14:2510–8.

16. Fiorini P, Folli F, Maffi P, et al. Islet transplantation improves vascular diabetic complications in patients with diabetes who underwent kidney transplantaion: a comparison between kidney–pancreas and kidney-alone transplantation. Transplantation 2003;14:1296–301.

17. Ryan EA, Germsheid J. Use of continuous glucose monitoring system in the management of severe hypoglycemia. Diabetes Technol Ther 2009;11(10):635–9.

18. Ryan EA, Shandro T, Green K, et al. Assessment of the severity of hypoglycaemia and glycaemic lability in type I diabetic subjects undergoing islet transplantation. Diabetes 2004;53:955–62.

19. Lakey JR, Warnock GL, Rajotte RV, et al. Variables in organ donors that affect the recovery of human islets of Langerhans. Transplantation 1996;61(7):1047–53.

20. O'Gorman D, Kin T, Murdoch T, et al. The standardization of pancreatic donors for islet isolations. Transplantation 2005;80(6):801–6.

21. Ihm SH, Matsumoto I, Sawada T, et al. Effect of donor age on function of isolated human islets. Diabetes 2006;55(5):1361–8.

22. Markmann JF, Deng S, Desai NM, et al. The use of non-heart-beating donors for isolated pancreatic islet transplantation. Transplantation 2003;75(9):1423–9.

23. Kenmochi T, Maruyama M, Saigo K, et al. Successful islet transplantation from the pancreata of non heart beating donors. Transplant Proc 2008;40(8):2568–70.

24. Liu X, Matsumoto S, Okitsu T, et al. Analysis of donor and isolation-related variables from non heart beating donors (NHBD) using the Kyoto isolation method. Cell Transplant 2008;17(6):649–56.

25. Saito T, Gotoh M, Satomi S, et al. Islet transplantation using donors after cardiac death: report of the Japan Islet Transplantation Registry. Transplantation 2010;90(7):74.

26. Zhao M, Muiesan P, Amiel SA, et al. Human islets derived from donors after cardiac death are fully biofunctional. Am J Transplant 2007;7(10):2318–25.

27. Lakey JR, Kneteman NM, Rajotte RV, et al. Effect of core pancreas temperature during cadaveric procurement on human islet isolation and functional viability. 1. Transplantation 2002;73(7):1106–10.

28. Deai T, Tanioka Y, Suzuki Y, et al. The effect of the two-layer cold storage method on islet isolation from ischemically damaged pancreas. Kobe J Med Sci 1999;45(3–4):191–9.

29. Tsujimura T, Kuroda Y, Kin T, et al. Human islet transplantation from pancreases with prolonged cold ischaemia using additional preservation by the two layer (UW solution/perfluorochemical) cold storage method. Transplantation 2002;74:1687–91.

30. Ricordi C, Fraker C, Szust J, et al. Improved human islet isolation from marginal donors following addition of oxygenated perfluorocarbon to the cold storage solution. Transplantation 2003;75:1524–7.

31. Ricordi C, Lacy PE, Scharp DW. Automated islet isolation from human pancreas. Diabetes 1989;38(Suppl. 1):140–2.

32. Lake SP, Bassett PD, Larkins A, et al. Large-scale purification of human islets utilizing discontinuous albumin gradient on IBM 2991 cell separator. Diabetes 1989;38(Suppl. 1):143–5.

33. Shapiro AM, Lakey JR, Rajotte RV, et al. Portal vein thrombosis after transplantation of partially purified pancreatic islets in a combined human liver/islet allograft. Transplantation 1995;59(7):1060–3.

34. Walsh TJ, Eggleston JC, Cameron JL. Portal hypertension, hepatic infarction, and liver failure complicating pancreatic islet autotransplantation. Surgery 1982;91(4):485–7.

35. Froberg MK, Leone JP, Jessurun J, et al. Fatal disseminated intravascular coagulation after autologous islet transplantation. Hum Pathol 1997;28(11):1295–8.

36. Gray DW, Sutton R, McShane P, et al. Exocrine contamination impairs implantation of pancreatic islets transplanted beneath the kidney capsule. J Surg Res 1988;45:432.

37. Alejandro JV, Ferreira A, Caulfield T, et al. Insulin independence in 7 patients following transplantation of cultured human islets. Am J Transplant 2002;2:227.

38. Gray DWR, Morris PJ. The use of fluorescein diacetate and ethidium bromide as a viability stain for isolated islets of Langerhans. Stain Technol 1987;62:379–81.

39. Hering BJ, Kandaswamy R, Harmon J, et al. Transplantation of cultured islets from two layer preserved pancreases in type I diabetes with anti CD3 antibody. Am J Transplant 2004;4:390–401.

40. Owen RJ, Ryan EA, O'Kelly K, et al. Percutaneous transhepatic pancreatic islet cell transplantation in type 1 diabetes mellitus: radiologic aspects. Radiology 2003;229:165–70.

41. Kemp C, Knight M, Scharp D, et al. Effect of transplantation site on the result of pancreatic islet isografts in diabetic rats. Diabetologia 1973; 9:486–91.

42. White SA, London NJ, Johnson PR, et al. The risks of total pancreatectomy and splenic islet autotransplantation. Cell Transplant 2000;9(1):19–24.

43. Menger MD, Vajkoczy P, Beger C, et al. Orientation of microvascular blood flow in pancreatic islet isografts. J Clin Invest 1994;93(5):2280–5.

44. Echeverri GJ, McGrath K, Bottino R, et al. Endoscopic gastric submucosal transplantation of islets (ENDO-STI): technique and initial results in diabetic pigs. Am J Transplant 2009;9(11):2485–96.

45. Qi Z, Yamamoto C, Imori N, et al. Immunoisolation effect of polyvinyl alcohol (PVA) macroencapsulated islets in type 1 diabetes therapy. Cell Transplant 2012;21(2–3):525–34.

46. Ryan EA, Paty BW, Senior PA, et al. Five-year follow-up after clinical islet transplantation. Diabetes 2005;54(7):2060–9.

47. Bellin MD, Barton FB, Heitman A, et al. Potent induction immunotherapy promotes long-term insulin independence after islet transplantation in type 1 diabetes. Am J Transplant 2012;12(6):1576–83.

48. Barton FB, Rickels MR, Alejandro R, et al. Improvement in outcomes of clinical islet transplantation: 1999–2010. Diabetes Care 2012;35(7):1436–45.

49. Casey JJ, Lakey JRT, Ryan EA, et al. Portal venous pressure changes following sequential clinical islet transplantation. Transplantation 2002;74:913–5.

50. Ryan EA, Lakey JR, Paty BW. Successful islet transplantation: continued insulin reserve provides long-term glycaemic control. Diabetes 2002;51:2148–57.

51. Takita M, Matsumoto S, Noguchi H, et al. Adverse events in clinical islet transplantation: one institutional experience. Cell Transplant 2012;21(2–3):547–51.

52. Dixon S, Tapping CR, Walker JN, et al. The role of interventional radiology and imaging in pancreatic islet cell transplantation. Clin Radiol 2012;67(9):923–31.

53. Ryan EA, Lakey JR, Rajotte RV, et al. Clinical outcomes and insulin secretion after islet transplantation with the Edmonton protocol. Diabetes 2001;50(4):710–9.

54. Bennet W, Groth CG, Larsson R, et al. Isolated human islets trigger an instant blood mediated inflammatory reaction: implications for intraportal islet transplantation as a treatment for patients with type 1 diabetes. Ups J Med Sci 2000;105:125–33.

55. Koh A, Senior P, Salam A, et al. Insulin–heparin infusions peritransplant substantially improve single-donor clinical islet transplant success. Transplantation 2010;89:465–71.

56. Soria B, Roche E, Berné G, et al. Insulin secreting cells from embryonic stem cells normalise glycaemia in streptozotocin-induced diabetic mice. Diabetes 2000;49(2):157–62.

57. Takahashi K, Yamanaka S. Induction of pluripotent stem cells from mouse embryonic and adult fibroblast cultures by defined factors. Cell 2006;126(4):663–76.

58. Zhou Q, Brown J, Kanarek A, et al. In vivo reprogramming of adult pancreatic exocrine cells to beta-cells. Nature 2008;455(7213):627–32.

59. Jiang FX, Morahan G. Pancreatic stem cells: from possible to probable. Stem Cell Rev 2012;8(3):647–57.

11

Cardiothoracic transplantation

Asif Hasan
John H. Dark

Introduction

The first successful heart transplantation undertaken on December 1967, at least in the public eye, represents a defining moment in surgical treatment of heart diseases in the 20th century. Since then heart transplantation has evolved from an experimental procedure to an effective therapeutic strategy for end-stage heart disease. In the current era the median survival or half-life (the time at which 50% of transplant recipients remain alive) is 11 years. For adult and paediatric patients surviving to 1 year after transplant, the median survival has reached 14 years. Many hundreds of patients have now lived past 25 years since their transplant procedure.[1]

Nevertheless, the success of heart transplantation has raised expectations that under present circumstances it cannot fulfil. On one hand, due to improved management of ischaemic heart disease and increased longevity, the number of patients with heart failure is growing.[2] On the other hand, there is a decrease in the number of cardiac transplantations due to donor organ constraints. This disparity between the number of donors and potential recipients has stimulated research to find new alternatives to transplantation. However, these have so far had little impact on the current practice of heart transplantation. The advent of novel therapeutics and surgical options for impaired ventricles may in selected patients defer consideration for transplantation, and clinical guidelines have been provided for this purpose.[3] The contemporary practice of heart transplantation with respect to indications, surgical

techniques, and donor and recipient management will now be reviewed.

Indications for heart transplantation

The reason for undertaking heart transplantation is to prolong life and to improve its quality. The indications for adult heart transplantation have remained essentially unchanged over the last three decades and at present are predominantly coronary artery disease-related ischaemic cardiomyopathy (38%) and non-ischaemic cardiomyopathies (53%). Adult congenital heart disease (3%), valvular heart disease (3%), repeat transplantation (2.6%) and miscellaneous diagnoses (1%) constitute the rest.[1]

The indications for paediatric heart transplantation (<18 years) are different to adults. In our series of 182 paediatric heart transplants (1987–2009), 64% were undertaken for cardiomyopathy and 36% for congenital heart disease.[4]

Aetiology of heart disease

Introduction

End-stage heart failure has become a major medical problem.[2] The increasing prevalence with the rising age of the general population in most societies accounts for a large proportion of healthcare spending due to frequent hospital admissions.[5] In the aetiology of congestive heart failure (CHF), we differentiate primarily ischaemic from other cardiomyopathies and congenital heart disease during transplant candidate assessment.

Ischaemic heart disease

This constitutes the largest group requiring heart transplantation. These patients can present in a variety of ways, from being acutely ill after myocardial infarction on mechanical support to being chronically ill with heart failure with or without previous surgical or catheter-based intervention. Unfortunately, there are no conclusive prospective studies comparing conventional treatment methods with heart transplantation to provide guidance in risk–benefit assessment. A digest of current thinking would indicate that heart transplantation would definitely be indicated in a patient with severe heart failure with poor ventricular function (ejection fraction <15%), symptoms of heart failure with little or no angina, diffuse coronary artery disease, absence of reversible ischaemia and/or poor right ventricular function (ejection fraction <35%). What is clear is that patients with ischaemic cardiomyopathy who develop heart failure are likely to have a worse prognosis than non-ischaemic patients.[6]

Non-ischaemic cardiomyopathy

This group includes a variety of aetiologies with marked left and/or right ventricular dysfunction. Disease processes that result in changes in heart muscle are classified as: (a) dilated cardiomyopathy; (b) hypertrophic cardiomyopathy; (c) restrictive cardiomyopathy; and (d) arrhythmogenic right ventricular dysplasia. In patients with non-ischaemic cardiomyopathy, transplantation is indicated if there is failure of aggressive medical treatment.

Certain types of cardiomyopathies can show reversibility, and a period of observation with medical treatment should be tried before listing. These include lymphocytic myocarditis, peripartum cardiomyopathy, hypertensive cardiomyopathy and alcoholic cardiomyopathy.[7]

Indications for paediatric patients are similar; however, the risk of death is highest during the first 3 months after presentation, therefore failure of aggressive medical treatment early in the course of the disease should lead to early assessment for transplantation. Acute myocarditis needs a special mention as the finding of acute inflammation on biopsy is a favourable prognostic sign for subsequent recovery.[8]

Congenital heart disease

An increasing number of patients with congenital heart disease and heart failure are now presenting in adulthood. This group is particularly challenging due to multiple comorbidities. These include previous complex surgeries, human leucocyte antigen (HLA) sensitisation, and presence of profound cyanosis and erythrocytosis.[9]

Recipient evaluation and selection

Patients are evaluated for transplantation once a referral has been made. We admit the patient for a few days for assessment. During this period there is a systematic evaluation of both the physical and psychological state of the patient; it also gives an opportunity to develop a rapport between the patient, relatives and the multidisciplinary team. The protocol used in our own centre for assessment is summarised in Box 11.1. The assessment process is designed to answer the following questions:

1. Does the patient fulfil the selection criteria for heart transplantation?
2. Are there any contraindications to transplantation?
3. Is there any possibility of any other treatment option?

Selection criteria

The process of selection of patients for transplantation remains an inexact science. In the majority of cases the referral for transplantation is of a patient with chronic heart failure. In these cases there is remarkable divergence of opinions when a patient should be listed for heart transplantation, further compounded by a paucity of evidence to guide day-to-day clinical practice. Avoidance of transplantation when a patient is 'too good' has important prognostic indications, as the 10-year survival after orthotopic heart transplantation remains 50% in most centres.

✔✔ Mancini et al.[8] and others[9–11] showed that patients with a peak exercise oxygen consumption of <14 mL/kg/min had a significantly higher mortality than patients with a peak exercise oxygen consumption of >14 mL/kg/min.

Box 11.1 • Recipient assessment protocol for heart transplantation

1. Full medical assessment

Full history and physical examination. Investigations include:

- Full blood count, platelets and coagulation screen
- Blood group
- Urea and electrolytes, liver function and thyroid function
- Microbiology – sputum, midstream specimen of urine (MSU), nose/throat/axilla/perineum swabs for culture
- Full viral screen (with patient consent)
- Fasting glucose and lipids
- Twelve-lead ECG
- Chest X-ray (posterior–anterior and lateral)
- Spirometry
- Echocardiogram
- Chromium EDTA glomerular filtration rate (GFR) (renal opinion and abdominal ultrasound would be required if GFR <32.5 mL/min)
- Estimation of peak oxygen consumption (VO_{2max})
- Right heart catheter to assess filling pressures and calculate pulmonary vascular resistance, after discussion with the transplant cardiologist (as per protocol)
- Bone density (if >50 years or symptoms)
- Urine flow rate/residual (if male >50 years or symptoms)
- Carotid/peripheral artery Doppler (if symptoms)

2. A structured educational package – provided by the transplant coordinator

Discussion points include:

- Patient's understanding of his or her illness
- Donor compatibility
- Introduction to the concept of transplantation
- Preparation for admission
- Reason for assessment
- Travelling arrangements
- Explain investigations and visits
- Accommodation
- Survival figures
- Outpatient routine
- Surveillance biopsies
- Waiting lists and waiting period
- Adjusting to family life
- Bleeper
- Driving
- Returning to work

3. Social assessment

This looks at both practical and emotional aspects of the transplant process with the patient and carer. Areas covered include:

- Feelings about what is happening to them
- Social security benefits
- Support networks
- Coping strategies

The aim is to evaluate whether the patient understands and whether he or she will cope with having a transplant and to prepare the ground for future involvement throughout the patient's contact with the transplant team

4. Physiotherapy assessment

An assessment and education package from the transplant physiotherapist with regard to exercise pre- and post-transplant, and postoperative chest care

The limitation of this technique is that it can be influenced by body composition, individual motivation or general deconditioning. Some centres have incorporated the heart failure survival score (HFSS) to their preoperative assessment. The score consists of seven variables – resting heart rate, left ventricular ejection fraction, mean arterial blood pressure, interventricular conduction delay, peak exercise oxygen consumption (VO_2), serum sodium and ischaemic cardiomyopathy. Using these variables Aaronson et al. developed a mathematical model to predict outcome with medical management.[10] This score, along with maximal oxygen consumption (VO_{2max}) and clinical assessment, can bring some rigour to the selection process for transplantation.

> ✅ Deng et al.[11] showed that cardiac transplantation does not benefit patients with medium and low mortality risk as assessed by calculation of heart failure survival score.

Patients who are inotrope dependent and in persistent circulatory shock due to primary cardiac disorder undergo urgent assessment. The aim in these patients is to list them for urgent transplantation or consider ventricular assist device implantation.

Contraindications

Contraindications to heart transplantation are summarised in Box 11.2. These can be classed in three groups:

1. Factors that increase perioperative mortality, e.g. elevated pulmonary vascular resistance.
2. Factors affecting long-term prognosis.
3. Factors related to life-threatening non-compliance.

These exclusion criteria have continued to change with improvement in medical treatment and increasing experience with heart transplantation, and now successful outcome can be obtained in cases previously excluded. Some of the contraindications deserve special mention.

Pulmonary vascular resistance (PVR) of more than 6 Wood units has been considered an absolute contraindication to heart transplantation but with the introduction of nitric oxide, use of a bicaval anastomotic technique, early implantation of ventricular

---

Box 11.2 • Contraindications for heart transplant

Factors increasing perioperative mortality

- Irreversible pulmonary hypertension:
  - PVR>6 Wood units despite standardised reversibility testing protocol
  - TPG>14 mmHg
- Active infection
- Recent peptic ulcer disease
- Severe obesity (>140% ideal body weight)
- Cachexia (<80% ideal body weight)
- Pulmonary infarction within 6–8 weeks

Factors affecting long-term prognosis

- Age >65 years
- Severe renal impairment measured by EDTA GFR and kidney biopsy
- Brittle diabetes
- Active or recent malignancy
- Significant chronic lung disease, FEV_1 <40% predicted, FVC <50% of normal and DL_{CO} <40% of predicted
- Severe peripheral vascular disease
- Significant hepatic impairment

Factors that impair compliance

- Active mental illness
- Drug abuse within last 6 months refractory to treatment
- Chronic illness affecting function

DL_{CO}, carbon monoxide diffusing capacity; FEV_1, forced expiratory volume in 1 second; FVC, forced vital capacity; GFR, glomerular filtration rate; PVR, pulmonary vascular resistance (see Box 11.3); TPG, transpulmonary gradient (see Box 11.3).

---

assist devices, and increasing use of perioperative phosphodiesterase inhibitors and isoprenaline, good results can be obtained in patients who formerly would not have been offered the opportunity of transplantation. Nevertheless, the presence of an elevated PVR should not be taken lightly as the donor right ventricle generally tolerates a systolic pressure of more than 50 mmHg poorly and would acutely fail. In our own practice a PVR >3 Wood units would be considered a relative contraindication to transplantation. The **transpulmonary gradient (TPG)** (see **Box 11.3**) represents the pressure gradient across the pulmonary vascular bed and is independent of the pulmonary blood flow. Some consider the elevation of this above 14 mmHg as a more useful indication of significantly raised PVR as this is independent of the cardiac output, which may be poor in these

Pulmonary vascular resistance

PVR (Wood units) = [PA mean – pulmonary capillary wedge pressure (PCW)/CO]

Pulmonary vascular resistance index

PVRI (Wood units/m²) = (PA mean – PCW)/CI = PVR BSA

Transpulmonary gradient

TPG (mmHg) = PA mean – PCW

PVR – Pulmonary Vascular Resistance; TPG – Trans Pulmonary Gradient in mmHg; Mean PA – Mean Pulmonary Artery Pressure in mmHg; PCW – Pulmonary Capillary Wedge Pressure in mmHg; CO – Cardiac Output in Litres per minute; PVRI - Pulmonary Vascular Resistance Index; BSA – Body Surface Area

patients. We rely more on this criterion and generally consider a fixed TPG of 12 mmHg and above as an absolute contraindication. In paediatric patients a higher TPG can be considered as it could be overcome with a larger sized donor heart.

Renal dysfunction is one of the most common problems encountered in the assessment of these patients. Multiple studies have shown that it is a major risk factor for mortality after heart transplantation. A common dilemma is to distinguish between renal dysfunction due to intrinsic renal disease or severe heart failure and aggressive diuretic therapy. It is essential to measure the glomerular filtration rate (GFR) and a low GFR may occasionally indicate renal biopsy to further elucidate the cause. Others have used measurement of effective renal plasma flow (ERPF) as an investigative modality, and less than 200 mL/min is considered indicative of major intrinsic renal dysfunction and an indication for combined heart and kidney transplantation, which can be peformed with good outcomes.[12]

Diabetic candidates have been shown to have good outcomes in the absence of significant end-organ damage (retinopathy, nephropathy, autonomic dysfunction and neuropathy or advanced peripheral vascular disease). Previously often excluded from heart transplantation, the 1- and 3-year survival, as well as rejection rates and infection prevalence achieved after transplantation, are comparable to non-diabetic recipients.

Compliance is the neurobehavioural capacity to adhere to a complex lifelong medical regimen. Non-compliance following heart transplantation can lead to major morbidity or death. Unfortunately, there are no proven psychological or sociological factors to predict poor compliance or adverse outcome after

transplantation. Adherence to medical treatment and ability to keep appointments can provide some pointers towards compliance. Psychiatric disorders that impair compliance, such as severe depression or untreated schizophrenia, are contraindications to heart transplantation.[13]

Other options

It is not unusual to find patients who have been referred for transplantation to be suitable for alternative treatments. In addition, there are newer methods of treatment of heart failure in both medical and surgical disciplines being developed, and some of these patients could derive benefit from them.[14] Some developments are worth mentioning.

Cardiac resynchronisation treatment (CRT)

In 20–30% of patients with symptomatic heart failure there is a prolonged PR interval, wide QRS complexes and intraventricular conduction disorders leading to a discoordinate contraction pattern. The result is earlier atrial contraction causing mitral regurgitation. This is further compromised by paradoxical septal motion due to wide QRS and conduction abnormalities. CRT should be undertaken in patients with severe heart failure prior to assessment for transplantation.[15] We have used biventricular pacing in several of our patients, with improvement in functional class and subsequent delisting from transplantation.

Implantable cardio defibrillators (ICDs)

Implantable defibrillators have had beneficial impact on survival of patients with heart failure due to systolic dysfunction, especially when the aetiology is ischaemic.[16] However, ICD treatment is unlikely to benefit patients who are confined to the hospital for refractory heart failure.

Ventricular assist devices

Over approximately 15 years, ventricular assist device support has developed into a realistic option for selected patients with refractory congestive heart failure of various aetiologies. This has been established in the REMATCH trial, where medical management of New York Heart Association (NYHA) class IV heart failure patients was inferior to mechanical assistance when comparing 1- and 2-year survival.[17,18] Current continuous flow devices with their low mechanical failure rate and fewer haematological complications are set to revolutionise our management of advanced heart failure.[19] Currently these devices are only available for bridge to transplantation in the UK; however, with the decline in the number of heart transplants these devices may have to be considered as final destination for some patients.[20]

Donor selection and matching

> ✓ Specific guidelines for optimal donor selection have been published by the International Society for Heart and Lung Transplantation and affiliated organisations.[21]

Management of the potential organ donor has evolved and requires a multidisciplinary approach.[22] Donor allocation for hearts in the UK is run by the Organ Donation and Transplantation arm (ODT) of NHS Blood and Transplant (NHSBT). The hearts are allocated on a pro-rata basis; however, a category of 'urgent' was created in 1999 to deal with acutely ill patients. Once a donor is identified, certain criteria apply before acceptance.

Donor age

An upper limit of 65 years is generally advocated and used by our own unit, but there is variation in other centres. The current mean age, including paediatric donors, at our programme currently is 44 years. It is important that donor age should not be viewed in absolute terms but should be considered along with other factors such as cardiac function, recipient urgency and projected ischaemic times. However, older donors are more likely to have coronary artery disease and there is increased mortality for the recipient if the heart has come from a donor over 40 years of age.[1] The presence of coronary artery disease should not be considered an absolute exclusion criterion as satisfactory outcomes can be achieved with concomitant coronary revascularisation.[23] United Network for Organ Sharing (UNOS) data from the USA show that in 1982 2.1% of donors were aged 50 years or greater but by 1994 this percentage had increased

to 8.9% and has remained the same over the last 10 years.[24] It remains difficult to evaluate pre-existing donor coronary artery disease at the time of organ procurement. Some centres advocate a single-plane coronary angiography (on table), but the availability and interpretation remain problematic.

Cardiac function

Brain death leads to myocardial changes with abnormalities seen on electrocardiogram (ECG) of ST segment elevation, T-wave inversion and Q waves, often signifying subendocardial ischaemia. Events following brain death, namely prolonged hypotension, cardiopulmonary resuscitation and high-dose inotropic support, also contribute to cardiac dysfunction, particularly acute right ventricular impairment. The assessment of cardiac function is undertaken by echocardiogram, Swan–Ganz catheter and finally by the surgeon procuring the organ. Troponin I may be useful in detecting donor myocardial injury and elevated levels are associated with impaired cardiac function.[25]

There is no consensus on what degree of inotropic support correlates with structural and functional damage sufficient to compromise graft function. It has been recommended that hearts should not be used if the inotropic requirements exceed 20 µg/kg/min of dopamine. Often, inotropes are used in conjunction with fluid infusions to fill a vasodilated circulation and bolster perfusion pressure. We utilise arginine vasopressin under these conditions and wean the inotropes. Failure to wean the inotropes under these conditions is a bad prognostic sign and suggests cardiac dysfunction. Donor hearts developing arrhythmias are not considered suitable.

Donor disease

Donors with an active infective focus are usually turned down. However, donors with a history of meningitis that has been adequately treated are considered for donation. Hepatitis C patients are not considered unless the recipient is positive for hepatitis C or is acutely ill on the urgent list. Hepatitis B donors with positive surface antigen are avoided, but core antibody-positive donors (surface antigen-negative) can be considered.

Donor hearts from donors with primary brain tumours should all be considered for transplantation.

The risk of transmission of the tumour to the recipient is very small ($\approx$1%) and only 1.5–2% for the more aggressive tumours or when there has been craniotomy or shunting.[26]

A history of intravenous drug abuse may disqualify the donor, but exceptions can be in the presence of negative serological viral testing. High-risk donors require careful evaluation as the routine enzyme-linked immunosorbent assay (ELISA) testing serology used does not achieve the same specificity as DNA-based tests.[27] Chronic cocaine use causes cardiomyopathic changes and caution should be used in accepting hearts from such donors.

Size matching

As a general rule for routine adult heart transplantation with a normal PVR, 10% undersizing is acceptable, although much smaller donors have been reported with satisfactory outcome.[28] In patients with a raised PVR deliberate oversizing is routinely undertaken to overcome pulmonary vascular resistance. In the paediatric group oversizing is often done to utilise all available hearts. In our last 30 consecutive paediatric transplants the average size discrepancy between donor and recipient was 150%, and in a cohort of patients who had a failing Fontan circulation as an indication for transplantation, the oversizing was 250%. The adverse consequences of oversizing are delayed sternal closure, collapse of the left lower lobe and systemic hypertension. However, all these factors can resolve with time and appropriate treatment.

ABO compatibility

ABO compatibility is required to avoid hyperacute or accelerated acute rejection. Rhesus incompatibility is acceptable. The only ABO exception would be the A_2 subgroup, as donors with this subgroup may be less prone to producing hyperacute rejection, because A_2 antigen is not readily displayed on the endothelial surface of the heart. However, in the paediatric group successful heart transplantation has been undertaken in the presence of ABO incompatibility.[29] This is possible as the immune system in infants is immature and their anti-A and anti-B titres remain low until 12–14 months of age. We have successfully undertaken 10 transplants in children with ABO incompatibility.[30]

Immunological matching

The rationale for undertaking immunological testing is to identify potential recipients with circulating anti-HLA antibodies to avoid mismatch between donor and recipient that could lead to hyperacute or accelerated acute rejection (see Chapter 4).

Common causes of sensitisation are pregnancy, prior blood transfusion or insertion of a ventricular assist device. Rarely, a patient may be sensitised for unknown reasons. Precise identification of existing anti-HLA antibody can easily be achieved. Donors with those types can be avoided by the 'virtual crossmatch' and a safe transplant achieved, although making timings of the transplant difficult.

Donor heart procurement

It is important to optimise the haemodynamic, metabolic and respiratory condition of the donor to maximise the yield of donor organs. This may entail using a multidisciplinary team to manage and optimise the donor before retrieval. Some poorly functioning hearts could be resuscitated by careful manipulation of inotropes and loading conditions of the heart. Using this strategy, up to 30% of such hearts can be successfully 'resuscitated' and used for transplantation.[31]

The thoracic organs are accessed by midline sternotomy; this might have already been performed by the liver retrieval team. It is important to secure haemostasis carefully and volume replacement should continue actively. This requires careful consideration of other organs procured, especially the lungs.

Whilst the abdominal dissection is being undertaken the pericardium is opened and the heart is inspected for its functional state, as well as the presence of any congenital abnormality. The heart is palpated to feel any thrill for valvular heart disease or any coronary plaques. When the mobilisation of abdominal organs is completed, heparin at a dose of 300 units/kg is administered. If a central line is in place, it is withdrawn. The superior vena cava is ligated and the inferior vena cava is completely divided. This allows the heart to exsanguinate into the right pleural cavity. The aorta is now clamped and cardioplegic solution is infused via the aortic root. We use 1 litre of St Thomas's cold crystalloid cardioplegic solution; this is augmented with cold topical saline. The dose for paediatric donors is 30 mL/kg. During the administration of cardioplegia the right superior pulmonary vein is incised to decompress the left side of the heart.

Once the cardioplegia has been given, the cardiectomy can proceed further. The superior vena cava is incised above the previous ligature. The aorta is now divided below the innominate artery; this exposes the pulmonary artery, which is divided on the left side where the left pulmonary artery is attached to the pericardial reflection and the right pulmonary artery is divided behind the aorta. The left atrium is now incised at the level of the pericardial reflection. Due consideration to leave sufficient left atrial tissue along each pulmonary vein is essential when lungs are procured for transplantation.

The heart is now inspected for the presence of a patent foramen ovale and, if found, is oversewn. The heart is now packed inside three bags with cold saline in the intervening bags. The heart is then placed in a transport cooler packed in ice to be transported.

Heart transplantation (Figs 11.1 and 11.2)

The classical technique of orthotopic heart transplantation as described by Lower et al.[32] and now modified to use the bicaval addition has remained the standard operation for 30 years.

> ✅✅ The most significant modification to heart transplant procedure has been the use of a bicaval technique. This results in less tricuspid regurgitation and better haemodynamic performance of the implanted heart.[33]

The operation is undertaken with a midline sternotomy. Cardiopulmonary bypass (CPB) is established with right atrial venous cannulation to allow decompression of the heart; this allows for easier cannulation of superior and inferior venae cavae. The patient is then cooled to 32 °C. The cavae are now snared and the aorta is clamped. To facilitate bicaval anastomosis it is recommended that at this stage the interatrial groove is dissected to develop a cuff of left atrium. The cardiectomy proceeds with a right atrial incision, which runs parallel to the atrioventricular groove; care is taken at the inferior caval end of this incision to preserve as much tissue as possible to facilitate inferior caval anastomosis. An incision is then

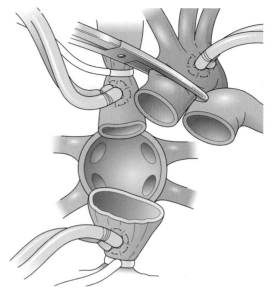

Figure 11.1 • Division of the right atrium to create superior and inferior vena caval cuffs for bicaval technique. The great vessels are divided as in the standard orthotopic method.

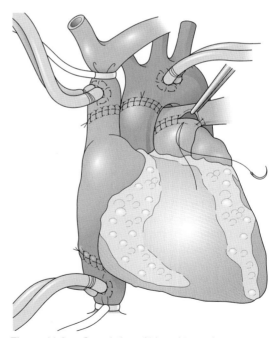

Figure 11.2 • Completion of bicaval transplant technique, showing the inferior vena caval, aortic and pulmonary artery anastomoses. Reproduced from Kirklin JK, Young JB, McGriffin DC. Heart transplantation. Edinburgh: Churchill Livingstone, 2002; Ch. 10.8, p. 343. With permission from Elsevier.

made in the roof of the left atrium to further decompress the heart before dividing the aorta just above the aortic valve. Retracting the heart downwards now exposes the pulmonary artery, which is again divided above the pulmonary valve. The superior vena cava is now divided just at its right atrial junction. The heart is now only attached to the pulmonary veins and via a small bridge of tissue to the inferior vena cava. The inferior caval attachment is divided, again being mindful of the inferior vena cava (IVC) cuff; the incision in the left atrium is now extended to encircle the pulmonary veins, leaving behind two pulmonary veins on each side attached with a bridge of tissue.

The donor heart is now prepared for implantation. The pulmonary veins are joined together by incisions removing any excess tissue, the pulmonary artery is cut back to its bifurcation, and a dose of blood cardioplegia is given in the aortic root. The donor and recipient atria are anastomosed with 3/0 polypropylene; care is taken not to leave excess tissue behind as it could be thrombogenic or can obstruct the pulmonary venous orifices. The suture line is not completed as a vent is left in the left atrium to take away the warm blood. The aortic anastomosis is now undertaken with a 4/0 polypropylene suture. At this stage the aortic cross-clamp can be removed to reduce the donor ischaemic time. De-airing is undertaken through the aortic root and a dose of steroids is given before the clamp is removed. This is a critical period as the heart has been reperfused after a prolonged period of ischaemia. The heart usually starts to beat, but if ventricular fibrillation occurs the heart is promptly defibrillated. Careful attention is paid to the perfusion pressures and the ventricle is kept decompressed; the atrial vent is left in until satisfactory contractility is resumed. The pulmonary artery anastomosis is next undertaken, care being taken in trimming of the pulmonary arterial cuff to avoid redundancy. The IVC and then the superior vena caval anastomoses are completed.

Once the implantation is complete the body temperature is brought back to normothermia. We would reperfuse the heart for at least 10 minutes of every hour of ischaemic time before making an attempt at weaning CPB. Weaning from CPB is undertaken carefully, avoiding distension of the right ventricle. Before closure of the chest, ventricular and atrial temporary pacing wires are attached, and a left atrial monitoring line is left in situ. Isoprenaline

is frequently used for rate control and initial right ventricular afterload reduction.

Special situations

Heart transplantation for congenital heart disease

This group of patients presents special technical challenges due to unusual anatomy, previous operations and raised pulmonary vascular resistance. Heart transplantation can be undertaken to overcome most structural abnormalities.[34]

Heterotopic heart transplantation

This describes the placement of the donor heart in parallel with the native heart. In the current era there are two possible indications for this procedure:

1. if the pulmonary vascular resistance is high (pulmonary artery pressure >60 mmHg) and cannot be manipulated by the use of nitric oxide;
2. if the donor is considerably smaller than the recipient.

The results of heterotopic transplantation have been generally inferior to orthotopic heart transplantation. However, this technique is occasionally considered.[35]

Perioperative management

The principles of early management of the heart transplant patient are: (a) to maintain graft function, specifically to recognise and manage right ventricular impairment early; (b) to establish adequate immunosuppression; (c) to prevent and treat early infections; and (d) to allow recovery of other system functions, such as renal function.

Graft function

Most patients will have reduced myocardial function after heart transplantation and would require inotropic support, which is usually weaned over 24–48 hours. However, some patients develop either right or left ventricular dysfunction. Development of right ventricular dysfunction is multifactorial. Initially, brain death-induced subendocardial ischaemia can occur in the donor. The right ventricle has a disposition to suffer the consequences of relative size mismatching of donor and recipient, especially related to the level of PVR after transplantation, inadequate myocardial preservation and discrepancy in size of the donor (smaller donor). The management of this would consist of adjusting preload, aggressive right ventricle (RV) afterload reduction and inotropic support. If the PVR is elevated, nitric oxide is added and in extreme cases a right ventricular assist device is used. It is important that an anastomotic complication is excluded by measuring the pressure gradient across the pulmonary artery suture line; surgical revision is indicated if the systolic gradient is >10 mmHg.

Left ventricular dysfunction is again managed with adjustment in inotropic support; under rare circumstances the dysfunction can be life threatening and left ventricular assist may be required.

Immunosuppression

Triple therapy consisting of ciclosporin, azathioprine or mycophenolate mofetil and steroids is the standard regimen used by most centres. We employ induction therapy using equine antithymocyte globulin (ATG) in the paediatric group and in patients with severe renal impairment who are intolerant of ciclosporin. Tacrolimus has been used as a substitute for ciclosporin in patients with persistent rejection and in children with side-effects of ciclosporin, i.e. gingival hypertrophy and hirsutism. Newer immunosuppressive agents, such as rapamycin and interleukin-2 receptor antibodies (basiliximab and daclizumab), are being used in heart transplant rejection prophylaxis and treatment but have not yet found their place in routine immunosuppression protocols, despite a number of promising studies.

Monitoring of rejection following heart transplantation is crucial to short- and long-term survival of patients. The gold standard of rejection monitoring is endomyocardial biopsy. However, the histological findings of rejection are not uniformly present throughout the myocardium, and a high degree of clinical vigilance is needed in post-transplant follow-up of these patients. Approximately 7% of patients have an early rejection episode within 30 days of transplantation and at least 15% receive treatment for acute rejection within the first year.

Infection prophylaxis and treatment

Significant progress has been made in both treatment and prophylaxis for heart transplant recipients. In most centres infective episodes have been reduced to <15% during the first year after transplantation. Notably, a dramatic reduction in cytomegalovirus (CMV), *Pneumocystis carinii* pneumonia (PCP) and toxoplasmosis infections has been achieved with strict prophylactic antimicrobial regimes. The most common type of infection is bacterial (50%), followed by viral (40%), fungal (5%) and protozoal (5%). The commonest single organism causing infection after heart transplantation is CMV.

Survival

The registry of the International Society for Heart and Lung Transplantation (ISHLT) collects data on heart transplantation performed worldwide. The data have been collected since 1980; in 2011 an important milestone was achieved, with 100 000 patients being registered.[1] The survival data show 5-year survival of approximately 65%, at 10 years approximately 50% and at 15 years 25–30%. The median survival time is now 10 years. For patients who are alive at 1 year, the median survival time is 14 years. Those who undergo transplantation for non-ischaemic cardiomyopathy have the best survival, followed by those with ischaemic cardiomyopathy. Survival of patients who receive heart transplantss because of congenital heart disease, valvular cardiomyopathy, and those in need of re-transplant is inferior to the former two groups, with the survival differences again being limited to the first post-transplant year.

Quality of life improves remarkably after transplantation. Some of our patients have lifetime ambitions of running marathons or climbing mountains. This improvement has been consistently shown in several studies.[36]

Cause of death after heart transplantation

This information is available from the ISHLT registry but needs to be considered in the context of inherent difficulties associated with registry information, namely non-uniformity of definitions, validity of information and other difficulties of collecting information. The distribution of causes, and modes and mechanisms of mortality after heart transplantation are time related. During the first 30 days after heart transplantation, graft failure accounts for 41% of the deaths, followed by non-CMV infection (14.2%) and multiorgan failure (13.9%). After 30 days and up to 1 year, non-CMV infection accounts for up to one-third of deaths (33%), followed by graft failure and acute rejection (together≈20%). Beyond 5 years, cardiac allograft vasculopathy (CAV) and late graft failure (possibly due to CAV) are the predominant causes of deaths. Malignancies are increasingly common after 10 years (>30%), and account for approximately 20% and non-CMV infections 10% of late deaths. Renal failure and multiorgan impairment are significant contributors.[1]

Cardiac allograft vasculopathy

This is an unusually accelerated and diffuse form of obliterative coronary artery arteriosclerosis and is the commonest cause of graft failure in the long term after heart transplantation. Coronary arterial disease begins to develop relatively early after heart transplantation and nearly all patients after 1 year show some histopathological evidence of this disease.[37] Two different types of lesions develop. Type A are discrete stenoses of proximal and middle thirds of epicardial arteries. Type B are present in the distal coronary arteries and consist of tubular constrictions. Small vessels of less than 100 μm in diameter are less frequently involved. CAV is probably due to a complex interplay between immunological and non-immunological factors. Viral infections, immunosuppressive drugs, dyslipidaemias and oxidant stress may all play a part.[38] Risk factors within 5 years of heart transplantation include pretransplant coronary artery disease, panel reactive antibody (PRA) positivity of >20% and donor hypertension. Female donors yield a weakly protective effect.[1] Beyond 5 years, hospitalisation for rejection within 5 years of transplantation and donor mass index also become additional risk factors.

Early identification of CAV is necessary as patients generally remain asymptomatic due to cardiac denervation; moreover, early recognition can improve long-term prognosis. Surveillance for CAV can be undertaken by several techniques, including intravascular ultrasound (IVUS), determination of coronary flow reserve and dobutamine stress echocardiography. However, coronary angiography remains the commonest form of investigation. IVUS is a much more sensitive tool in the detection of early intimal thickening.[39] However, it suffers from theoretical shortcomings of a lack of universal grading system and absence of an initial estimate of intimal thickening of donor arteries. In addition, the size of available catheters means that they can only be used in vessels exceeding 1.5 mm in diameter. Dobutamine stress echocardiography has the advantage of non-invasive monitoring of CAV but its reported sensitivity of 72%[38] does not make it a suitable tool for replacement of angiography. Angiography is generally undertaken on an annual basis but if new lesions are identified it can be repeated more frequently. We would also perform a baseline study if the presence of atherosclerosis is suspected in the donor heart at the time of transplant operation.

There is no conventional treatment for CAV and the emphasis has been on tertiary prevention of progression. The usual preventative measures of coronary artery disease have limited value in this setting. Calcium channel blockers, especially diltiazem and statins, have been shown to be effective.[40,41]

> ✔ Newer immunosuppressive agents like rapamycin and everolimus, due to their proliferation inhibitor properties, also offer hope for the future.[42] In a prospective randomised study comparing everolimus with azathioprine, the incidence of CAV was significantly lower in the group receiving everolimus.

Malignancy

The incidence of malignancy after heart transplantation is three to four times higher than in the general population. The three common cancers after heart transplantation in order of frequency are cutaneous malignancies, post-transplant lymphoproliferative disorder (PTLD) and lung cancers. The risk factors for development of malignancies are presence of pretransplant malignancy, pretransplant coronary artery disease and increasing age. Female gender, use of mycophenolate mofetil and tacrolimus seem to have protective effects.[1] The probability of dying from malignancy (other than lymphoma) after heart transplantation after 10 years is≈18%.

The incidence of PTLD with ciclosporin-based immunosuppression is 2–4% and the incidence is highest≈3–5 years after transplantation.[43]

Epstein–Barr virus-negative PTLD has been described after heart transplantation but is considerably less common. There is a wide spectrum of presentation of PTLD from pulmonary, gastrointestinal, tonsillar, to central nervous system involvement. Disseminated PTLD is associated with a poor prognosis. PTLD may respond to reduction of immunosuppression, and lymphomas showing CD20 expression can be successfully treated with CD20 antibody (rituximab)[44] (see Chapter 12).

Hypertension

Most patients will develop arterial hypertension after heart transplantation. It is of interest to note that in the pre-ciclosporin era the incidence of hypertension was 20%; now, more than 60% will have elevated systemic blood pressure at 1 year and virtually all patients are expected to have it within 5 years following transplantation.[45] Hypertension needs to be aggressively treated in these patients to prevent CAV and renal dysfunction. The treatment consists of sodium restriction with addition of calcium channel blockers and angiotensin-converting enzyme (ACE) inhibitors.

Chronic renal dysfunction

Chronic renal failure is a well-recognised complication after heart transplantation. The incidence of this is 5–10% at 60 months after transplantation in most series.[46] Our incidence of dialysis is 10% at 10 years. The causation is multifactorial, with preoperative renal dysfunction, perioperative haemodynamic insult, hypertension and diabetes mellitus all contributing in some measure, but the principal cause is calcineurin inhibitor treatment. The major decline in renal function occurs during the first 12 months after transplantation; thereafter there is gradual worsening of dysfunction. Unless there is pre-existing intrinsic renal disease, early renal dysfunction following transplantation is not a predictor of chronic renal failure. The management of chronic renal impairment consists of preventative measures with close monitoring of calcineurin inhibitor levels, treatment of hypertension and avoidance of other nephrotoxic agents. It is hoped that the use of newer immunosuppressive agents such as sirolimus may lead to less renal toxicity.

Heart and lung transplantation (HLT)

This form of pulmonary transplantation has had a transformation in its indications and the frequency with which it is done since it was first undertaken in 1982. At its inception it was the commonest form of pulmonary transplantation but with the success of isolated lung transplantation the indications are now mainly confined to pulmonary hypertension without congenital heart disease and pulmonary hypertension associated with Eisenmenger's syndrome and congenital heart disease.[47]

Recipient selection criteria

The selection criteria for patients requiring HLT are similar to isolated lung transplantation. We have an upper limit of 60 years for acceptance to the transplant list. Specific guidelines for selection of patients in this group are as follows.

Pulmonary hypertension without congenital heart disease

These patients have either pulmonary hypertension as a result of thromboembolic disease, veno-occlusive disease or collagen vascular disease. Patients are considered for transplantation when they become symptomatic and in spite of medical or surgical treatment remain in NYHA grade III or IV. They should be resistant to vasodilator treatment with either prostacyclin or calcium channel blockers. Useful parameters for acceptance include cardiac index $<2\,L/min/m^2$, right atrial pressure of $>15\,mmHg$ and a mean pulmonary artery pressure of $>55\,mmHg$.[48] Most of these patients now receive bilateral lung transplants. Only if right ventricular dysfunction is so severe that inotrope infusions are needed does combined heart–lung transplantation have a regular role.

Eisenmenger's syndrome

These patients behave differently from the above group in several ways. With a similar degree of pulmonary hypertension these patients have better cardiac function and better prognosis. The predictors of survival are also less reliable. The selection criteria are unclear but severe progressive symptoms with NYHA grade III or IV symptoms despite optimum medical treatment would constitute an indication for transplantation.

Heart–lung operation

The operation is undertaken via sternotomy. Cardiopulmonary bypass is similar to heart implantation. The heart is excised first as it improves visualisation for pneumonectomy. Both the phrenic and vagus nerves are carefully preserved while pneumonectomy is undertaken. The recurrent laryngeal nerve is particularly at risk while the left pulmonary artery is being divided as the pulmonary artery is markedly enlarged due to pulmonary hypertension. A cuff of pulmonary artery can be left around the ligamentum arteriosum region to add to protection. The trachea is divided two rings above the carina.

The implantation proceeds with tracheal anastomosis, which is similar to bronchial anastomosis as described with lung transplantation (see below). The left and right lungs are carefully placed in their respective cavities behind the phrenic nerves, taking care to avoid hilar torsion. The aortic and caval anastomoses are undertaken to complete the operation. Often the donor atrial appendage has been divided at the time of procurement of organs to decompress the heart and requires securing.

The postoperative care is similar to patients who have had lung transplantation (see below).

Survival

The results of HLT are not dissimilar to pulmonary transplantation. Survival at 1 and 5 years is 61% and 40%, respectively.[46] Recipients with Eisenmenger's syndrome have a better prognosis than patients with primary pulmonary hypertension.[47]

Future direction in heart transplantation

It is gradually being recognised that, due to donor limitations, the number of heart transplant procedures is unlikely to exceed the present numbers of <3000 in the USA and <300 in the UK. Unfortunately, the demand for donor hearts continues to escalate.

Alternatives to heart transplantation are being explored worldwide, with research programmes exploring novel strategies including cell transplantation and regrowth of heart muscle, mechanical circulatory support and use of neurohumoral blockers to treat end-stage heart failure.

Xenotransplantation has continued to raise hopes for an unlimited supply of donor hearts. However, the feasibility of translating this technology into good long-term outcome in the foreseeable future looks rather remote. The median time of survival of transgenic pig hearts in baboon is only a few months.[49] According to a committee of the ISHLT, the current experimental results do not justify initiating a clinical trial.[50] The future of xenotransplantation for hearts is still indeterminate.

Lung transplantation

The first lung transplant was performed as long ago as 1963, by Hardy.[51] Subsequent early attempts were marred by frequent bronchial anastomotic breakdown. Reliable airway healing, and a clear understanding of the indications and choice of procedure led to an explosion of activity from the late 1980s onwards. Chronic small airways narrowing, entitled obliterative bronchiolitis, remains an unsolved problem that limits long-term survival.

An improvement of the quality of life is reported by most lung transplant recipients, and prolonged survival has now been shown in most subgroups of patients with end-stage respiratory failure.

Demographically, the ISHLT registry indicates that 78% of recipients in Europe were between 35 and 65 years of age, with the majority receiving their transplant for chronic obstructive pulmonary disease, cystic fibrosis (CF) or pulmonary fibrotic disease (**Fig. 11.3**). Only 4.1% were re-transplant procedures.[47]

Choice of lung transplant procedure

It is possible to transplant lungs singly or sequentially as a bilateral lung transplant, depending on patient characteristics and the nature of the pathological lung condition present. In some situations combined transplantation of the heart and lungs en bloc is necessary, as described previously.

Bilateral sequential lung transplantation (BSLT) is performed where it is clinically necessary to remove all native lung tissue. In the context of chronic lung sepsis in CF or bronchiectasis, single lung transplantation would fail as infection may cross-contaminate from the native remaining lung into the graft. Similarly, extensive destruction of both lungs in

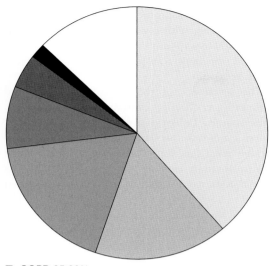

□ COPD 35.30%
▨ Cystic fibrosis 15.40%
▨ Pulmonary fibrosis 16.30%
■ Alpha 1 antitrypsin deficiency 7.40%
■ Primary pulmonary hypertension 3.70%
■ Re-transplant 1.90%
□ Other 11.70%

Figure 11.3 • Indications for lung transplantation.

emphysema may suggest the need for bilateral replacement to avoid air trapping in a remaining overly compliant native lung, resulting in mediastinal shift and compromise of the contralateral graft.

Single lung transplantation (SLT) is an attractive approach to the treatment of lung failure. The operation can often be performed without the potential for acute lung injury and other attendant risks associated with cardiopulmonary bypass. Most transplant centres experience an increasing disparity between the numbers of patients added to the waiting list for lung transplantation and stagnating numbers of suitable donors providing allografts; therefore, there is an economy in the use of scarce donor organs, with two lung recipients benefiting from each donor, and in the event of acute or chronic injury to the graft some viable native lung tissue will remain. Fibrotic lung conditions with normal pulmonary vasculature, a relatively immobile mediastinum and no significant native lung overinflation are most suited to this type of pulmonary transplant procedure. However, SLT is still used with varying enthusiasm between centres for selected patients with emphysema (with or without α_1-antitrypsin deficiency) and sarcoidosis. In the

past, most patients with emphysema received single lung transplants. There is increasing evidence that the bilateral procedure gives better short- and long-term results, better functional capacity and improved quality of life.[52]

A controversial area is lung transplantation for primary pulmonary hypertension. Here, in the absence of structural problems in the heart, SLT may suffice, although many centres still advocate bilateral lung transplantation or occasionally combined heart–lung transplantation with respect to potential cardiac involvement. Some centres are performing SLT alone in these circumstances.[53] Survival for all three modalities of treatment for primary pulmonary hypertension is similar.

Transplantation of both lungs en bloc with the heart for pulmonary pathology is now less frequent, although this was the early means of lung replacement. Few centres use this approach in circumstances where total lung replacement is required (the same indications as for bilateral lung transplantation). Although at first sight this may seem wasteful of scarce donor hearts where sequential lung transplantation will suffice, the structurally normal recipient heart is harvested and used for a heart transplant candidate (the 'domino' operation).[54]

Lung recipient assessment and selection

The general aspects of assessment for lung transplantation are identical to those for heart assessment. A detailed history of the patient's overall status and comorbidites as well as baseline evaluation of organ functions is essential. In view of the adverse effects of potent immunosuppressive regimens, a glomerular filtration rate (GFR) to determine renal function is performed routinely.

Again, after inpatient assessment, a recommendation is made to the patient by the surgeon after ensuring that all conventional treatments have been exhausted and, in terms of patient prognosis, that the timing for listing for transplantation is appropriate. Lung transplant assessment tests will typically also include specific sputum tests for otherwise difficult to eradicate pathogens, including *Aspergillus* species and certain *Pseudomonas* species.

✔✔ A 6-minute walk test is performed, which measures the distance a patient is able to walk in a given time and the degree of arterial desaturation that results during this exertion. Not only does this give a measure of symptomatic restriction, it also has prognostic value. Values of less than 300 m are seen in patients in end-stage pulmonary failure.[55]

Computed tomography (CT) is used to study the texture of lung parenchyma and identify areas of maximal lung destruction or bullous disease accurately. This, along with the results of ventilation–perfusion scanning, assists with the decision of whether to perform BSLT or SLT in those conditions where either might be considered and, if SLT is selected, which side should be transplanted. For SLT it is usual to replace the lung that has the poorer perfusion. It is always preferable to explant a lung if there is evidence of chronic sepsis within it or if there is a bulla that is likely to rupture. These investigations also help to identify those emphysematous patients who might be suitable for lung volume reduction surgery as an alternative to transplantation, with the aim of improving their ventilatory mechanics with symptomatic relief.

Detailed microbiological screening is an essential part of the assessment, with attention also paid to cultures performed over the preceding months and years at the referring centre. This information identifies patients likely to be colonised with multiply resistant organisms (multi- or pan-resistant pseudomonads in the cystic population) and helps direct antibiotic prophylaxis in the perioperative period.

Patients with some particularly resistant organisms are known to do badly after transplant. In this respect, *Burkholderia cenocepacia* is regarded as a contraindication.[56]

In CF patients with chronic sepsis and malabsorption, a nutritional assessment is vital since wound healing is impaired and the loss of muscle bulk may result in insufficient respiratory effort to permit weaning from the ventilator in the postoperative period.

Cardiopulmonary bypass is often needed for BSLT but in less than half of cases undergoing SLT. This depends mostly on patient oxygenation during single lung ventilation and haemodynamic stability after pulmonary artery clamping during the SLT procedure. Therefore, identifying coincidental cardiac disease is important. Older patients and those with relevant risk profiles should undergo cardiac catheterisation with coronary angiography. Right heart catheterisation is undertaken in patients considered for lung transplantation for pulmonary hypertension.

The remainder of the assessment is designed primarily to identify contraindications to organ replacement. Unlike patients with cardiac failure most candidates for lung replacement have preserved renal function. The incidence of post-lung transplantation renal failure requiring dialysis is a major source of mobility and has been reported in up to 15% at 3 years post-transplantation. The pretransplant creatinine clearance (<15 mL/min per 1.73 m²), as well as recipient height and the calcineurin inhibitor load after transplantation, correlate with higher risk of dialysis.[57]

Absolute contraindications to pulmonary transplantation include multiorgan failure and ongoing sepsis. Current malignancy, active peptic ulceration and inadequate conventional therapy are also important. Relative contraindications include peripheral and cerebral vascular disease, advanced diabetes, morbid obesity, osteoporosis and ischaemic heart disease.

The ISHLT has produced guidelines for the selection of lung transplant candidates that have been accepted in most centres.[58] On occasion, patients who have acute pulmonary failure – e.g. acute respiratory distress syndrome – and are ventilator dependent are referred to be considered for transplantation.[59] Pulmonary transplantation is less successful under these circumstances as sepsis and multiorgan failure are common and may not be reversible. Recent reports suggest better outcomes.[60]

No universally accepted assist device technology has been established for patients with potential for 'bridge to lung transplantation'. Extracorporeal membrane oxygenation (ECMO) has been advocated by some centres but utilises considerable resources in this setting. NovaLung®, a pumpless arteriovenous CO_2 elimination device, has been used successfully by some centres for this purpose and may find more frequent application in the future.[61] There have been rapid advances in ECMO for the patient who requires more than CO_2 removal. Technology now exists for the support of such patients that is less invasive, and permits the patient to be awake and ambulant.[62]

Lung donor criteria and selection

The majority of lung allografts are from declared brain-dead donors according to strict criteria (deceased heart-beating donors, DBDs). Specific considerations for lung donation must include a demonstration of good gas exchange with no evidence of aspiration, embolism or pneumonia. Smokers and patients with a history of mild asthma may still be considered as potential lung donors. In practice, only a minority of multiorgan donors are suitable for lung donation, as potential lung injury may arise in a number of ways. After chest trauma, a haemothorax and fractured ribs may indicate parenchymal damage, but this is not always so and the contralateral lung may be uninjured and available for use. Aspiration of gastric contents at the time of injury or cardiac arrest is not uncommon.

In addition, it is increasingly recognised that brain stem death is itself a specific and major cause of lung injury. There is both a haemodynamic stress injury, which can result in reversible capillary disruption, and a global inflammatory up-regulation.[63,64]

In many circumstances donors that do not meet the strict brain death criteria may be declared non-heart-beating donors (donation after circulatory death, DCD). Such DCD lung allografts have recently been shown to provide very acceptable early and midterm lung function after transplantation.[65] There is some evidence that inflammatory up-regulation is less in DCD lungs.[66] The transfusion of blood and blood products in large volumes predisposes to lung injury (sometimes becoming apparent only after implantation). Fat embolus from long-bone fractures with catastrophic results has also been reported. In all these circumstances, infection in the donor is more likely and will compound the injury to the lung.

Examination of the chest radiograph is essential. Aspirates taken from the endotracheal tube should be examined microscopically and Gram stained at the donor hospital. Only culture results from a donor bronchoalveolar lavage are of significance in affecting early outcome.[67] Flexible bronchoscopy and recruitment manoeuvres are important to facilitate full expansion of the lungs.

> ✔ Lung function is assessed by gas exchange. A useful standardised measure is the P_aO_2 with the donor ventilated on 100% oxygen and with 8 mmHg of positive end-expiratory pressure to optimise ventilation. A value of <30 kPa is an indicator of possible lung injury, and many centres will not use lungs where a value of <40 kPa is recorded. The aspiration of blood from individual upper and lower lobe pulmonary veins is often useful when evaluating single lungs, where 40 kPa is a reasonable level of acceptability.[68]

Final assessment of the lungs is performed by the donor surgeon, who can see bullae and traumatised lung and feel areas of consolidation. Oedematous lungs feel heavy and spongy and may lead the donor team to reject the organs for use.

Ex vivo lung perfusion

A new technique to both aid in the subjective assessment of the DCD donor lung and also to improve the function of the damaged lung from the DBD donor has recently been introduced. It involves placing the retrieved donor lungs on an apparatus which allows perfusion with a solution mainly comprising dextrans and albumin (Steen solution). The lung is carefully rewarmed, then ventilated in a protective fashion. The perfusate is free of white cells, platelets and complement. It is hyperosmolar, to encourage resorption of fluid, and contains high-dose steroids and antibiotics. Initial use in a DCD donor[69] led to the realisation that traditionally unacceptable lungs from DBD donors could be 'reconditioned'. The initial very encouraging results[70] have led other centres to utilise this technique of 'ex vivo lung perfusion' (EVLP) with excellent outcomes. Lungs that were initially not accepted can be successfully used (assuming they come up to standard criteria of gas exchange, vascular resistance and airway characteristics), and appear to have at least comparable and possibly superior results.[71] EVLP is currently the subject of a multicentre UK trial.

Lung recipient–donor matching

As with heart donors, matching of donor and recipient for lung transplantation is a relatively crude process, focusing on blood group and dimensions with no prospective match for tissue typing due to time constraints.

Size can be assessed in a number of ways, including comparison of measurements taken from donor and recipient chest radiographs. Donor and recipient heights are a useful guide to matching, with a 10–15% mismatch permissible. However, it is now generally recognised that donors should be matched to the predicted lung size of the recipient rather than the pathological size, since thoracic capacity and chest wall mechanics will often normalise after transplantation.

CMV status of donor and recipient is an important consideration. CMV mismatch here has greater implications for a lung recipient in the event of seroconversion or reactivation in the grafted tissue.

Lung retrieval and preservation

As with heart retrieval, the median sternotomy is completed after initial mobilisation of the liver. Both pleurae are now opened widely and the lungs inspected. Any adhesions between visceral and parietal pleura are divided with electrocautery. The inferior pulmonary ligament on each side is divided up to the inferior pulmonary vein. The innominate vein is now ligated between ligatures and the pericardium is opened with the incision being continued up along the innominate artery, which is similarly divided. For this reason central venous access must be via the right internal jugular vein and arterial monitoring from the left radial artery. The pericardium is now opened and the aorta, superior vena cava (SVC) and inferior vena cava (IVC) are mobilised as before. Once the SVC has been mobilised the azygos vein can be identified, ligated and divided behind the SVC to facilitate the future removal of the bloc. It is now possible to mobilise the trachea above the aortic arch. It is important not to denude the trachea of its blood supply and a tape is simply passed around it. Perfusion cannulae are now inserted into the ascending aorta and into the main pulmonary artery.

When systemic heparinisation is administered and the perfusion apparatus has been set up for perfusion of the abdominal organs, removal of the heart and lung bloc can proceed. The SVC is divided between ligatures and the IVC is clamped above the diaphragm. The aorta is now cross-clamped and the heart is cardcopleged

as described above for solitary heart transplant organ retrieval. However, under these circumstances the cardioplegia is vented from the heart by incision of the tip of the left atrial appendage, leaving the pulmonary veins intact. Once electromechanical arrest has been achieved, infusion of preservative into the lungs can proceed through the pulmonary artery catheter. Simultaneous topical cooling of heart and lungs with cold saline solution proceeds throughout this time.

> ✅ Pulmonary preservative solutions exist in many forms. Traditionally Eurocollins solution has been used, which essentially has an intracellular fluid electrolyte composition. Recently, other preservatives based on extracellular fluids have been used, such as low-potassium dextran, with more encouraging results and the potential to extend organ ischaemic times.[72]

Prostaglandins may help prevent leucocyte sequestration and also optimise perfusion of the pulmonary capillary bed, and are given before infusion of the pulmoplegic solution. Preservation is achieved by cooling with extracorporeal circulation in some centres but most units use a hypothermic cold flush perfusion technique. Ischaemic times of 6–8 hours can be safely achieved.

The anaesthetist is now asked to ventilate the lungs by hand with air to prevent alveolar collapse. Occasional cessation of ventilation will facilitate excision of the bloc, which is undertaken when cardioplegia and pulmonary preservative solutions have both been given. The heart is elevated and the pericardium incised posteriorly below the inferior pulmonary veins joining right and left pleural spaces. It is now possible to elevate the heart, the back of the left atrium and both hila, dividing the connective tissue between these structures and the descending aorta and oesophagus and vertebral column posteriorly. As the surgeon proceeds up the descending aorta the ligamentum arteriosum is encountered and divided. On the right-hand side, the divided azygos vein is seen as dissection proceeds in a cephalad direction. At this point the heart–lung bloc is placed back in the chest and attention turned to the aorta, which is divided below the cross-clamp. The anaesthetist is now asked to withdraw the endotracheal tube into the upper trachea whilst still ventilating. A clamp can now be placed across the trachea below the endotracheal tube and the trachea divided above. All that remains is to divide the connective tissue behind the ascending aorta and trachea and remove the entire heart–lung bloc. The trachea is stapled to allow removal of the clamp whilst leaving the lungs inflated for transfer.

If the lungs are to be sent to a different destination from the heart, it is now necessary to split the bloc. This is performed by incising the left atrium anterior to the hilum on each side to separate pulmonary veins from the left atrium. It is important to leave a small cuff of left atrium on the pulmonary veins to facilitate implantation in the lung recipient. The pulmonary artery is divided at its bifurcation, leaving a good length of pulmonary artery attached to each lung. All that remains now is to separate the ascending aorta and heart from the pulmonary arteries on each side and from loose connective tissue connecting it to the carina posteriorly. Lungs and heart can now be transported separately to different destinations as required.

Single lung implantation

Anaesthesia is established with a double-lumen endotracheal tube to permit ventilation of the native lung whilst implantation proceeds. A pulmonary artery flotation catheter is often used to monitor pulmonary artery pressure during implantation, and full arterial and venous monitoring is established. Facilities for cardiopulmonary bypass are made available but are used only if unacceptable desaturation during implantation occurs or if systemic hypotension or pulmonary hypertension develop.

A lateral thoracotomy is performed and the native lung is excised with ligation of inferior and superior pulmonary veins and pulmonary artery. The bronchus is divided and the native organ removed. Care is taken not to contaminate the pleural space with endobronchial secretions. Meticulous haemostasis at the hilum is established. The pericardium is now incised adjacent to the pulmonary veins and these are mobilised to develop a cuff of left atrium. The pulmonary artery is mobilised in a similar fashion. The donor lung is now prepared by trimming the left atrial cuff, cutting the pulmonary artery to length and excising the stapled end of the bronchus to deflate the lung.

Implantation commences with the bronchial anastomosis. The membranous part of the bronchus is anastomosed with a continuous 4/0 Prolene suture. A series of figure-of-eight interrupted sutures is

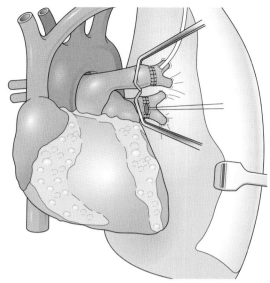

Figure 11.4 • The technique of vascular anastomosis in lung transplantation.

now placed on the anterior cartilaginous part of the bronchus to complete the anastomosis. Loose connective tissue at the hilum of donor lung can now be used to cover the anastomosis. A long side-biting clamp is next placed across the native left atrial cuff, which encompasses the pulmonary veins; the cuff is then opened longitudinally. The left atrial anastomosis is now performed with a continuous 4/0 Prolene suture and the clamp is left applied. The pulmonary artery anastomosis is performed in the same fashion and the donor organ is now de-aired by partially releasing the clamp from the pulmonary artery and de-airing through the left atrial anastomosis. The left atrial clamp can now be removed. Ventilation of the new lung commences (**Fig. 11.4**).

Apical and basal chest drains are now inserted. The thoracotomy is closed and the patient is returned to the intensive care unit for further monitoring and care. It is usually possible to extubate the stable patient after the insertion of an epidural analgesic catheter. Typically the patient will return to the ward after approximately 24–48 hours.

Bilateral sequential lung implantation

Single-lumen intubation for anaesthesia is performed. At many centres, this procedure is undertaken as sequential single lung transplants to avoid the perceived increase in acute lung injury postoperatively that is said to accompany extracorporeal perfusion. At our institution and others, cardiopulmonary bypass is routinely used and seems to have little impact on lung function following surgery.[73]

The operation is approached through a submammary 'clam shell' incision that divides the sternum transversely. A median sternotomy is a less painful incision that can be used in some cases, although access can sometimes be more of a challenge.

The patient is fully heparinised, the pericardium is opened and the patient is placed on cardiopulmonary bypass with an ascending aortic inflow cannula and venous drainage from individual cannulation of the caval veins. Excision of each lung now proceeds with electrocautery division of adhesions. Care is taken to preserve the phrenic nerve while mobilising structures at each hilum, especially in patients with septic lung disease where large lymph nodes and dense hilar adhesions make excision of the lung difficult. Excision of each lung proceeds in turn, and in cases of pulmonary sepsis the pleural cavities are irrigated thoroughly with the antiseptic Taurolin. Implantation of the donor lungs is performed in exactly the fashion described for single lung transplantation, the right side being anastomosed first. The patient is usually cooled to 32 °C during implantation, the heart being allowed to continue to beat and eject in sinus rhythm. After implantation, de-airing and reperfusion are performed and ventilation is recommended. At normothermia cardiopulmonary bypass can be weaned.

✔ It is important that the pulmonary artery (PA) pressure at reperfusion is controlled. A number of experimental studies have shown reduced lung reperfusion injury when this is practised – even a short period of controlled pressure reperfusion is beneficial.

We keep the mean PA pressure at less than 20 mmHg for at least 10 minutes while reperfusing a lung transplant.

Each thoracic cavity is drained with basal and apical drains and the wound is closed. The patient is then returned to the intensive care unit for further monitoring and can usually be extubated at 8–12 hours postoperatively. Epidural analgesia is essential following the 'clam shell' incision. Return to the ward is usually at about 24–48 hours.

Peri- and postoperative care for lung transplants

On notification of a possible donor the selected recipient is admitted and reassessed for deterioration or unexpected infection.

Infection and colonisation of the airway and lung is a major feature of lung transplant and a leading cause of morbidity and mortality in the postoperative period. Antibiotic prophylaxis is largely directed by the known flora of the recipient but flucloxacillin is used for Gram-positive cover and metronidazole for Gram-negative cover in the absence of other positive cultures. Colomycin is administered by nebuliser in the immediate postoperative period. Antibiotic therapy is modified in the first few days after transplant as the results of perioperative donor and recipient bronchoalveolar lavages become available. In the absence of infection, antibacterial agents are stopped after the first routine bronchoscopy and biopsy at 1 week, provided airway anastomoses appear healthy. Aciclovir, antifungal agents and pneumocystis prophylaxis are used routinely, as in cardiac transplantation.[74]

Immunosuppression, as in heart transplantation, commences preoperatively with the administration of azathioprine and ciclosporin A. In patients with normal GFR, calcineurin inhibitor doses require adjustment to avoid postoperative renal impairment. Methylprednisolone is administered at reperfusion and continued intravenously for 24 hours in three divided doses, after which oral steroids may be commenced. However, since many pulmonary recipients have malabsorption and early ciclosporin levels may be erratic, antithymocyte globulin (ATG) remains an important modality to reduce acute rejection rates after lung transplantation and its use is reflected in the incidence of bronchiolitis obliterans syndrome. ATG is administered routinely for the first 3 days as induction therapy, with dosage and timing being regulated by daily flow cytometry lymphocyte counts. With this exception, immunosuppression is managed in an identical fashion with the same dosage regimens as in cardiac transplantation.

In recent years, other immunosuppressants have been put forward for use in postoperative immunosuppressive regimens. In particular, the use of induction therapy with ATG has been questioned due to concerns over increased rates of infection and of post-transplant lymphoma, though this remains controversial. Tacrolimus, mycophenolate mofetil and rapamycin have been investigated but no conclusive advantages have been demonstrated, although side-effect profiles may be subject to some improvements.[75]

If acute lung injury is present in the immediate postoperative period, ventilation can present great difficulties. Such reperfusion injury results from the sequestration of neutrophils in the lung parenchyma, with release of injurious enzymes and oxygen free radicals. Lungs may be oedematous or infected, with poor gas exchange. Meticulous control of fluid balance, optimisation of ventilation and microbiological control are needed in this situation. ECMO has been shown to improve survival in patients severely affected by primary graft dysfunction, but this requires early institution and has significant resource implications.[76]

> ✅ Nitric oxide administration has many benefits in reperfusion injury and is distributed preferentially to ventilated areas of the lung. It improves ventilation–perfusion matching and lowers pulmonary artery pressures. It reduces the adhesion of neutrophils to the endothelium and so alleviates reperfusion injury.[77,78]

A number of other interventions (controlled pressure reperfusion, pentoxifylline, extracorporeal filters, adhesion molecule modulators) affecting neutrophil sequestration in the lung have been put forward to try to combat this problem postoperatively but have not been widely evaluated in clinical practice.[79]

In the case of the single lung transplant for emphysema, the residual overcompliant lung can inflate excessively, with air trapping and resultant mediastinal shift if the expiratory period of ventilation is insufficient. Modification of the ventilatory cycle can help but sometimes independent ventilation of each lung through a double-lumen endotracheal tube is needed. When the time comes to wean the recipient from the ventilator an epidural catheter to administer analgesics is essential. Epidural infusions can be continued for some days after extubation to assist expectoration of secretions.

Transbronchial biopsy and bronchoalveolar lavage with a flexible bronchoscope under sedation are performed at 1 week, 1 month and then every 3 months before reverting to annual biopsies to detect rejection and direct antimicrobial intervention. Additional biopsies are taken if rejection is suspected on the grounds of unexplained fever, symptomatic deterioration with arterial desaturation or a fall in pulmonary function tests, including spirometry and transfer factor.

Rejection is graded according to a standard system adopted by the ISHLT. Treatment is by augmentation of steroid therapy – 3 days of intravenous methylprednisolone (500 mg) and subsequent augmentation of oral steroids. Treatment is required for grades 3 and 4 and for grade 2 if there is clinical concern.

Outcomes and complications of lung transplantation

Generally, the 30-day survival is approximately 85%, with 75% surviving to 1 year. In the past, at 5 years 45% remained alive and after a decade 25%. More recently there has been a progressive improvement, with survival for some groups significantly better. Recent outcomes for CF patients have identified a median survival now exceeding 11 years.[80] Survival curves for bilateral lung transplantation are a little better than for unilateral procedures. The early decline in survival mirrors that seen in heart transplantation and reflects operative mortality and donor organ dysfunction. The causes of perioperative mortality include unsuspected donor allograft injury (infection, oedema, embolic disease or poor preservation) and reperfusion injury with subsequent multiorgan failure complications.

Specific technical difficulties include anastomotic stenoses with pulmonary oligaemia (pulmonary arterial obstruction) or pulmonary oedema (venous stenosis),[81] and airway ischaemia and dehiscence with resultant mediastinitis and pleural sepsis.

The vascular supply of bronchial and tracheal anastomoses is compromised and early dehiscence with ischaemia is a life-threatening complication with prolonged air leak and mediastinitis. Attention to detail when the anastomosis is performed, with care not to denude the airway, minimises this risk. It is no longer thought necessary to wrap the anastomosis in a vascularised pedicle or omentum. Concurrent steroid therapy (once considered a contraindication to lung transplantation) may even reduce dehiscence, as development of capillaries at the anastomosis is enhanced. Some early in-hospital deaths result from infection and acute rejection episodes.

> ✅✅ Quality of life is significantly improved by transplantation for pulmonary failure. Studies in lung transplant patient groups consistently show improvements in functional status and the perception of symptoms, irrespective of the type of transplant performed or the primary pathology.[82]

Diagnosis of acute rejection is often made more difficult by concurrent infection, and the decision to treat can also be problematic because of the fear of resulting uncontrollable sepsis. Persistent or repeated episodes of rejection are managed with cytolytic therapy (ATG), monoclonal therapy or a change in immunosuppressive agent, perhaps to one of the newer agents (Box 11.4).

Fungal and viral infections are seen commonly in the early postoperative period (*Aspergillus* and CMV) and carry a significant morbidity. *Pseudomonas* colonisation is common in the CF population. If preoperative data suggest that multiresistant pseudomonads are present, antibacterial therapy is kept to a minimum to allow growth of sensitive organisms.

CMV infection can be a major clinical problem. Diagnosis is by immunofluorescence at lavage, by transbronchial biopsy, estimation of antigenaemia and culture on bronchoalveolar lavage samples and quantitative CMV-PCR (polymerase chain reaction). Performed on a weekly basis to estimate viral load and identify those requiring treatment, this has provided improved treatment strategies with novel antiviral agents such as valganciclovir. Infection is common in all except the donor-negative/recipient-negative transplants (see Chapter 12).

Lymphoproliferative disease and other malignancies are seen as in cardiac transplantation, although lymphomas are more common (one series reports an incidence of 3.4% in heart recipients and 7.9% in lung recipients). Mortality is significantly higher in lymphomas appearing after the first year after transplantation. Reduction in immunosuppression can be highly effective in early disease but later conventional chemotherapy may be required.

Longer-term airway complications can arise with overgrowth of granulation tissue at the anastomosis, especially in the presence of chronic infection, or fibrotic stricture formation, which is usually ischaemic in origin. Treatment is local with dilatation or laser therapy, sometimes augmented with expandable stenting devices.

Chronic rejection in lung transplantation manifests itself as obliterative bronchiolitis or vascular atherosclerosis, the former being the greatest cause of long-term morbidity and mortality in recipients. Gradual deterioration in exercise tolerance and lung function arouse suspicion. Characteristic appearances are seen on the chest radiograph and CT scan, and the diagnosis is confirmed by transbronchial biopsy. Predisposing factors may include the occurrence of reperfusion injury and multiple episodes of acute rejection in the postoperative period, and CMV infection may be an aetiological factor. Treatment is directed towards decreased intensity of immunosuppression and total lymphoid irradiation may also help in some cases.

Recent advances and controversies

Over the last decade the outcomes in lung transplantation have significantly improved (**Fig. 11.5**).[1]

Recent changes in practice in lung transplantation are driven by a need to optimise the donor pool and reduce the impact of primary graft dysfunction in recipients. To this end, donation has been considered from both older and more marginal donors, and in attempting to prolong the permissible ischaemic time. Encouraging results have been obtained and expansion of the donor pool through these methods has been achieved.[83] A further increase of donor organs available is now possible with the use of DCD donor lungs. In practice realistic only with controlled donors (category III of the Maastricht criteria for DCDs), this has achieved very acceptable early outcomes.[84]

Living-related donation of lungs by blood relatives of patients needing pulmonary transplantation has been performed with reasonable results. This technique is most applicable to paediatric transplantation for CF or small recipients, where lobar donation by relatives alone may provide

---

Box 11.4 • Grading of pulmonary allograft rejection

A. Acute rejection

0   None
1   Minimal – scattered mononuclear infiltrates
2   Mild – frequent infiltrates of activated lymphocytes: 'endotheliitis'
3   Moderate – vascular cuffing, alveolar macrophages, extension of infiltrate into perivascular and air spaces
4   Severe – intra-alveolar necrosis, hyaline membrane, haemorrhage

B. Airway inflammation

0–4   According to severity

C. Chronic airway rejection

A   Active
B   Inactive

D. Chronic vascular rejection

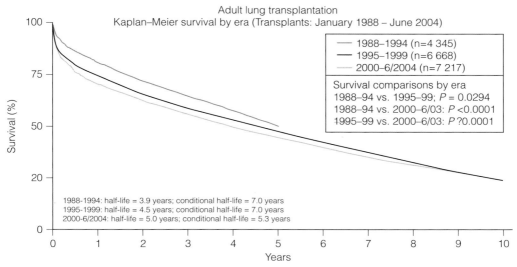

Figure 11.5 • Significant improvement of lung transplantation outcomes. Reproduced from Trulock EP, Edwards LB, Taylor DO et al. Registry of the International Society for Heart and Lung Transplantation: twenty-third official adult lung and heart–lung transplantation report – 2006. J Heart Lung Transplant 2006; 25:880–92. With permission from Elsevier.

sufficient lung tissue to fill the recipient chest. Donor morbidity, reported even in experienced centres (up to 20% of lobectomies), can also be significant and this raises difficult ethical dilemmas.[85] Lung volume reduction surgery for symptomatic, non-prognostic emphysematous disease has diverted away from transplant lists some patients who might otherwise have been transplanted on the grounds of symptomatic restriction.

Lung volume reduction surgery selectively excises the overexpanded, underventilated and underperfused parenchyma. The reduction in lung volume permits better ventilatory performance and ventilation–perfusion matching.

> ✅ The specific subgroups of emphysema patients who are most likely to benefit from such lung volume reduction surgery have been established with the help of the NETT trial.[86,87]

Future developments may include the utilisation of lungs from Maastricht category II donors.[88] EVLP is the key to this sort of technique. However, perfusion of the lungs, perhaps for 12–24 hours, gives further and very exciting scope for manipulation with gene transfer.[89] In contrast to the situation with the heart, the far more complex lung cannot be replaced by machines at present, but the prospects for expanding lung transplantation are very exciting indeed.

Key points

- Heart transplantation improves survival and quality of life for selected patients with end-stage heart failure.
- Heart transplantation is most beneficial in patients with greatest risk of dying.
- More specific immunosuppression agents continue to decrease the impact of acute and chronic rejection and immunosuppression-related side-effects.
- Lung transplantation outcomes have improved significantly in recent times, with good survival and functional improvement in many forms of end-stage lung disease.
- Single or bilateral lung transplantation is possible depending on the underlying pathology.
- Colonisation with *Burkholderia cepacia* in cystic fibrosis patients is an important adverse prognostic marker.
- Reperfusion injury is a major challenge postoperatively but nitric oxide administration has the potential to limit this in clinical practice.

References

1. Stehlik J, Edwards LB, Kuchervavaya AY, et al. Registry of the International Society for Heart and Lung Transplantation: twenty-eighth official adult heart transplant report – 2011. J Heart Lung Transplant 2011;30(10):1078–94.

2. McMurray JJ, Stewart S. Epidemiology, aetiology, and prognosis of heart failure. Heart 2000;83(5):596–602.

3. Jessup M, Banner N, Brozena S, et al. Optimal pharmacologic and non-pharmacologic management of cardiac transplant candidates: approaches to be considered prior to transplant evaluation: International Society for Heart and Lung Transplantation guidelines for the care of cardiac transplant candidates. J Heart Lung Transplant 2006;25(9):1003–23.

4. Irving AC, Kirk R, Parry G, et al. Outcomes following more than two decades of paediatric cardiac transplantation. Eur J Cardiothorac Surg 2011;40:1197–202.

5. McCullough PA, Philbin EF, Spertus JA, et al. Confirmation of a heart failure epidemic: findings from the Resource Utilization Among Congestive Heart Failure. J Am Coll Cardiol 2002;39(1):60–9.

6. Figulla HR, Rahlf G, Nieger M, et al. Spontaneous hemodynamic improvement or stabilization and associated biopsy findings in patients with congestive cardiomyopathy. Circulation 1985;71(6):1095–104.

7. Matitiau A, Perez-Atayde A, Sanders SP, et al. Infantile dilated cardiomyopathy. Relation of outcome to left ventricular mechanics, hemodynamics, and histology at the time of presentation. Circulation 1994;90(3):1310–8.

8. Mancini DM, Eisen H, Kussmaul W, et al. Value of peak exercise oxygen consumption for optimal timing of cardiac transplantation in ambulatory patients with heart failure. Circulation 1991;83(3):778–86.
This clinical study nicely demonstrated the value of measurement of peak oxygen consumption during maximal exercise testing and has brought some objectivity in assessment of patients for heart transplantation.

9. Simmonds J, Burch M, Dawkins H, et al. Heart transplantation after congenital heart surgery: improving results and future goals. Eur J Cardiothorac Surg 2008;34:313–7.

10. Aaronson KD, Schwartz JS, Chery TM, et al. Development and prospective validation of a clinical index to predict survival in ambulatory patients referred for cardiac transplant evaluation. Circulation 1997;95(12):2660–7.

11. Deng MC, De Meeste JM, Smits JM, et al. Effect of receiving a heart transplant: analysis of a national cohort entering a waiting list, stratified by heart failure severity. Comparative Outcome Clinical Profiles in Transplantation (COCPIT) Study Group. Br Med J 2000;321(7260):540–5.

12. Hermsen JL, Nath DS, del Rio AM, et al. Combined heart–kidney transplantation: the University of Wisconsin experience. J Heart Lung Transplant 2007;26(11):1119–26.

13. Olbrisch ME, Levenson JL. Psychosocial evaluation of heart transplant candidates: an international survey of process, criteria, and outcomes. J Heart Lung Transplant 1991;10(6):948–55.

14. Mehra MR, Kobashigawa J, Starling R, et al. Listing criteria for heart transplantation: International Society for Heart and Lung Transplantation guidelines for the care of cardiac transplant candidates. J Heart Lung Transplant 2006;25(9):1024–42.

15. Dickstein K, Vardas PE, Auricchio A, et al. 2010 focused update of ESC guidelines on device therapy in heart failure: an update of the 2008 ESC guidelines for the diagnosis and treatment of acute and chronic heart failure and the 2007 ESC guidelines for cardiac and resynchronization therapy. Developed with the special contribution of the Heart Failure Association and the European Heart Rhythm Association. Eur Heart J 2010;31:2677–87.

16. Moss AJ, Zareba W, Hall WJ, et al. Prophylactic implantation of a defibrillator in patients with myocardial infarction and reduced ejection fraction. N Engl J Med 2002;346:877–83.

17. Rose EA, Moskowitz AJ, Packer M, et al. The REMATCH trial: rationale, design, and end points. Ann Thorac Surg 1999;67(3):723–30.

18. Rose EA, Gelijns AC. Moskowitz AJ, for the REMATCH Study Group. Long-term mechanical left ventricular assistance for end-stage heart failure. N Engl J Med 2001;345:1435–43.

19. Rogers JG, Aaronson KD, Boyle AJ, et al. Continuous flow left ventricular assist device improves functional capacity and quality of life of advanced heart failure patients. J Am Coll Cardiol 2010;55:1826–34.

20. Macgowan GA, Parry G, Schueler S, et al. The decline in heart transplantation in the UK. Br Med J 2011;342:d2483.

21. Rosengard BR, Feng S, Alfrey EJ, et al. Report of the Crystal City meeting to maximize the use of organs recovered from the cadaver donor. Am J Transplant 2002;2(8):701–11.

22. Wood KE, Becker BN, McCartney JG, et al. Care of the potential organ donor. N Engl J Med 2004;351:2730–9.

23. Marelli D, Laks H, Bresson S, et al. Results after transplantation using donor hearts with preexisting coronary artery disease. J Thorac Cardiovasc Surg 2003;126(3):821–5.

24. Kirklin JK, Naftel DC, Kormos RL, et al. The Fourth INTERMACS Annual Report: 4,000 implants and counting. J Heart Lung Transplant 2012;31(2):117–26.

25. Potapov EV, Ivanitskaia EA, Loebe M, et al. Value of cardiac troponin I and T for selection of heart donors and as predictors of early graft failure. Transplantation 2001;71(10):1394–400.

26. Watson CJE, Roberts R, Wright KE, et al. Use of organs from donors with primary intracranial malignacy. Am J Transplant 2010;10:1–8.

27. Advisory Committee on the Safety of Blood Tissues and Organs (SaBTO). Guidance on the microbiological safety of human organs, tissues and cells used in transplantation, http://www.dh.gov.uk/en/Publicationsandstatistics/Publications/PublicationsPolicyAndGuidance/DH_121497; [accessed 15.11.12].

28. Sethi GK, Lanause P, Rosado LJ, et al. Clinical significance of weight difference between donor and recipient in heart transplantation. J Thorac Cardiovasc Surg 1993;106(3):444–8.

29. West LJ, Pollock-Barziv SM, Dipchard AI, et al. ABO-incompatible heart transplantation in infants. N Engl J Med 2001;344(11):793–800.

30. Roche SL, Burch M, O'Sullivan J, et al. Multicenter experience of ABO-incompatible pediatric cardiac transplantation. Am J Transplant 2008;8(1):208–15.

31. Wheeldon DR, Potter CD, Odano A, et al. Transforming the 'unacceptable' donor: outcomes from the adoption of a standardized donor management technique. J Heart Lung Transplant 1995;14(4):734–42.

32. Lower RR, Stofer RC, Shumway NE. Homovital transplantation of the heart. J Thorac Cardiovasc Surg 1961;41:196–204.

33. Aziz TM, Burgess AI, Rahman A, et al. Risk factors for tricuspid valve regurgitation after orthotopic heart transplantation. Ann Thorac Surg 1999;68(4):1247–51.

34. Hasan A, Au J, Hamilton JR, et al. Orthotopic heart transplantation for congenital heart disease. Technical considerations. Eur J Cardiothorac Surg 1993;7(2):65–70.

35. Bleasdale RA, Bannen NR, Anyanwu AC, et al. Determinants of outcome after heterotopic heart transplantation. J Heart Lung Transplant 2002;21(8):867–73.

36. Kugler C, Tegtbur U, Gottlieb J, et al. Health-related quality of life in long-term survivors after heart and lung transplantation: a prospective cohort study. Transplantation 2010;90:451–7.

37. Johnson DE, Gao SZ, Schroeden JS, et al. The spectrum of coronary artery pathologic findings in human cardiac allografts. J Heart Transplant 1989;8(5):349–59.

38. Spes CH, Klauss V, Mudra H, et al. Diagnostic and prognostic value of serial dobutamine stress echocardiography for noninvasive assessment of cardiac allograft vasculopathy: a comparison with coronary angiography and intravascular ultrasound. Circulation 1999;100(5):509–15.

39. St Goar FG, Pinto FJ, Alderman EL, et al. Detection of coronary atherosclerosis in young adult hearts using intravascular ultrasound. Circulation 1992;86(3):756–63.

40. Wenke K, Meiser B, Thiery J, et al. Simvastatin reduces graft vessel disease and mortality after heart transplantation: a four-year randomized trial. Circulation 1997;96(5):1398–402.

41. Schroeder JS, Gao SZ, Alderman EL, et al. A preliminary study of diltiazem in the prevention of coronary artery disease in heart-transplant recipients. N Engl J Med 1993;328(3):164–70.

42. Eisen HJ, Tuzai EM, Dorent R, et al. Everolimus for the prevention of allograft rejection and vasculopathy in cardiac-transplant recipients. N Engl J Med 2003;349(9):847–58.

43. Penn I. Tumors after renal and cardiac transplantation. Hematol Oncol Clin North Am 1993;7(2):431–45.

44. Zilz ND, Olson LJ, McGregor CG. Treatment of post-transplant lymphoproliferative disorder with monoclonal CD20 antibody (rituximab) after heart transplantation. J Heart Lung Transplant 2001;20(7):770–2.

45. Corcos T, Tamburino C, Leger P, et al. Early and late hemodynamic evaluation after cardiac transplantation: a study of 28 cases. J Am Coll Cardiol 1988;11(2):264–9.

46. Ojo AO, Held PJ, Port FK, et al. Chronic renal failure after transplantation of a nonrenal organ. N Engl J Med 2003;349(10):931–40.

47. Christie JD, Edwards LB, Kuchervaya AK, et al. The Registry of the International Society for Heart and Lung Transplantation: 29th Adult Lung and Heart–Lung Transplant Report – 2012. J Heart Lung Transplant 2012;31:1073–86.

48. D'Alonzo GE, Barst RJ, Ayres SM. Survival in patients with primary pulmonary hypertension. Results from a national prospective registry. Ann Intern Med 1991;115(5):343–9.

49. Cooper DK. Clinical xenotransplantation – how close are we? Lancet 2003;362(9383):557–9.

50. Cooper DK, Keogh AM, Brink J, et al. Report of the Xenotransplantation Advisory Committee of the International Society for Heart and Lung Transplantation. The present status of xenotransplantation and its potential role in the treatment of end-stage cardiac and pulmonary diseases. J Heart Lung Transplant 2000;19(12):1125–65.

51. Hardy JD, Alican F. Lung transplantation. Adv Surg 1966;2:235–64.

52. Thabut G, Christie JD, Ravaud P, et al. Survival after bilateral versus single lung transplantation for patients with chronic obstructive pulmonary disease: a retrospective analysis of registry data. Lancet 2008;371(9614):744–51.

53. Bando K, Armitage J, Paradis IL, et al. Indications for and results of single, bilateral, and heart–lung

transplantation for pulmonary hypertension. J Thorac Cardiovasc Surg 1994;108(6):1056–65.

54. Anyanwu AC, Banner NR, Radley-Smith R, et al. Long-term results of cardiac transplantation from live donors: the domino heart transplant. J Heart Lung Transplant 2002;21(9):971–5.

55. Kadikar A, Maurer J, Kesten S. The six-minute walk test: a guide to assessment for lung transplantation. J Heart Lung Transplant 1997;16(3):313–9.

56. De Soyza A, McDowell A, Archer L, et al. *Burkholderia cepacia* complex genomovars and pulmonary transplantation outcomes in patients with cystic fibrosis. Lancet 2001;358(9295):1780–1.

57. Mason DP, Solovera-Rozas M, Feng J, et al. Dialysis after lung transplantation: prevalence, risk factors and outcome. J Heart Lung Transplant 2007;27:1155–62.

58. Orens JB, Estenne M, Arcasoy S, et al. International Guidelines for the Selection of Lung Transplant Candidates: 2006 Update – A Consensus Report from the Pulmonary Scientific Council of the International Society for Heart and Lung Transplantation. J Heart Lung Transplant 2006;25(7):745–55.

59. Flume PA, Egan TM, Westerman JH, et al. Lung transplantation for mechanically ventilated patients. J Heart Lung Transplant 1994;13(1):15–23.

60. Mason DP, Thuita L, Nowicki ER, et al. Should lung transplantation be performed for patients on mechanical respiratory support? The US experience. J Thorac Cardiovasc Surg 2010;139:304–6.

61. Fischer S, Simon AR, Welte T, et al. Bridge to lung transplantation with the novel pumpless interventional lung assist device NovaLung. J Thorac Cardiovasc Surg 2006;131(3):719–23.

62. Garcia JP, Iacono A, Kon ZN. Ambulatory extracorporeal oxygenation; a new approach to bridge to lung transplantation. J Thorac Cardiovasc Surg 2010;139:137–9.

63. Fisher AJ, Donnelly SC, Hirani N, et al. Enhanced pulmonary inflammation in organ donors following fatal non-traumatic brain injury. Lancet 1999;353(9162):1412–3.

64. Avlonitis VS, Wigfield CH, Golledge HD, et al. Early hemodynamic injury during donor brain death determines the severity of primary graft dysfunction after lung transplantation. Am J Transplant 2007;7(1):83–90.

65. Van Raemdonck DE, Rega FR, Neyrinck AP, et al. Non heart beating donors. Semin Thorac Cardiovasc Surg 2004;16:309–21.

66. Yeung JC, Cypel M, Waddell TK, et al. Update on donor assessment, resuscitation, and acceptance criteria, including novel techniques – non-heart-beating donor lung retrieval and ex vivo donor lung perfusion. Thorac Surg Clin 2009;19(2):261–74.

67. Avlonitis VS, Krause A, Luzzi L, et al. Bacterial colonization of the donor lower airways is a predictor of poor outcome in lung transplantation. Eur J Cardiothorac Surg 2003;24(4):601–7.

68. Aziz TM, El-Gamel A, Saad RA, et al. Pulmonary vein gas analysis for assessing donor lung function. Ann Thorac Surg 2002;73(5):1599–605.

69. Steen S, Sjöberg T, Pierre L, et al. Transplantation of lungs from a non-heart-beating donor. Lancet 2001;357(9259):825–9.

70. Ingemansson R, Eyjolfsson A, Mared L, et al. Clinical transplantation of initially rejected donor lungs after reconditioning ex vivo. Ann Thorac Surg 2009;87(1):255–60.

71. Cypel M, Yeung JC, Liu M, et al. Normothermic ex vivo lung perfusion in clinical lung transplantation. N Engl J Med 2011;364(15):1431–40.

72. Rabanal JM, Ibaanez AM, Mons R, et al. Influence of preservation solution on early lung function (Euro-Collins vs Perfadex). Transplant Proc 2003;35(5):1938–9.

73. Szeto WY, Kreisel D, Karakousis GC, et al. Cardiopulmonary bypass for bilateral sequential lung transplantation in patients with chronic obstructive pulmonary disease without adverse effect on lung function or clinical outcome. J Thorac Cardiovasc Surg 2002;124(2):241–9.

74. Chan KM, Allen SA. Infectious pulmonary complications in lung transplant recipients. Semin Respir Infect 2002;17(4):291–302.

75. Lama R, Santos F, Algar FJ, et al. Lung transplants with tacrolimus and mycophenolate mofetil: a review. Transplant Proc 2003;35(5):1968–73.

76. Wigfield CH, Lindsey JD, Steffens TG, et al. Early institution of extracorporeal membrane oxygenation for primary graft dysfunction after lung transplantation improves outcome. J Heart Lung Transplant 2007;26:331–8.

77. Adatia I, Lillemei C, Arnolds JH, et al. Inhaled nitric oxide in the treatment of postoperative graft dysfunction after lung transplantation. Ann Thorac Surg 1994;57(5):1311–8.

78. Bacha EA, Hervae P, Murakami S, et al. Lasting beneficial effect of short-term inhaled nitric oxide on graft function after lung transplantation. Paris-Sud University Lung Transplantation Group. J Thorac Cardiovasc Surg 1996;112(3):590–8.

79. Clark SC, Sudarshan CD, Dark JH, et al. Controlled reperfusion and pentoxifylline modulate reperfusion injury after single lung transplantation. J Thorac Cardiovasc Surg 1998;115(6):1335–41.

80. Meachery G, De Soyza A, Nicholson A, et al. Outcomes of lung transplantation for cystic fibrosis in a large UK cohort. Thorax 2008;63(8):725–31.

81. Clark SC, Levine AJ, Hasan A, et al. Vascular complications of lung transplantation. Ann Thorac Surg 1996;61(4):1079–82.

82. Charman SC, Sharples LD, McNeil AD, et al. Assessment of survival benefit after lung transplantation by patient diagnosis. J Heart Lung Transplant 2002;21(2):226–32.

This review of 653 patients undergoing lung transplantation used Cox regression analysis to demonstrate the survival advantages of postoperative patients irrespective of their primary pathology. There was no survival difference between patients having single or bilateral lung transplantation.

83. Meyer DM, Bennett LE, Novick RJ, et al. Effect of donor age and ischemic time on intermediate survival and morbidity after lung transplantation. Chest 2000;118(5):1255–62.

84. Dark JH. Lung transplantation from the non-heart beating donor. Transplantation 2008;86(2):200–1.

85. Bowdish ME, Barr ML, Schenkel FA, et al. A decade of living lobar lung transplantation; peri-operative complications after 253 donor lobectomies. Am J Transplant 2004;4:1283–8.

86. National Emphysema Treatment Research Group. A randomised trial comparing lung volume reduction surgery with medical therapy for severe emphysema. N Engl J Med 2003;348:2059–73.

87. Tutic M, Lardinois D, Imfeld S, et al. LVRS as an alternative or bridging procedure to lung transplantation. Ann Thorac Surg 2006;82:208–13.

88. Gámez P, Córdoba M, Ussetti P, et al. Lung transplantation from out-of-hospital non-heart-beating lung donors. one-year experience and results. J Heart Lung Transplant 2005;24(8):1098–102.

89. Cypel M, Liu M, Rubacha M, et al. Functional repair of human donor lungs by IL-10 gene therapy. Sci Transl Med 2009;1(4):4ra9.

12

Transplant infectious disease

Camille Nelson Kotton

Introduction and general concepts

Immunosuppression makes organ transplantation possible, while increasing the risk of infections, both routine and opportunistic. Understanding how to optimally prevent, diagnose and treat infection after organ transplantation can greatly enhance outcomes. New infections result from acquisition of infections in the hospital (i.e. nosocomial infections), from the organ transplant or blood product donor, or in the community; reactivation of latent infections encompasses another significant number of infections. Viruses are the most common cause of infections; bacterial, fungal and parasitic infections also occur. In general, the intensity of immunosuppression is considered highest for a year after solid-organ transplant, with more of the opportunistic infections occurring in the first 6 months. This chapter will cover such infections by category, including optimal prophylaxis, diagnosis and management. In addition, the best possible pre-transplant evaluation and preparation methods will be reviewed, lifestyle issues covered and emerging topics such as donor-derived infections will be discussed.

Infections are among the most common complications after transplantation, and greatly increase the morbidity and mortality of transplantation, while decreasing graft and patient survival. New infections occur from acquisition of infections in the hospital (i.e. nosocomial infections), from the organ transplant or blood product donor, or in the community. Reactivation of latent infections encompasses another significant number of infections. In general, the intensity of immunosuppression is considered highest for a year after solid-organ transplant, and for 2 years after hematopoietic stem cell transplant.[1,2] Clinically focused guidelines on diagnosis, treatment and prevention of many infections after solid-organ transplants have recently been published by the Infectious Disease Community of Practice of the American Society of Transplantation.[3]

A timeline of infection after transplantation has been described (**Fig. 12.1**).[1] In the first month after organ transplantation, infections tend to be related to the surgical procedure and hospital stay, and include wound infection, anastomotic leaks and ischaemia, aspiration pneumonia, catheter infection and *Clostridium difficile* colitis. In this population with frequent healthcare setting exposure, such infections are more likely to be due to resistant pathogens, including methicillin-resistant *Staphylococcus aureus* (MRSA), vancomycin-resistant *Enterococcus faecalis* (VRE) and non-*albicans Candida*. Donor-derived infections and recipient-derived infection, due to prior colonisation with agents such as *Aspergillus* or *Pseudomonas*, may present in this phase.

Months 1–5 after transplant are often the period when the classic opportunistic infections occur; their risk can be mitigated or delayed by prophylaxis, and increased by intensified immunosuppression, leucopenia or immunomodulatory viral infections. While relatively standard

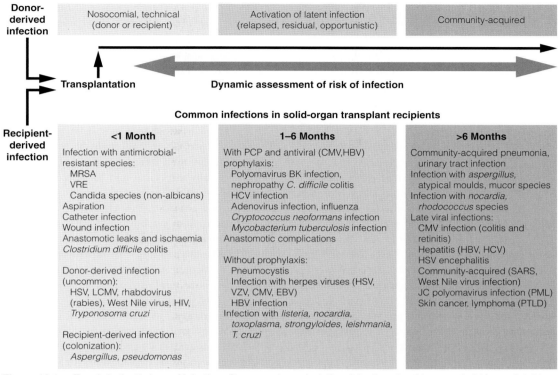

| Donor-derived infection | Nosocomial, technical (donor or recipient) | Activation of latent infection (relapsed, residual, opportunistic) | Community-acquired |

Transplantation   **Dynamic assessment of risk of infection**

Common infections in solid-organ transplant recipients

	<1 Month	1–6 Months	>6 Months

Recipient-derived infection	Infection with antimicrobial-resistant species:
	  MRSA
	  VRE
	  Candida species (non-albicans)
	Aspiration
	Catheter infection
	Wound infection
	Anastomotic leaks and ischaemia
	Clostridium difficile colitis
	
	Donor-derived infection (uncommon):
	  HSV, LCMV, rhabdovirus (rabies), West Nile virus, HIV, *Tryponosoma cruzi*
	
	Recipient-derived infection (colonization):
	  Aspergillus, pseudomonas
		With PCP and antiviral (CMV,HBV) prophylaxis:
		  Polyomavirus BK infection, nephropathy *C. difficile* colitis
		  HCV infection
		  Adenovirus infection, influenza
		  Cryptococcus neoformans infection
		  Mycobacterium tuberculosis infection
		  Anastomotic complications
		
		Without prophylaxis:
		  Pneumocystis
		  Infection with herpes viruses (HSV, VZV, CMV, EBV)
		  HBV infection
		Infection with *listeria, nocardia, toxoplasma, strongyloides, leishmania, T. cruzi*
			Community-acquired pneumonia, urinary tract infection
			Infection with *aspergillus,* atypical moulds, mucor species
			Infection with *nocardia, rhodococcus* species
			Late viral infections:
			  CMV infection (colitis and retinitis)
			  Hepatitis (HBV, HCV)
			  HSV encephalitis
			  Community-acquired (SARS, West Nile virus infection)
			  JC polyomavirus infection (PML)
			  Skin cancer, lymphoma (PTLD)

Figure 12.1 • Trends in the timings of infection after organ transplantation. Infections tend to occur in fairly predictable phases after solid-organ transplant. While many of the classic opportunistic infections occur in the first 6 months, during what is usually the period of most intense immunosuppression, the risk of such infection remains for the duration of time that the recipients are on immunosuppressive medications. The risk of infection is decreased by the use of prophylaxis, and augmented by the use of more potent immunosuppression (both in the induction and maintenance phases as well as during treatment of rejection), allograft rejection, concomitant infections, leucopenia, and technical surgical issues. HBV, hepatitis B virus; HIV, human immunodeficiency virus; HSV, herpes simplex virus; LCMV, lymphocytic choriomeningitis virus; MRSA, methicillin-resistant *Staphylococcus aureus*; PCP, *Pneumocystis carinii* pneumonia; PML, progressive multifocal leucoencephalopathy; PTLD, post-transplantation lymphoproliferative disorder; SARS, severe acute respiratory syndrome; VRE, vancomycin-resistant *Enterococcus faecalis*; VZV, varicella–zoster virus. Reproduced from Fishman JA. Infection in solid-organ transplant recipients. N Engl J Med 2007; 357:2601–14. With permission from the Massachusetts Medical Society. © 2007 Massachusetts Medical Society.

prophylaxis such as trimethoprim/sulfamethoxa-zole and an antiviral (aciclovir or ganciclovir or related products) mitigates the risk of many infections, certain infections are still seen, including BK reactivation, hepatitis C virus (HCV) infection, adenovirus and influenza infections (especially seasonally), and *Cryptococcus neoformans* infection. Without prophylaxis, numerous additional infections are seen (especially those in the herpes virus family and hepatitis B virus (HBV)), as well as *Pneumocystis jiroveci* pneumonia and infections with *Listeria, Nocardia, Mycobacterium tuberculosis, Toxoplasma, Strongyloides, Leishmania* and *Trypanosoma cruzi.*

The stable and relatively healthy organ transplant recipient who is more than 6 months out from transplant tends to develop community acquired or routine infections, including urinary tract infections, upper respiratory infections and pneumonia, gastroenteritis and varicella zoster. Infections with unusual and opportunistic pathogens such as *Aspergillus*, unusual moulds, *Nocardia* and *Rhodococcus* are still seen. In the era of effective prophylaxis with valganciclovir, an increased risk of late cytomegalovirus (CMV; occurring more than 6 months after organ transplant) has been noted, primarily in the few months after prophylaxis has been stopped.[4] Other late viral infections include polyomavirus infections (from BK, causing nephropathy primarily in renal transplant recipients, or JC, causing progressive multifocal leucoencephalopathy) and Epstein–Barr virus (EBV)-related post-transplant lymphoproliferative disease.

Pre-transplant evaluation can help mitigate the risk of some infections, especially latent ones. Knowledge of serostatus for CMV, EBV, HBV and HCV can help optimise post-transplant management. Potential transplant recipients and donors are typically screened for latent tuberculosis, by history and sometimes by chest X-ray and either by skin testing or use of an interferon-gamma release assay-based blood test such as the T-SPOT. TB® or Quantiferon® TB Gold. Recipients from or in endemic regions should be screened for latent infections such as *T. cruzi*, *Coccidioides* and *Strongyloides*. Those seronegative for measles, mumps, rubella, hepatitis A and B, and varicella should undergo important pre-transplant vaccination, as some are with live viral vaccines that cannot be given after transplant when a recipient is significantly immunosuppressed,[5] as shown in Table 12.1, leaving them potentially permanently vulnerable to potentially life-threatening infection(s).

Atypical presentation of infection is more common in immunosuppressed hosts. Clinical presentations may be subtler, yet the patients more ill compared with normal hosts. For example, transplant recipients with West Nile virus infection are much more likely to have clinical illness and succumb to infection. Clinicians need to expand their differential diagnoses when caring for transplant recipients. Diagnosis of emerging, novel and atypical pathogens is especially challenging in this vulnerable population, as has been seen with cases of lymphocytic choriomeningitis virus, tuberculosis, Chagas' disease, strongyloidiasis and numerous others.

The importance of donor-derived infections has been increasingly recognised in recent times. Such infection occurs in up to 1% of deceased donor organ transplants.[6] While transmission of some infections is expected, such as CMV and EBV, others have been a surprise to clinicians caring for patients. Such unanticipated donor-derived infections range from viruses such as rabies, lymphocytic choriomeningitis and West Nile virus, to bacteria including bacteraemias and tuberculosis,

fungi including cryptococcosis and histoplasmosis, and parasites including *Trypanosoma cruzi* (causing Chagas' disease) and *Strongyloides*.[6] Enhanced appreciation of donor-derived infections has resulted in better screening and diagnosis.

The specific immunosuppressive agents used can potentially alter the risk of certain infections. For example, ciclosporin may have some anti-hepatitis C properties, and might be preferable to using tacrolimus in infected patients. Ciclosporin has been shown in vitro and in animals to have anti-schistosomal properties, especially with *Schistosoma mansoni*; this effect has never been confirmed in humans, but could affect risk of disease.[7] Although data have been somewhat conflicting, the mammalian target of rapamycin (mTOR) inhibitors (sirolimus, everolimus) may have an impact on various viral infections, including human herpes virus 8 (HHV-8) and risk of developing Kaposi's sarcoma,[8] as well as the risk of developing EBV-mediated post-transplant lymphoproliferative disorder (PTLD) and active CMV. Whether there are mechanistic explanations, or this just reflects the net potency of the immunosuppression used, remains to be determined.

Transplant clinicians should be aware of the long-term impact of the use of anti-T-cell cytolytic induction therapies such as alemtuzumab, thymoglobulin, OKT3 and others. While these may decrease the risk of rejection, they often result in a prolonged period of lymphopenia, often lasting many months to over a year or two,[9,10] which may render the host more vulnerable to infection. When such therapies are used to treat organ rejection, clinicians should remember to restart prophylaxis therapies (i.e. antiviral, antibacterial, antifungal and antiparasitic) and reinitiate local screening protocols for BK, CMV and EBV viruses, and other infections.

Post-transplant infections can be mitigated by preventative methods, as described below in individual sections, as well as routine vaccinations, consumption of clean food and water, preventative measures during times of outbreaks (as with severe acute respiratory syndrome (SARS) and H1N1 influenza), safer sexual practices for non-monogamous recipients, visits with travel medicine specialists prior to visiting high-risk regions, and guidance on better tattoo acquisition.

Table 12.1 • Vaccines that might be indicated for adults, based on medical and other indications[1]—United States, 2012

VACCINE ▼ / INDICATION ▶	Pregnancy	Immuno-compromising conditions (excluding human immunodeficiency virus [HIV])[4,6,7,10,15]	HIV infection CD4+ T lymphocyte count[4,6,7,10,14,15] <200 cells/µL	HIV infection ≥200 cells/µL	Men who have sex with men (MSM)	Heart disease, chronic lung disease, chronic alcoholism	Asplenia (including elective splenectomy and persistent complement component deficiencies)[10,14]	Chronic liver disease	Kidney failure, end-stage renal disease, receipt of hemodialysis	Diabetes	Healthcare personnel
Influenza[2,*]	1 dose IIV annually	1 dose IIV annually	1 dose IIV annually	1 dose IIV annually	1 dose IIV or LAIV annually	1 dose IIV annually	1 dose IIV annually	1 dose IIV annually	1 dose IIV annually	1 dose IIV annually	1 dose IIV or LAIV annually
Tetanus, diphtheria, pertussis (Td/Tdap)[3,*]	1 dose Tdap each pregnancy	Substitute 1-time dose of Tdap for Td booster; then boost with Td every 10 yrs									
Varicella[4,*]	Contraindicated	Contraindicated	Contraindicated	2 doses	2 doses	2 doses	2 doses	2 doses	2 doses	2 doses	2 doses
Human papillomavirus (HPV) Female[5,*]	3 doses through age 26 yrs	3 doses through age 26 yrs	3 doses through age 26 yrs	3 doses through age 26 yrs	3 doses through age 26 yrs	3 doses through age 26 yrs	3 doses through age 26 yrs	3 doses through age 26 yrs	3 doses through age 26 yrs	3 doses through age 26 yrs	3 doses through age 26 yrs
Human papillomavirus (HPV) Male[5,*]	3 doses through age 26 yrs	3 doses through age 26 yrs	3 doses through age 26 yrs	3 doses through age 26 yrs	3 doses through age 26 yrs	3 doses through age 21 yrs	3 doses through age 21 yrs	3 doses through age 21 yrs	3 doses through age 21 yrs	3 doses through age 21 yrs	3 doses through age 21 yrs
Zoster[6]	Contraindicated	Contraindicated	Contraindicated	1 dose	1 dose	1 dose	1 dose	1 dose	1 dose	1 dose	1 dose
Measles, mumps, rubella (MMR)[7,*]	Contraindicated	Contraindicated	Contraindicated	1 or 2 doses	1 or 2 doses	1 or 2 doses	1 or 2 doses	1 or 2 doses	1 or 2 doses	1 or 2 doses	1 or 2 doses
Pneumococcal polysaccharide (PPSV23)[8,9]		1 or 2 doses	1 or 2 doses	1 or 2 doses	1 or 2 doses	1 or 2 doses	1 or 2 doses	1 or 2 doses	1 or 2 doses	1 or 2 doses	
Pneumococcal 13-valent conjugate (PCV13)[10,*]		1 dose	1 dose	1 dose			1 dose		1 dose		
Meningococcal[11,*]	1 or more doses	1 or more doses	1 or more doses	1 or more doses	1 or more doses	1 or more doses	1 or more doses	1 or more doses	1 or more doses	1 or more doses	1 or more doses
Hepatitis A[12,*]	2 doses	2 doses	2 doses	2 doses	2 doses	2 doses	2 doses	2 doses	2 doses	2 doses	2 doses
Hepatitis B[13,*]	3 doses	3 doses	3 doses	3 doses	3 doses	3 doses	3 doses	3 doses	3 doses	3 doses	3 doses

*Covered by the Vaccine Injury Compensation Program

For all persons in this category who meet the age requirements and who lack documentation of vaccination or have no evidence of previous infection; zoster vaccine recommended regardless of prior episode of zoster

Recommended if some other risk factor is present (e.g., on the basis of medical, occupational, lifestyle, or other indications)

No recommendation

Available online, www.cdc.gov/vaccines/schedules/downloads/adult/mmwr-adult-schedule.pdf, accessed December 17, 2012.

Viruses: epidemiology, prophylaxis, diagnosis and treatment

Epidemiology

Viral infections are the most common infection after transplantation. They encompass a broad array of viruses, ranging from herpes to respiratory to hepatitis and other viruses. In addition to the direct effects (i.e. clinical syndromes) caused by viruses, they can be quite immunomodulatory, especially CMV, HCV or EBV, resulting in inflammation (potentially mitigating graft tolerance) as well as increased immunosuppression (increasing the risk of infection from other opportunistic pathogens). Since many of the important viruses after transplantation are latent (i.e the herpes viruses), their ongoing prevention and management is a fine balance between optimal levels of immunosuppression and reactivation of infection.

The human herpes viruses are the most common aetiological agents of infection after transplantation. The family includes eight viruses: herpes simplex type 1 and type 2 (HSV-1, -2), varicella, EBV, CMV, the roseola-like human herpes virus 6 and 7 (HHV-6, -7), and human herpes virus 8 (HHV-8, the aetiological agent of Kaposi's sarcoma). The alpha herpes virus family (HSV-1, -2, varicella) establishes latent infections primarily in sensory ganglia, while the beta herpes viruses (CMV, HHV-6, -7) maintain latency in leucocytes, endothelium and other tissues, and the gamma herpes viruses (EBV and HHV-8) are latent in lymphoid tissue. Disseminated infection from any of the human herpes viruses can be life threatening; recipients who acquired de novo infection from their donors, who did not have prior immunity to these viruses, are at higher risk for infection.

Numerous other types of viruses cause disease in transplant recipients. Respiratory viruses such as influenza, respiratory syncitial virus (RSV), adenovirus, parainfluenza and human metapneumovirus are common and may present more subtly or with fulminate disease. Hepatitis viruses (primarily B and C) are common causes for liver transplantation and can be common complications after transplant, predominantly as reactivation of latent infections; in addition, the primarily zoonotic hepatitis E has been reported as an emerging pathogen that may cause chronic hepatitis in transplant recipients.[11] Most adults have latent infection with the polyoma viruses BK and JC, which can reactivate in the setting of immunosuppression, causing primarily kidney and brain disease, respectively. While BK is predominantly a pathogen in kidney transplant recipients, it can cause disease in other transplant recipients. Risk of BK reactivation relates directly to the intensity of the immunosuppression; early diagnosis of BK replication and subsequent reduction in the immunosuppressive regimen largely abrogates the risk of BK nephropathy, which generally has poor outcomes in kidney transplant recipients, with high rates of graft loss. JC virus causes progressive multifocal leucoencephalopathy, which is often mortal but fortunately fairly rare. A multicentre, retrospective cohort study of progressive multifocal leucoencephalopathy after solid-organ transplant found a median time to development of first symptoms of 27 months, with a median survival of 6.4 months, with a rough incidence of 0.1%.[12] Numerous other viruses have been shown to cause disease in transplant recipients, including parvovirus B19, West Nile virus, lymphocytic choriomeningitis virus and others.

Hundreds of patients with human immodeficiency virus (HIV) infection have undergone organ transplant, primarily kidney but also liver and other organs. In a large multicentre trial between November 2003 and June 2009, a total of 150 HIV-positive patients underwent kidney transplantation: patient survival rates at 1 and 3 years were 94.6 ± 2.0% and 88.2 ± 3.8%, respectively, while the corresponding graft survival rates were 90.4% and 73.7%.[13] These outcomes fall somewhere in the national database between kidney transplant recipients who are 65+ years old and those reported for all kidney transplant recipients. Multivariate analysis showed that the risk of graft loss was increased among patients treated for rejection and those receiving antithymocyte globulin induction therapy, while living-donor transplants were protective. A higher than expected rejection rate was observed, with 1- and 3-year estimates of 31% and 41%, respectively. HIV infection remained well controlled, with stable CD4-positive T-cell counts and few HIV-associated complications.

> ✔ Such data suggest that in appropriately chosen HIV-positive candidates, renal transplant may be an appropriate therapy.

Prophylaxis

Prevention of viral infections is paramount for renal transplant patients. Prevention of viral infections can be achieved by the use of antiviral medications, judicious use of immunosuppression, occasional use of immunoglobulins, careful monitoring and vaccination. Since the severity of many viral infections relates to the intensity of immunosuppression, careful reduction of the immunosuppressive regimen can result in a decreased risk of viral infections, especially with latent viruses. The most common antiviral medications used for prevention include the aciclovir family (including famciclovir and valaciclovir), primarily for HSV and varicella prophylaxis, and ganciclovir (with the oral prodrug, valganciclovir), which is targeted at CMV prevention but also successfully decreases the rates of other herpes virus infections to varying extents, as well as anti-hepatitis B agents. Prophylaxis against hepatitis C is not usually given, due to toxicities that outweigh benefits.

> ✓✓ The duration of prevention varies considerably among institutions, but many programmes use antivirals for 3–6 months after organ transplant (especially with high-risk situations where the donor is CMV seropositive and the recipient seronegative, or with lung transplant),[4] often with either ganciclovir or valganciclovir to prevent CMV, or an aciclovir-type drug to prevent disseminated varicella infection, as well as HSV; use of such prophylaxis is a strong recommendation.[1]

While some organ transplant centres use antiviral agents in certain cohorts of patients at risk for CMV (termed 'universal prophylaxis'), others use 'pre-emptive therapy' where treatment is begun only when routine monitoring tests show evidence of active infection. Guidelines for optimal management of CMV after solid-organ transplantation have been published.[4] CMV immunoglobulin and HBV and varicella hyperimmune globulins have been shown to be effective in preventing infection in certain settings, and repleting recipients with hypogammaglobulinaemia (often defined as <400 IU/mL) with intravenous immunoglobulin can reduce their risk of infection.[14] In addition, periodic monitoring has been shown to be helpful, as with CMV, EBV and BK viruses.

In the immediate post-transplant period, universal prophylaxis and pre-emptive therapy comprise the two main methods for CMV prevention. Universal prophylaxis involves giving antiviral medication at prophylaxis dose for a defined period of time to a cohort (i.e. when either donor and/or recipient are seropositive for CMV) or defined subset of a cohort (i.e. given only to the highest risk subset, thus just when donors are seropositive and recipients are negative for CMV, hereafter referred to as D+/R−). Pre-emptive therapy is defined as serial testing done for the first few months after transplant or after treatment of rejection, and use of treatment dose antivirals is initiated once a certain test threshold is achieved.

> ✓ While some programmes elect not to utilise either of these methods of prevention and to observe clinically with a plan to test and treat based on signs and symptoms of active CMV, this should be strongly discouraged, as this is likely to result in high rates of symptomatic CMV infection, ranging from CMV syndrome to end-organ disease (colitis, hepatitis, pneumonitis, encephalitis, retinitis and others), and clinical outcomes are likely to be inferior to programmes using either pre-emptive therapy or universal prophylaxis, with higher rates of graft dysfunction and loss, more opportunistic infections and a great risk of post-PTLD.[1,4]

The two methods of prevention each have their merits and disadvantages. While large, randomised trials have not been conducted, numerous studies suggest that universal prophylaxis may convey better outcomes compared with pre-emptive therapy, especially in the higher risk D+/R−population, as summarised in recent guidelines.[4] Benefits of universal prophylaxis include lower drug cost, fewer opportunistic infections (including Kaposi's sarcoma and PTLD), improved graft and patient survival, lower rates of rejection, easier logistics, and lower monitoring costs. Negatives include higher rates of late CMV, resistant virus, and higher drug costs and toxicities. Advantages of pre-emptive therapy include lower drug cost, reduced drug exposure, lower rates of late CMV (possibly due to enhanced immunological priming[15]), lower drug cost, reduced drug exposure and theoretically lower risk of resistant CMV due to lower rates of drug exposure. Disadvantages include lower rates of graft and patient survival, higher rates of opportunistic infections and more complex logistics (organising weekly testing for several months after transplant and managing results). Whether to initiate secondary chemoprophylaxis or viral monitoring after treatment of active CMV infection has not been well studied. Experts vary in their range of practice.[4] Institutions should develop local protocols, based on previous clinical outcomes, use of cytolytic induction therapies, the net state of immunosuppression, type of organ(s) transplanted, costs, ability to do periodic testing and other factors.

> ✅ Outcomes with 'pre-emptive therapy' may not be as optimal as with universal prophylaxis, especially in high-risk transplants (i.e. CMV D+/R–), and transplant centres may wish to use universal prophylaxis, especially in high-risk transplants.[4]

Perhaps some of the more compelling data come from a randomised clinical trial of oral ganciclovir prophylaxis (n=74) versus pre-emptive therapy with intravenous ganciclovir (n=74), where prophylaxis significantly increased long-term graft survival 4 years after transplant (92.2% vs. 78.3%; P=0.0425).[16] Patients with CMV donor seropositive/recipient seropositive (D+/R+) status had the lowest rate of graft loss following prophylaxis (0.0% vs. 26.8%; P=0.0035), suggesting that perhaps the prophylaxis strategy can be tailored according to serostatus. Recent work demonstrated an unexpected and higher risk of antiviral resistance in those D+/R−renal recipients on pre-emptive therapy;[17] prior work had shown an increased risk of resistance for those on universal prophylaxis, suggesting that perhaps both methods convey some risk of resistance.

There has long been concern about the 'direct' and 'indirect' effects of CMV on transplant recipients. The direct effects, which are the manifestations of infection, are clinically obvious. The indirect effects are more insidious and may have negative impacts on both the organ graft outcome and the recipient, and include increased rates of bacterial, viral and fungal infections, more aggressive recurrent HCV after liver transplantation, higher rates of acute rejection and increased graft dysfunction and failure, chronic allograft nephropathy, vascular disease (coronary, aortic and transplant), cancer (especially PTLD) and diabetes.[18]

Costs are an important part of transplant care throughout the world, and may have a significant influence on choice of prevention method. Costs of serial testing (including personnel and laboratory monitoring costs) may be somewhat similar to the costs of medications (i.e. with 'universal prophylaxis') in some settings, although the net costs to the patient (i.e. co-payments for medication) or to the transplant programme or healthcare system may be different. Nonetheless, it is important to remember to focus on long-term outcomes and overall cost and benefit to the patient and to the programme. In one recent study, the incidence of CMV infection in seropositive kidney transplant recipients was 4.1% and 55.5% within the first year after transplant while under universal prophylaxis and pre-emptive therapy, respectively.[19] Universal prophylaxis incurred $1464 more in direct cost compared with pre-emptive therapy, while saving $7309 in indirect cost, and resulted in a net gain of 0.209 in quality-adjusted life-years per patient over a 10-year period. Thus, universal prophylaxis resulted in a cost saving of $27 967 for 1 quality-adjusted life-year gained when compared with pre-emptive therapy, and the authors concluded that universal prophylaxis in CMV-seropositive kidney transplant patients is clinically effective and cost saving.

Evidence from the Improved Protection Against CMV in Transplant (IMPACT) trial demonstrated that prolonged prophylaxis of 200 days with valganciclovir compared with 100 days significantly reduces the incidence of CMV in high-risk kidney transplant (D+/R−) recipients, as shown in **Fig. 12.2**.[20] Subsequent researchers

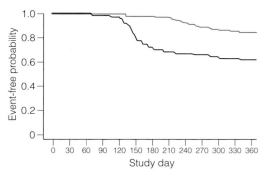

Number of patients left													
— 100 days	163	161	161	157	151	125	110	104	102	101	95	94	83
— 200 days	155	154	152	150	149	147	145	143	136	130	125	122	120

Figure 12.2 • From the IMPACT trial in D+/R−kidney transplant recipients, the Kaplan–Meier plot of time to cytomegalovirus disease up to month 12 post-transplant, comparing 100 versus 200 days of valganciclovir prophylaxis.[20] Reproduced from Humar A, Lebranchu Y, Vincenti F et al. The efficacy and safety of 200 days valganciclovir cytomegalovirus prophylaxis in high-risk kidney transplant recipients. Am J Transplant 2010; 10(5):1228–37. With permission from John Wiley and Sons.

developed a cost-effectiveness model to evaluate prolonged prophylaxis of 200 days with valganciclovir in D+/R−kidney transplant recipients and its long-term economic impact from the US healthcare payer perspective.[21] They found that for the 5-year time horizon, the incremental cost-effectiveness ratio of US $14 859/quality-adjusted life-year suggests that 200-day valganciclovir prophylaxis is cost-effective over the 100-day regimen considering a threshold of US $50 000 per quality-adjusted life-year. The 10-year analysis revealed the 200-day prophylaxis as cost saving with a 2380 quality-adjusted life-year gain (per 10 000 patients) and simultaneously lower costs. The authors concluded that prolonged prophylaxis with valganciclovir reduces the incidence of events associated with CMV infection in high-risk kidney transplant recipients and is a cost-effective strategy in CMV disease management. Another single-centre, retrospective study reached the same conclusion, that 6 months of prophylaxis in those who are CMV D+/R−was more cost-effective than 3 months, with an incremental cost of $34 362 and $16 215 per case of infection and disease avoided, respectively, and $8304 per one quality-adjusted life-year gained.[22]

> ✔ Based on the lower risk of CMV infection and disease, as well as cost-effectiveness, expert opinion suggests that in D+/R−transplants, 200 days of prophylaxis with valganciclovir may be optimal, compared with 100 days.[20–22]

Polyoma viruses, especially BK virus, can result in significant graft dysfunction and loss. Numerous studies show that routine monitoring for BK for the first 12–18 months after transplant, with early detection of viral replication and subsequent reduction of immunosuppression, is likely to provide the best clinical outcomes. Once BK nephropathy has become established, salvage of the kidney is less likely to be successful. Antiviral therapy, including cidofovir and leflunomide, has shown fairly limited success, and with potentially significant toxicity. Limited data suggest that fluoroquinolones (such as ciprofloxacin or levofloxacin) after renal transplant may decrease the risk of BK viraemia; additional data suggest that they may reduce the incidence of severe BK haemorrhagic cystitis after allogeneic hematopoietic stem cell transplantation. While generally considered antibacterial agents, fluoroquinolones seem to have some activity against large T-antigen helicase activity in polyomavirus, and may also inhibit cellular enzymes; thus, they inhibit but do not eradicate BKV replication.

> ✔✔ It should be emphasised that BK viraemia and nephropathy appear to be consequences of excessively potent immunosuppression, that the primary method of prevention is screening, and that the primary method of treatment is reduction in immunosuppression with subsequent monitoring.

Hepatitis B is a common indication for cirrhosis and liver transplantation; post-transplant management may include antiviral agents such as lamivudine, entecavir, adefovir and others, as well as the use of hyperimmune hepatitis B globulin. Other organ transplant recipients may have latent hepatitis B, which can reactivate in the setting of immunosuppression, especially in those who have a positive hepatitis B surface antigen, and much less commonly in those who have a negative surface antigen but a positive core antibody. When they are non-immune, all patients undergoing dialysis and organ transplantation should undergo vaccination in the pre-transplant period; some patients may benefit from a higher dose of vaccine and accelerated vaccine series, especially if they are to undergo organ transplantation soon.

EBV is mainly an issue for those who were seronegative before transplant and for those who are very potently immunosuppressed (lung, intestinal, composite tissue transplants). EBV replication increases the risk of PTLD, 90% of which are EBV mediated. An analysis of the SRTR National Registry Data in the United States found that the unadjusted hazard ratio (HR) for PTLD (if recipient EBV seronegative) was 5.005 for kidney transplant, 6.528 for heart transplant and 2.615 for liver transplant ($P < 0.001$ for all).[23] Some centres screen periodically in the first year after transplant in EBV D+/R−, and reduce the immunosuppression with significant viraemia.[24,25] In a recent series, 34 D+/R−adult renal transplant recipients at a single institution were prospectively monitored for EBV during the first year post-transplant.[24] Twenty (60.6%) of the 34 recipients developed viraemia during the first year post-transplant, of which six were given rituximab and did not develop PTLD; of the six recipients who were not monitored, three (50%) developed PTLD and lost their grafts. It was concluded that recipients who were not monitored on the protocol were more likely to have PTLD and graft loss compared to those who were monitored ($P = 0.008$). There are no data to suggest that antiviral agents can prevent or decrease EBV viraemia; ganciclovir only works in the very small percentage of virus that is in the lytic phase. Belatacept, one of the newer immunosuppressive medications, is approved only for use in EBV-seropositive recipients, due to a higher risk of PTLD in seronegative recipients.[26]

✔ Monitoring of EBV viral load after EBV D+/R−transplants, with careful adjustment of immunosuppression, may be helpful in reducing the risk of PTLD.

Interestingly, replicating EBV is not always a marker for poor outcomes. In a cohort of 31 lung transplant recipients followed for up to 2 years after transplantation with EBV viral loads performed on plasma and whole blood, patients with positive whole blood EBV viral loads had a statistically significant lower incidence (45% vs. 83%) of grade 2 or higher acute allograft rejection compared with patients with no positive assays, but did not have an increased risk for infectious complications followed longitudinally, suggesting that whole-blood EBV viral loads may represent an important functional measure of the net state of immunosuppression in solid-organ transplant patients.[25] None of these patients developed PTLD.

The term post-transplant lymphoproliferative disorder (PTLD) describes lymphoproliferations, which, in contrast with lymphomas, are not always monoclonal and whose morphological features often differ from those of lymphomas. While not truly an infection, they are a hybrid between infection and malignancy. PTLDs are the second most frequent neoplasia in transplant patients after skin carcinomas, with a risk 10–20 times higher compared to the general population. Approximately 90% of PTLD cases are EBV related. The risk of PTLD is much higher in those who are EBV D+/R−, or on more potent suppression, such as after lung transplant. In a recent series from the French national registry of adult renal transplant recipients, the cumulative incidence was 1% after 5 years, and climbed to 2.1% after 10 years, and multivariate analysis showed that PTLD was significantly associated with older

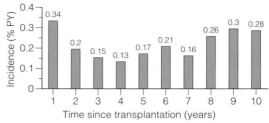

Figure 12.3 • Histogram of occurrence of PTLD in adult kidney and kidney–pancreas recipients as a function of time since transplant.[27] Reproduced from Caillard S, Lamy FX, Quelen C et al. Epidemiology of posttransplant lymphoproliferative disorders in adult kidney and kidney pancreas recipients: report of the French registry and analysis of subgroups of lymphomas. Am J Transplant 2012; 12(3):682–93. With permission from John Wiley and Sons.

age of the recipient, simultaneous kidney–pancreas transplantation, earlier year of transplant (1998–9 and 2000–1 versus 2006–7), EBV mismatch, five or six HLA mismatches, and induction therapy.[27] The risk of PTLD was fairly continuous and significant, as shown in **Fig. 12.3**.

Zoonotic infections such as lymphocytic choriomeningitis virus and rabies have also resulted in life-threatening donor-derived infections in transplant recipients.[28,29] Other zoonotic viral infections that have caused significant infections in transplant recipients include hepatitis E, parapoxvirus and SARS.[30] Mosquito-borne infections such as West Nile virus, dengue fever, Eastern equine encephalitis, chickungunya and others can cause significant disease in transplant recipients. Avoidance of insect bites via the use of protective clothing, insect repellant and screens or sleeping nets when necessary will decrease risk of transmission. West Nile virus infections in both blood and organ donors have caused infections in transplant recipients.[31]

✔✔ Vaccination against influenza, hepatitis A and B, measles, mumps, rubella, human papillomavirus, varicella/zoster and other viral pathogens can provide additional protection; it is strongly recommended that protection be optimised prior to transplantation, as the immunological response is likely to be augmented, compared with after transplantation.

Certain viral vaccines have live attenuated virus and cannot be used after transplantation, such as varicella/zoster, measles, mumps, rubella and yellow fever, as shown in Table 12.1. In general, transplant centres are much more inclined to administer vaccines to transplant patients compared to previously, and annual influenza vaccine is recommended by numerous experts.[32] Surveys in 1999 and 2009 of United Network for Organ Sharing-certified kidney and kidney–pancreas transplant centres in the United States regarding their influenza vaccination practices established that the 2009 respondents, compared with 1999, were more likely to recommend vaccination for kidney (94.5% vs. 84.4%, $P = 0.02$) and kidney–pancreas recipients (76.8% vs. 48.5%, $P < 0.001$), and family members of transplant recipients (52.5% vs. 21.0%, $P < 0.001$).[33] While there has been some concern that vaccines could disrupt tolerance or increase the risk of rejection, this has not been borne out in trials to date.

> ✔ When possible, transplant recipients should avoid the adjuvants in some vaccines, and be given unadjuvanted vaccines; adjuvants are immunostimulatory molecules that could cause harm.[32]

Diagnosis

Viral diagnostics have improved exponentially with the onset of molecular techniques. Viral culture is progressively being replaced by more rapid and specific molecular assays. Within a matter of hours, various amplification methods can precisely document active replicating viral infections. In the era of quantitative assays, trends in viral load can be followed over time, as is seen with serial assays for response to CMV treatment, or for BK viraemia/viruria or EBV viraemia. Molecular diagnostics have given us powerful assays for infections that were previously very challenging (or even impossible) to diagnose in this population, such as parvovirus B19, HHV-6 and -7, and others. Knowledge of pre-transplant serostatus (i.e. antibody titre) for some viruses, such as CMV, EBV and the hepatitis viruses, can be helpful in guiding diagnosis and management; in general, serology is much less helpful in the immunosuppressed population, as they are much less likely to seroconvert to acute illness, and molecular diagnostics may have a much higher yield. Immunohistochemistry on biopsy specimens can be very helpful for various herpes infections, including HSV, varicella, EBV, CMV and HHV-8,

and for other viruses including BK virus; the appropriate diagnosis of BK virus nephropathy can only be made by biopsy, as viraemia alone is not diagnostic of nephropathy. The recent development of an international standard by the WHO for CMV viral load testing may revolutionise our ability to diagnose and manage CMV across all testing platforms, thus enabling development of multicentre protocols. Assays for cellular immunity, such as interferon-gamma enzyme-linked immunospot assay (ELISpot), intracellular cytokine staining, major histocompatibility complex (MHC) multimer-based assays and Quantiferon-CMV, are emerging as technologies that may be able to predict an individual's risk of developing viral diseases.

Treatment

Effective treatment of viral infections may involve a multi-pronged approach: use of antiviral agents, reduction of immunosuppression when possible, and augmentation of immunity through the use of immunoglobulins and sometimes infusions of virus-specific T-cells. Common antiviral treatments include the aciclovir family (including famciclovir and valaciclovir, primarily for HSV and varicella infections), ganciclovir (with the oral prodrug, valganciclovir, for CMV and other infections), foscarnet (predominantly for resistant CMV), cidofovir (for resistant CMV, BK virus and others) and ribavirin (for RSV and other less common infections). Hepatitis B has numerous antiviral agents for treatment, and hepatitis C is primarily treated with ribavirin and interferon; although there are newly released protease inhibitors (telaprevir and boceprevir) with anti-HCV activity, data are lacking in transplant patients, and drug interactions are profound. Reducing the intensity of immunosuppression (even transiently) may allow for more rapid clearance of a viral infection. Although not always evidence based, repleting recipients who have hypogammaglobulinaemia with intravenous immunoglobulin may help clear infection.[14] Some centres use CMV immunoglobulin in seronegative recipients with serious active disease. The novel use of adoptive infusions of CMV or EBV-specific T-cells has been shown to be effective, especially in hematopoietic stem cell recipients and increasingly in organ transplant recipients.

Bacteria: epidemiology, prophylaxis, diagnosis and treatment

Epidemiology

Bacterial infections occur at increased frequency in the vulnerable transplant recipient. They range from routine infections such as urinary tract infections, pneumonias and bacteraemias to more exotic infections with *Nocardia*, *Rhodococcus*, *Listeria* and other pathogens. Their more frequent exposure to healthcare settings increases the risk of resistant pathogens, including methicillin-resistant and vancomycin-intermediate *Staphylococcus aureus* (MRSA and VISA, respectively), vancomycin-resistant *Enterococcus faecalis* (VRE), *Pseudomonas*, *Stenotrophomonas* and others. Latent infections such as *Mycobacterium tuberculosis* reactivate at much higher rates in those with renal and hepatic failure, as well as in the post-transplant period.

Prophylaxis

Prevention of bacterial infection requires review of the risk factors in the individual patient, i.e. recurrent urinary tract infections, prior pneumonias or episodes of cellulitis, poorly drained collections (ascites, pleural fluid), etc.

> ✔ The use of trimethoprim/sulfamethoxazole after transplant to prevent *Pneumocystis* has the additional advantage of preventing other bacterial infections, ranging from *Streptococcus* to *Listeria* to *Nocardia* and many others, and is widely recommended.[1]

Vaccination against *Streptococcus pneumoniae*, *Clostridium tetani* (tetanus), *Corynebacterium diphtheriae*, *Bordetella pertussis* (whooping cough) and other bacterial pathogens may provide additional protection.

Recurrent urinary tract infections are common in transplant recipients. Investigation of the anatomical aetiology for recurrent infection is paramount; many transplant recipients often have abnormal bladder, prostate or other genitourinary anatomy that predisposes them to recurrent infection. While some clinicians use long-term antibiotics to prevent recurrent infections, this approach is less successful in the era of antibiotic resistance and increased rates of

Clostridium difficile; although not studied, rotating antibiotics may alter the risk of antibiotic resistance. This author strongly encourages further anatomical investigation whenever possible. Use of vaginal oestrogen replacement (i.e. local, not necessarily systemic) in post-menopausal women may be helpful.

Diagnosis

Diagnosis of bacterial infections still relies heavily on culture techniques. In order to optimise the diagnostic yield of cultures, clinicians should notify the laboratory when unusual organisms are suspected, such as *Listeria*, *Rhodococcus*, mycobacteria and *Nocardia*. Expanding the standard panel of antibiotic sensitivity at the time of initial diagnosis may help with subsequent therapy, especially given the increased risk of drug interactions and side-effects, partly due to concomitant use of multiple medications (i.e. increased risks of leucopenia, nephrotoxicity, etc.). Histopathology, especially with special stains for micro-organisms, can sometimes be helpful in achieving a diagnosis; examples include the Fite stain for mycobacteria, the May–Grunwald Giemsa stain, and the Warthin–Starry or Steiner stain for spirochetes, among others. Molecular diagnostics are emerging as a diagnostic methodology for bacterial infections. Serological techniques tend to yield diagnoses less frequently in this population due to more muted immunological responses.

Treatment

Treatment often begins in febrile or ill-appearing transplant recipients with empirical antibacterial therapy, which should be chosen based on local epidemiology. This approach appears to be justified by the significant incidence of bacteraemia in the post-transplant period and by the concomitant high mortality rate when appropriate treatment is delayed, especially when infections are caused by certain pathogens. Transplant patients are at higher risk for resistant pathogens, and the empirical antibiotic choice should reflect this. Once a culture diagnosis has been made and antibiotic susceptibilities are available, the antibiotic regimen may be tailored. Optimal duration of therapy has usually not been well studied in this population, but often is the same or somewhat longer than in normal hosts.

Certain antibiotic types should be avoided when possible due to toxicities and side-effects, including aminoglycosides (which can increase the risk of renal toxicity) and rifamycins (rifampin/rifampicin or rifabutin, which have profound interactions with tacrolimus, ciclosporin A, sirolimus, prednisone and others).

Because of the increased rates of resistance resulting in decreased susceptibility to oral antibiotics, intravenous therapy is more common in this population, which requires the use of prolonged intravenous access, sometimes through peripherally inserted central catheters (PICCs or PIC lines). In general, arm veins should be avoided and preserved for future haemodialysis access in those at higher risk for chronic kidney disease, and small-bore tunnelled central venous catheters have grown increasingly popular.[34] Optimising the drainage of collections via the use of radiographically or surgically placed drains may help clear infection and prevent recurrent infection; appropriately drained infections do not necessarily need long-term antibiotics while the drain stays in place. Preventative measures include eliminating any nidus of infection (such as intravascular catheters, indwelling urinary catheters, stents, skin defects that encourage abscess formation, etc.) and optimising foci of recurrent infections (i.e. urinary tract infections).

Fungi: epidemiology, prophylaxis, diagnosis and treatment

Epidemiology

While infections from *Candida* tend to be more manageable, infections such as invasive aspergillosis and zygomycosis (due to *Rhizopus*, *Absidia*, *Rhizomucor*, *Mucor*, *Cunninghamella* and numerous others) have very high mortality rates and are among the most dreaded of infectious complications. While these have a predilection to occur in the early post-transplant period, especially *Candida* infections, they may also occur years later. For example, *Cryptococcus neoformans* is among the most common causes of meningitis in organ transplant recipients. *Pneumocystis jiroveci* (formerly *P. carinii*) is also a fungus, previously classified as a protozoan.

Prophylaxis

Preventing *Candida* and other yeast infections requires judicious use of antibiotics and immunosuppression. Spontaneous *Candida* infections (without risk factors) are quite rare on their own. They often follow broad antibiotic exposure, decreasing normal flora and increasing *Candida* colonisation of the gut, urinary system and upper respiratory tract, which increases the risk of translocation from a non-sterile site to a sterile site, such as the bloodstream, pleural or peritoneal spaces, or elsewhere. Urinary catheters greatly increase the risk of urinary *Candida* colonisation and subsequent invasive infection. *Cryptococcus neoformans* spores live in bird droppings (especially pigeon droppings) and in soil contaminated with bird droppings; humans can get cryptococcal infection by inhalation of airborne fungi from such sources, and it is recommended that transplant patients avoid bird contact.

Mould spores are ubiquitous in the environment. Preventing mould infections involves a combination of avoidance measures, including filtered air systems in hospitals, recognition of existing infection or colonisation, and targeted antifungal prophylaxis. It is very rarely possible to reliably distinguish community-acquired from nosocomial aspergillosis. Transplant recipients should wear gloves while gardening, or touching plants or soil, and they should avoid inhaling or creating soil or dust aerosols that may contain mould spores. They may wish to wear N95 masks in some unavoidable situations, and should always wash their hands after such contact, and care for skin abrasions or cuts sustained during soil or plant contact. They should not have birds as pets. Invasive mould infections in the explanted lungs, more common in those with cystic fibrosis, are often not recognised before lung transplantation and have been associated with poor outcomes; similarly, airway colonisation with mould in other organ recipients may blossom into a full infection after transplant; thus, knowledge of culture data at or before the time of transplant may

---

✔ Many centres recommend prophylaxis against *P. jiroveci*, often with trimethoprim/sulfamethoxazole, atovaquone or dapsone; it should be noted that trimethoprim/sulfamethoxazole has the broadest spectrum of prevention of infection, and is most preferable for that reason compared with the other agents.

help target therapy and mitigate infection. Antifungal prophylaxis varies broadly among transplant centres; in general, most renal centres would rarely give prophylaxis against *Aspergillus* and other moulds.

Adherence to avoidance measures, acknowledging their limitations, combined with antifungal prophylaxis, is likely to be the most effective approach to prevent invasive mould diseases.

Demographic fungi such as *Coccidioides* or *Histoplasma* are also seen at elevated rates in transplant patients. Interestingly, coccidiomycosis occurs more commonly than histoplasmosis in transplant patients, with higher rates of reactivation of latent infection. Transplant patients who travel to endemic areas are also at risk for acquisition of de novo infection, and should be cautioned about this. Rare cases of donor-derived infection from demographic fungi have also been described; in some cases, since these infections were not expected in non-endemic regions where the transplant occurred, there were high mortality rates.

Fungal infections may be due to animal exposure.[30] *Cryptococcus* species are the third most common cause of invasive fungal infection in organ transplant recipients after *Candida* species and *Aspergillus* species.[35] Birds and their droppings are the most commonly perceived risk. Some authors suggest that immunocompromised hosts should not keep cockatoos, given their association with cryptococcosis.[36] Sporotrichosis due to *Sporothrix schenckii* infection can be connected to animal contact, especially contact with cats. Dermatophytes are common in both regular and exotic animals and can cause both superficial and invasive disease in humans.

Diagnosis

Fungal diagnostics utilise dedicated fungal stains and culture as well as detection of fungal antigens in blood, urine and other fluids. Fungi may be harder to grow in culture and harder to diagnose than other pathogens. A high level of suspicion, as well as multiple diagnostic approaches, is imperative in the diagnosis of these potentially more elusive pathogens. Some pathogens such as *Candida* will usually grow on routine culture, while others require dedicated fungal culture media to promote growth. *Candida* will grow from regular blood cultures, while filamentous fungi (such as *Aspergillus*,

very rarely found by blood culture, i.e. in less than 1% of cases of aspergillosis) need fungal isolators.

Fungal antigens, including the 1,3-β-D-glucan, galactomannan and cryptococcal assays, have increased the diagnostic capacity in recent times. The 1,3-β-D-glucan assay, tested in blood, can be positive with a variety of fungal pathogens, ranging from *Candida* to *Aspergillus* and numerous others, including *Fusarium* spp., *Trichosporon* spp., *Saccharomyces cerevisiae*, *Acremonium*, *Coccidioides immitis*, *Histoplasma capsulatum*, *Sporothrix schenckii*, *Blastomyces dermatitidis* and *Pneumocystis carinii*. The galactomannan antigen has been used on a variety of specimens and is relatively specific for *Aspergillus*; both blood and body fluids can be tested. Cryptococcal antigen testing of blood or spinal fluid is both very sensitive and specific for cryptococcosis.

For pulmonary lesions that may be fungal in nature, bronchoscopy with bronchial alveolar lavage and transbronchial biopsy, or radiographically guided transthoracic biopsy, or further lung biopsy is often imperative in making the diagnosis. Delays in diagnostic procedures in patients on empirical antifungal regimens greatly decrease the diagnostic outcomes of such procedures, and should be avoided. Galactomannan antigen testing on bronchial alveolar lavage fluid can be diagnostically helpful for *Aspergillus* when it is positive. Special stains for *Pneumocystis jiroveci* should be included. *Pneumocystis jiroveci* may also have elevated lactate dehydrogenase (LDH) and a positive 1,3-β-D-glucan assay.

Serology and urinary antigen testing may sometimes be helpful (i.e. *Coccidioides*). When biopsy material or tissue is available, histopathology can also provide diagnostic input, especially with special stains for fungi, including Gomori's metanamine silver, periodic acid–Schiff staining, mucicarmine for *Cryptococcus*, and immunohistochemistry for *Pneumocystis jiroveci*.

Treatment

Treatment of fungal infections may involve use of one or more antifungal agents, as well as surgical debulking (especially with mucormycosis and sometimes aspergillosis). *Candida* infection may be treated with an azole (primarily fluconazole) or with an echinocandin (i.e. micafungin, caspofungin, anidulafungin). Depending on the individual pathogen, the filamentous mould infections are treated with an amphotericin B product, often a lipid-based one for better tolerability (such as Ambisome® or Abelcet®), or with a higher level azole such as voriconazole or posaconazole. The echinocandins are sometimes used in salvage regimens, or as part of a multidrug regimen, albeit with very few available data for multidrug regimens in this setting. Antifungal susceptibilities are increasingly being used to guide optimal treatment, as is therapeutic drug monitoring, especially for the higher level azoles, voriconazole and posaconazole. There are important drug interactions between the immunosuppressive agents (especially tacrolimus, ciclosporin and sirolimus) and the azoles (especially the higher level ones), necessitating reductions in doses of the immunosuppressive agents. Most of the endemic fungal and cryptococcal infections respond to treatment with an amphotericin product or fluconazole. *Pneumocystis jiroveci* is treated (and prevented, using lower doses) with agents such as trimethoprim/sulfamethoxazole, clindamycin, primaquine, atovaquone and others.

Parasites: epidemiology, prophylaxis, diagnosis, and treatment

Epidemiology

Parasitic infections are less common than the previously mentioned pathogens. The more clinically significant parasites in transplant recipients include *Toxoplasma gondii*, *Strongyloides stercoralis*, *Trypanosoma cruzi* (the aetiological agent of Chagas' disease), *Leishmania* and intestinal parasites (*Cryptosporidium*, *Giardia* and others). The incidence of parasitic infection is anticipated to increase in transplant recipients due to multiple factors, including: increases in active organ transplant programmes in geographical areas where parasitic infections are endemic; increases in travel and migration of donors and recipients from endemic areas, with latent or asymptomatic infections, as well as patients from developed countries undergoing transplantation in endemic areas (transplant tourism, with associated significant infectious disease risks;[37] increases in leisure tourism to endemic regions by transplant recipients; and decreases in

ciclosporin-based immunosuppressive regimens as they are replaced by newer drugs that lack the antiparasitic effects of ciclosporin metabolites. Specific guidelines regarding parasitic infections in transplant recipients have recently been published.[7]

Numerous zoonotic parasites have been shown to cause disease in transplant recipients.[30] Blood-borne and organ-borne infection may be transmitted at the time of transplantation; enteric pathogens are less likely to be transmitted during the peritransplantation period, although this could potentially occur with intestine and liver transplantation. Depending on the location and circumstances, toxoplasmosis, babesiosis, Chagas' disease and leishmaniasis are among the more common zoonotic parasite-related infections observed in transplant recipients.

Prophylaxis

Parasitic infections can be prevented by avoiding ingestion of contaminated food and water (predominantly for intestinal pathogens and *Toxoplasma gondii*), by avoiding skin contact with soil harbouring pathogens (*Strongyloides*) and by avoiding insect bites (*Plasmodium* (malaria), *Babesia*, *T. cruzi* and *Leishmania*). In addition, recipients with epidemiological risk factors should be screened for latent infection prior to transplant, as should organ and blood product donors in endemic regions (i.e. *T. cruzi*/Chagas' disease, malaria, babesiosis, *Leishmania*). Preventative medications such as trimethoprim/sulfamethoxazole (used to prevent *T. gondii* infection, both de novo and reactivation disease) or ivermectin (to treat active or latent *Strongyloides*) are effective methods of prevention. Toxoplasmosis, once a more common infection after solid-organ transplant, has become a largely preventable disease in the era of trimethoprim/sulfamethoxazole (or atovaquone, or dapsone) prophylaxis. Use of antimalarial prophylaxis in endemic regions is recommended for all transplant recipients travelling to such regions.

Diagnosis

Diagnosis of parasitic infections in solid-organ transplant recipients can be complex. Depending on the parasite suspected, a variety of techniques may be used, ranging from rapid diagnostics on stool by microscopic examination for ova and parasites, peripheral blood smears (*Babesia*, malaria, *T. cruzi*), special stains and microscopic examination of various specimens or tissues (blood, stool, biopsy), culture, serology (which may be less helpful in this population, as they are less likely to seroconvert) and histopathology. Molecular diagnostics, when available, can be quite helpful; examples would include rapid malaria diagnostics and polymerase chain reaction (PCR) testing for *T. cruzi* and *Toxoplasma*. Use of clinical markers such as eosinophilia may be muted in this population, where the immunosuppressive regimen (especially steroids, for eosinophilia) may cause false-negative results.

Certain diseases may require monitoring after transplant, or after treatment of infection. For example, pre-transplant treatment of Chagas' disease has not been shown to decrease the risk of reactivation disease after transplant; since the minority of infected patients will experience reactivation with immunosuppression, and the medications are toxic, many experts recommend monitoring in the post-transplant period, and treating with any evidence of parasitaemia or clinical disease. Similarly, treatment of donor or recipients with positive *Leishmania* serologies is not necessarily indicated in the absence of clinical disease. Some parasites such as *Schistosoma* species die after several years, although the recipients may have a positive serology for much longer; it is not known whether they need treatment, where the parasites would be predicted to be defunct.

Treatment

Treatment of individual parasitic infections may involve medications with significant side-effects and toxicities or that interact with transplant medications, and should be used carefully. Immunocompromised hosts are more likely to have relapses of certain parasitic infections (i.e. *Babesia*, *T. cruzi*, *Strongyloides*) and should be monitored after treatment. Clinicians may wish to lengthen the treatment course in certain infections, especially with more readily tolerated antiparasitic medications and for diseases at higher risk of relapse, i.e. with treatment for *Babesia*, *Strongyloides* and others. Whether reduction of immunosuppression may be helpful in clearing such infections has not been studied.

Pre-transplant infectious disease evaluation

✅ Pre-transplant evaluation by an infectious disease specialist familiar with organ transplantation is a window of opportunity to mitigate the risk of infection.

Epidemiology and medical history should be evaluated for risk of latent infections (tuberculosis, histoplasmosis, coccidiomycosis, cryptococcus, Chagas' disease, hepatitis B and others); if testing is positive or history strongly suggestive, centres may wish to initiate prophylaxis or screening for reactivation. Potential transplant recipients and donors are typically screened for latent tuberculosis, by history and sometimes by chest X-ray and either by skin testing or use of an interferon-gamma release assay-based blood test such as the T-SPOT.TB® or Quantiferon® TB Gold. Those with latent tuberculosis should likely be given chemoprophylaxis, although the optimal timing around transplant has not been determined, but it usually does not have to delay the transplant, as it could be given after transplant. Patients with *Staphylococcus aureus* colonisation may undergo a decolonisation protocol shortly before surgery, which can decrease the chance of surgical site infection; such protocols may include the use of intranasal mupirocin, chlorhexidine washes, oral doxycycline, and rifampin/rifampicin.

Vaccination status should be reviewed and updated, both for routine vaccines and for more exotic vaccines if the recipient is planning on high-risk exposures (i.e. vaccinating a veterinarian against rabies, or vaccinating a Brazilian native against yellow fever, who is living abroad but plans to return home after transplant). Those seronegative for measles, mumps, rubella, hepatitis A and B, and varicella should undergo important pre-transplant vaccination, as some are with live viral vaccines (varicella/zoster, measles, mumps, rubella, yellow fever, BCG) that cannot be given after transplant when a recipient is significantly immunosuppressed,[5] as shown in Table 12.1, leaving them potentially permanently vulnerable to potentially life-threatening infection(s). When live viral vaccines are given, a minimum of 1 month should pass before the recipient undergoes organ transplantation, in order for the live virus to be cleared from the system.

An optimal prophylaxis regimen for each recipient after transplant should be developed. Antiviral prevention would usually be determined by local protocols. Recipients with possible trimethoprim/sulfamethoxazole allergies (or other significant antibiotic allergies, especially when multiple) could be seen by an allergist to determine whether such agents could be used after transplant. Antifungal protocols are usually fairly limited except for lung transplant recipients. Antituberculosis prophylaxis may be needed in those who did not get pre-transplant treatment, or who are at higher risk of relapse. While histoplasmosis does not usually require chemoprophylaxis, many clinicians in endemic regions do give chemoprophylaxis to those recipients with evidence of coccidiomycosis in either the donor or recipient.

Donor-derived infections

Donor-derived infections are an emerging topic in transplant infectious disease. While some infections are known and anticipated to be transmitted from donor to recipient (i.e. CMV, EBV), many others are unexpected, and result in much higher morbidity and mortality in the transplant recipients. From the published literature and reports to the Organ Procurement and Transplant Network (OPTN), which are reviewed and categorised by the ad hoc Disease Transmission Advisory Committee (DTAC), it is estimated that donor-derived disease transmission complicates less than 1% of all transplant procedures, but when a transmission occurs, a higher rate of adverse outcomes may result.[6] Since data collection began in 2005, the number of cases has increased significantly, from seven reports in 2005 (less than 0.5% of all organ transplant donors) to 152 reports in 2009 (close to 3% of all transplant donors); this large increase likely suggests a lack of prior reporting of cases, rather than a true increased incidence of disease transmissions.

Viral transmissions are the most frequent cause of donor reports, at almost three times the number of other types of infections (although less frequently confirmed as cases). Reported and/or confirmed viral transmissions occurred with adenovirus, hepatitis B, hepatitis C, herpes simplex, HIV, human T-lymphotropic virus (HTLV), influenza, lymphocytic choriomeningitis virus (LCMV), parainfluenza-3, parvovirus B19, rabies and West Nile virus.[6] Unfortunately, treatment for many of these viral infections is not available; reduction in immunosuppression in hopes of clearing the infection, with potentially negative impact on the transplanted graft, remains a common therapeutic modality.

Bacterial infections and colonisation in the donor, with bacterial contamination of organs (or preservation fluid), occurs frequently but rarely results in transmission of infection.[38] Interestingly, *Mycobacterium tuberculosis* has been the most commonly transmitted bacterial infection, with potentially devastating consequences when the infection is not expected.[6]

Bacteria reported to the OPTN from 2005 to 2009 include a broad range of pathogens, all numbering five reports or less, including *Acinetobacter*, *Brucella*, *Enterococcus*, *Ehrlichia*, *E. coli*, *Klebsiella*, *Legionella*, *Listeria*, Lyme disease, *Nocardia*, *Pseudomonas*, Rocky Mountain spotted fever, *Serratia*, *S. aureus*, *Streptococcus*, *Treponemapallidum* and *Veillonella*.[6] Such a broad array of pathogens suggests clinicians should be vigilant in recognising unexpected donor-derived infections.

Fungi and parasites can have significant complication rates, especially when unexpected and in immunocompromised hosts. Therapies can be less readily available, and sometimes more toxic, especially given the potential for drug interactions in more medically complex transplant recipients. Reported fungi include *Aspergillus*, *Candida*, *Coccidioidesimitis*, *Cryptococcus neoformans*, *Histoplasma capsulatum* and zygomyces, while reported parasites include *Babesia*, *Balamuthia mandrillaris*, Chagas (*Trypanosoma cruzi*), *Naegleria fowleri*, *Schistosoma* and *Strongyloides*.[6]

> ✔✔ Organ procurement organisations and transplant clinicians must be vigilant about the potential for such transmissions. Case review of the donor epidemiology is critical.

Lapses in testing accuracy due to haemodilution, 'window periods' (during which a recipient is infected, but has not yet seroconverted) and human error have all contributed to these transmissions. After transplantation, the team caring for the recipients must notify the organ procurement organisation and/or national transplant authorities if there is concern about a donor-derived event.

While many of these are not preventable, some could be avoided through further testing, such as certain geographic infections (e.g. *Trypanosoma cruzi* (the aetiological agent of Chagas' disease), *Coccidioides immitis*, *Strongyloides* and numerous others).

Lifestyle and infection: food, pets, travel and sexuality

Companion animals provide numerous benefits, along with some zoonotic risk. Discussions about pet ownership should optimally occur prior to transplantation. Pets may enhance health and well-being, and many people would welcome advice and support to enable them to reconcile or manage pet ownership. Guidance on pet choice can decrease zoonotic risk. In general, mature pets from reputable sources provide lower zoonotic risk. Fish are the least likely pets to be associated with illness (especially if aquarium cleaning by the transplant recipient is avoided). Animals that should be avoided as pets include birds, reptiles (lizards, snakes and turtles), baby chicks and ducklings, and exotic pets (chinchillas and monkeys); contact with stray and wild animals should also be avoided. The individual risk of acquiring an infection from an animal is hard to calculate, and little work has been done in this field.

Careful handwashing after any animal contact is imperative. Routine veterinarian care, with frequent stool examination for parasites, administration of routine vaccines and evaluation when an animal is sick (especially with diarrhoea), can reduce the risks of pet ownership to a transplant recipient. Immunocompromised hosts should avoid direct contact with any live viral vaccines that are administered to their pets and animals (i.e. kennel cough/*Bordetella* vaccine). In addition, contact with animal excreta or saliva should be avoided. Good-quality animal food should be given (not raw eggs or meat) and animals should not drink toilet bowl water. Humans should avoid flea and tick bites, as well as animal-related scratches and bites. Because small children are more likely to be bitten by pets and are less likely to practise good hand hygiene, pet ownership should potentially be deferred for very young transplant recipients. Pet therapy should potentially be avoided in hospitalised patients during the immediate post-transplant period, when the patient is most immunosuppressed. The US Centers for Disease Control and Prevention's report on 'Pets and Organ Transplant Patients' provides both general and animal-specific guidelines.[39]

Food-borne illnesses are among the most common sources of infection. *Salmonella*, *Campylobacter*, *E. coli*, *Listeria* and toxoplasmosis can cause significant disease in transplant recipients. The two most significant risks include those from uncooked fresh fruits and vegetables, and those from animal products, such as unpasteurised milk, soft cheeses, raw eggs, raw meat, raw poultry, raw fish, raw seafood and their juices.[40] Many transplant programmes recommend very careful intake for the first 3–6 months after transplant, during the period of greatest vulnerability. Unfortunately, transplant patients should probably always avoid raw animal products, including soft cheese, sushi and other frequently desired foods. Careful food preparation in the home kitchen can greatly decrease the risk of food-borne illness.

International travel exposes travellers to a variety of pathogens that are absent or uncommon in their country of residence, and increases the potential for exposure to familiar pathogens such as those transmitted through food and water, mosquito bites, and other modes of transmission. The level of risk depends on the location of travel, types of food and accommodation, activities pursued, and length of stay. In general, travel within developed countries poses minimally increased risk for travellers. Travel to developing countries, particularly those in tropical or subtropical regions, exposes travellers to greater risks. Areas in the yellow fever zones, as shown in **Fig. 12.4**,[41] are of special concern to this more vulnerable transplant population, as they cannot be vaccinated with the live viral yellow fever vaccine, and should generally be avoided except under extenuating circumstances. All transplant recipients travelling to areas of increased infection risk should be educated about the risk of food- and water-borne illness, optimal sun protection (especially given their increased rates of skin cancer), management of diarrhoea and other common infections, and avoidance of mosquito- and blood-borne infections. All should travel with antibiotics in case of gastroenteritis or other common infections. Transplant recipients should be encouraged to see a travel medicine specialist with expertise in immunocompromised hosts prior to travel. Those travelling for the main purposes of undergoing

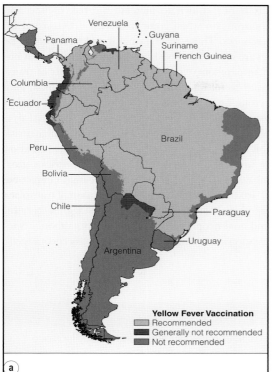

Figure 12.4 • Yellow fever zones of South America and Africa.[41] Transplant recipients should generally defer travel to these regions. For more detail see http://wwwnc. cdc.gov/travel/images/map3-19-yellow-fever-vaccine-recommendations-americas-2010.jpg http://wwwnc. cdc.gov/travel/images/map3-18-yellow-fever-vaccine-recommendation-in-africa-2010-large.jpg

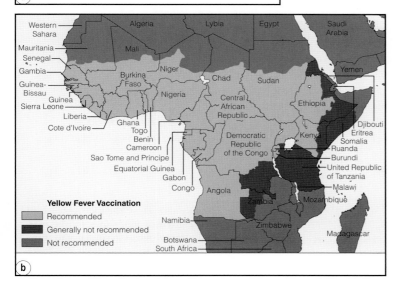

organ transplantation (often commercial in nature) should be cautioned about the risks of infectious disease (and ethical concerns).[37]

Travellers may need vaccines for safer travel. Certain live vaccines should not be given to transplant recipients, including vaccines against yellow fever, *Salmonella typhi* (as oral Ty21a), polio (oral vaccine only), measles, varicella, mumps, rubella and tuberculosis. Additionally, vaccines may not afford as much protection due to the attenuated immune system. Sometimes gamma-globulin is given in lieu of hepatitis A vaccine; it may provide protection against other types of infection as well. Yellow fever vaccine should not be given to transplant recipients on active immunosuppression.[2] If travel to an area with yellow fever is necessary and immunisation is not performed, the traveller should be advised of the risks, instructed in methods to avoid mosquito bites, and provided with a vaccination waiver letter. Travellers whose destinations or transit stops include countries requiring yellow fever vaccination should also carry such a letter. A yellow fever vaccination waiver letter is available through a yellow fever vaccination centre and must be signed by a physician.

Healthy sexuality after organ transplantation should be encouraged. Safer sex techniques, such as condoms and other barrier methods, should be encouraged to avoid transmission of infection, especially with new partners or in non-monogamous relationships. Oral sex is not known to increase the risk of infection transmission when compared with heterosexual intercourse. Those having anal intercourse should be aware of the increased oncogenic potential with human papilloma virus infection. In a cohort of transplant recipients at the Royal London Hospital, anal cytology and polymerase chain reaction were used to assess anal HPV disease; they found that anal dysplasia was associated with HPV strains at higher risk for anal oncogenisis ($P < 0.001$), longer duration of immunosuppression ($P = 0.050$), previous genital warts ($P = 0.018$) and receptive anal intercourse ($P = 0.013$).[42] Whether HPV vaccination of transplant recipients may provide protection against cervical and anal neoplasia is not yet known, although vaccination according to local guidelines is encouraged.

Key points

- Infections are among the most common complications after transplantation, and greatly increase the morbidity and mortality of transplantation, and decrease graft survival.
- Improved understanding of various infections, diagnostics, therapeutics and prevention has allowed for improvement of outcomes after infection in transplant recipients.
- Prophylactic measures and medications can significantly decrease the risk of infection after transplantation.
- Pre-transplant evaluation for latent infections and optimisation of vaccination can help mitigate the risk of infection after transplantation.
- Donor-derived infections have been increasingly recognised in recent times; expecting the unexpected may enhance diagnostics and outcomes.
- Lifestyle issues after transplantation are very important to the recipient. Optimal knowledge regarding vaccines, pets, travel, food and sexual behaviour may decrease the risk of infection.

References

1. Fishman JA. Infection in solid-organ transplant recipients. N Engl J Med 2007;357(25):2601–14.
2. Jong EC, Freedman DO. 2012 Health information for international travel, Chapter 8: Advising travelers with specific needs: immunocompromised travelers. Atlanta: Centers for Disease Control and Prevention; 2012. Available at http://wwwnc.cdc.gov/travel/yellowbook/2012/chapter-8-advising-travelers-with-specific-needs/immunocompromised-travelers.htm accessed December 17, 2012.
3. American Society of Transplantation Infectious Diseases guidelines. 2nd edition. Am J Transplant 2009;9(Suppl. 4):S1–281.
4. Kotton CN, Kumar D, Caliendo AM, et al. International consensus guidelines on the management of cytomegalovirus in solid organ transplantation. Transplantation 2010;89(7):779–95.
5. Jong EC, Freedman DO. 2010 Health information for international travel, Chapter 8: Advising travelers with specific needs: the immunocompromised traveler. Atlanta: Centers for Disease Control and Prevention; 2010. Available at http://wwwnc.cdc.gov/travel/yellowbook/2012/chapter-8-advising-travelers-with-specific-needs/immunocompromised-travelers.htm accessed December 17, 2012.
6. Ison MG, Nalesnik MA. An update on donor-derived disease transmission in organ transplantation. Am J Transplant 2011;11(6):1123–30.

7. Kotton CN, Lattes R. Parasitic infections in solid organ transplant recipients. Am J Transplant 2009;9(Suppl. 4):S234–51.

8. Monaco AP. The role of mTOR inhibitors in the management of posttransplant malignancy. Transplantation 2009;87(2):157–63.

9. Muller TF, Grebe SO, Neumann MC, et al. Persistent long-term changes in lymphocyte subsets induced by polyclonal antibodies. Transplantation 1997;64(10):1432–7.

10. Hanaway MJ, Woodle ES, Mulgaonkar S, et al. Alemtuzumab induction in renal transplantation. N Engl J Med 2011;364(20):1909–19.

11. Kamar N, Garrouste C, Haagsma EB, et al. Factors associated with chronic hepatitis in patients with hepatitis E virus infection who have received solid organ transplants. Gastroenterology 2011;140(5):1481–9.

12. Mateen FJ, Muralidharan R, Carone M, et al. Progressive multifocal leukoencephalopathy in transplant recipients. Ann Neurol 2011;70(2):305–22.

13. Stock PG, Barin B, Murphy B, et al. Outcomes of kidney transplantation in HIV-infected recipients. N Engl J Med 2010;363(21):2004–14.

14. Mawhorter S, Yamani MH. Hypogammaglobulinemia and infection risk in solid organ transplant recipients. Curr Opin Organ Transplant 2008;13(6):581–5.

15. Abate D, Saldan A, Fiscon M, et al. Evaluation of cytomegalovirus (CMV)-specific T cell immune reconstitution revealed that baseline antiviral immunity, prophylaxis, or preemptive therapy but not antithymocyte globulin treatment contribute to CMV-specific T cell reconstitution in kidney transplant recipients. J Infect Dis 2010;202(4):585–94.

16. Kliem V, Fricke L, Wollbrink T, et al. Improvement in long-term renal graft survival due to CMV prophylaxis with oral ganciclovir: results of a randomized clinical trial. Am J Transplant 2008;8(5):975–83.

17. Couzi L, Helou S, Bachelet T, et al. High incidence of anticytomegalovirus drug resistance among D+R− kidney transplant recipients receiving preemptive therapy. Am J Transplant 2012;12(1):202–9.

18. Freeman Jr RB. The 'indirect' effects of cytomegalovirus infection. Am J Transplant 2009;9(11):2453–8.

19. Luan FL, Kommareddi M, Ojo AO. Universal prophylaxis is cost effective in cytomegalovirus serology-positive kidney transplant patients. Transplantation 2011;91(2):237–44.

20. Humar A, Lebranchu Y, Vincenti F, et al. The efficacy and safety of 200 days valganciclovir cytomegalovirus prophylaxis in high-risk kidney transplant recipients. Am J Transplant 2010;10(5):1228–37.

21. Blumberg EA, Hauser IA, Stanisic S, et al. Prolonged prophylaxis with valganciclovir is cost effective in reducing posttransplant cytomegalovirus disease within the United States. Transplantation 2010;90(12):1420–6.

22. Luan FL, Stuckey LJ, Park JM, et al. Six-month prophylaxis is cost effective in transplant patients at high risk for cytomegalovirus infection. J Am Soc Nephrol 2009;20(11):2449–58.

23. Dharnidharka VR, Lamb KE, Gregg JA, et al. Associations between EBV serostatus and organ transplant type in PTLD risk: an analysis of the SRTR National Registry Data in the United States. Am J Transplant 2012;12(4):976–83.

24. Martin SI, Dodson B, Wheeler C, et al. Monitoring infection with Epstein–Barr virus among sero-mismatch adult renal transplant recipients. Am J Transplant 2011;11(5):1058–63.

25. Ahya VN, Douglas LP, Andreadis C, et al. Association between elevated whole blood Epstein–Barr virus (EBV)-encoded RNA EBV polymerase chain reaction and reduced incidence of acute lung allograft rejection. J Heart Lung Transplant 2007;26(8):839–44.

26. Larsen CP, Grinyo J, Medina-Pestana J, et al. Belatacept-based regimens versus a cyclosporine A-based regimen in kidney transplant recipients: 2-year results from the BENEFIT and BENEFIT-EXT studies. Transplantation 2010;90(12):1528–35.

27. Caillard S, Lamy FX, Quelen C, et al. Epidemiology of posttransplant lymphoproliferative disorders in adult kidney and kidney pancreas recipients: report of the French registry and analysis of subgroups of lymphomas. Am J Transplant 2012;12(3):682–93.

28. Fischer SA, Graham MB, Kuehnert MJ, et al. Transmission of lymphocytic choriomeningitis virus by organ transplantation. N Engl J Med 2006;354(21):2235–49.

29. Srinivasan A, Burton EC, Kuehnert MJ, et al. Transmission of rabies virus from an organ donor to four transplant recipients. N Engl J Med 2005;352(11):1103–11.

30. Kotton CN. Zoonoses in solid-organ and hematopoietic stem cell transplant recipients. Clin Infect Dis 2007;44(6):857–66.

31. Iwamoto M, Jernigan DB, Guasch A, et al. Transmission of West Nile virus from an organ donor to four transplant recipients. N Engl J Med 2003;348(22):2196–203.

32. Kumar D, Blumberg EA, Danziger-Isakov L, et al. Influenza vaccination in the organ transplant recipient: review and summary recommendations. Am J Transplant 2011;11(10):2020–30.

33. Chon WJ, Kadambi PV, Harland RC, et al. Changing attitudes toward influenza vaccination in U.S. kidney transplant programs over the past decade. Clin J Am Soc Nephrol 2010;5(9):1637–41.

34. Sasadeusz KJ, Trerotola SO, Shah H, et al. Tunneled jugular small-bore central catheters as an alternative to peripherally inserted central catheters for intermediate-term venous access in patients with hemodialysis and chronic renal insufficiency. Radiology 1999;213(1):303–6.

35. Vilchez RA, Fung J, Kusne S. Cryptococcosis in organ transplant recipients: an overview. Am J Transplant 2002;2(7):575–80.

36. Rosen T, Jablon J. Infectious threats from exotic pets: dermatological implications. Dermatol Clin 2003;21(2):229–36.

37. Kotton CN. Transplant tourism and donor-derived parasitic infections. Transplant Proc 2011;43(6):2448–9.

38. Lumbreras C, Sanz F, Gonzalez A, et al. Clinical significance of donor-unrecognized bacteremia in the outcome of solid-organ transplant recipients. Clin Infect Dis 2001;33(5):722–6.

39. Healthy Pets Healthy People: Organ Transplant Patients. Atlanta, GA: Centers for Disease Control; updated 26 January 2010. Available at www.cdc.gov/healthypets/bonemarrow_transplant.htm [accessed 15.08.12]

40. Food Safety for Transplant Recipients. Washington DC: United States Department of Agriculture; 2006. Available at http://www.fda.gov/downloads/Food/ResourcesForYou/Consumers/SelectedHealthTopics/UCM312793.pdf accessed December 17, 2012.

41. Gershman M, Staples JE. 2012 Health information for international travel, Chapter 3: Infectious diseases related to travel. Available at wwwnc.cdc.gov/travel/yellowbook/2012/chapter-3-infectious-diseases-related-to-travel/yellow-fever.htm accessed December 17, 2012. Atlanta: Centers for Disease Control and Prevention; 2012.

42. Patel HS, Silver AR, Levine T, et al. Human papillomavirus infection and anal dysplasia in renal transplant recipients. Br J Surg 2010;97(11):1716–21.

13

Chronic transplant dysfunction

Shikha Mehta
Roslyn B. Mannon

Introduction

Solid-organ transplantation provides life-saving and rejuvenating therapy for those with end-organ damage. Initial functional success is at an all-time high for all organs, including cellular transplants such as islets. However, long-term outcomes have been less positive, in spite of improvements in immunosuppressive therapy for both prophylaxis and treatment of acute cellular rejection. Specifically, 10-year graft survival of deceased donor kidneys is about 48%, in hearts and liver 53%, and in lung a dismal 25%. Thus, long-term graft dysfunction has become the critical issue in patient management and there is renewed focus on finding mechanisms not only to develop interventions, but also to discover critical biomarkers that will identify those at risk for the disease.

Chronic transplant dysfunction (CTD) is a disorder of transplanted organs in which there is progressive functional decline over a period of months to years after transplantation. There are no uniform features across all organs, but the pathology is typified by interstitial fibrosis (IF) and tubular atrophy (TA) in kidney allografts, by airway obstruction with inflammatory cells and matrix in the lung (bronchiolitis obliterans syndrome, BOS), graft fibrosis in the liver, and arteriosclerosis in the heart (cardiac allograft vasculopathy, CAV). Both immune-dependent and immune-independent factors may lead to allograft failure. Often, it is difficult to identify those at risk; moreover, diagnosis typically occurs when there is symptomatic graft dysfunction,

a time so late in disease development that graft failure becomes a fait accompli. In this chapter, we will review the presentation and diagnosis of CTD in all organs. Further, we will adopt renal transplantation as the paradigm for our understanding of CTD. By improving our understanding of what promotes graft failure, we may develop better insight into biomarkers and treatment.

Organ-specific findings

The development of CTD varies in each organ. Epithelial injury is the primary cell target in the kidney and lung, although more recent data have implicated microvascular injury as the target of both organs. In the heart, however, endothelial cells are the primary target of injury, which may be mediated by both immune- and non-immune-dependent phenomena.[1] Immune-mediated injury may occur by cellular- and/or antibody-mediated pathways, the latter becoming more frequently recognised in all solid organs with our expanded understanding of the humoral immune response. Due to the differences in allograft injuries, we will discuss each organ separately and compare the presentations and outcomes when relevant.

Heart

In cardiac allografts, CTD is a disorder manifested by clinical dysfunction and accelerated cardiac allograft arteriosclerosis, known as cardiac allograft vasculopathy (CAV). CAV is extremely common, seen in ~7% of recipients at 1 year, 32% at 5 years and in more than half at 10 years post-transplant.[2] CAV and late graft failure (i.e. unrecognised CAV) account for about 31% of deaths at 5 years post-transplant. Risk factors include the more traditional associations with hypertension, diabetes and dyslipidaemia, with transplant-related risks that include cytomegalovirus (CMV) infection, donor cause of death, number of human leucocyte antigen (HLA) mismatches between donor and recipient and the number of allograft rejection episodes.[3] The pathognomonic lesion of CAV is concentric intimal thickening affecting the coronary vessels, particularly the smaller distal intramyocardial vessels. Myocardial fibrosis may also be seen in some cases. However, until recently, there were disparate definitions of CAV based on the histology, angiographic findings and findings on intravascular ultrasound. In 2010, the International Society of Heart and Lung Transplantation (ISHLT) published guidelines for the terminology of cardiac allograft vasculopathy with the goal of having a more universal and prognostically significant definition that would also serve as an end-point of clinical trials. The consensus of the ISHLT working group was to base the definition and diagnosis of CAV on conventional invasive coronary angiography. A grading system based on angiographic findings and graft function (evaluated by echocardiography or invasive haemodynamic data) was established (Box 13.1).[4] This new definition was based on evidence from a large population study performed by Costanzo et al., in which 4637 postoperative angiograms were performed to look for CAV. The study demonstrated an overall likelihood of death or re-transplantation secondary to CAV of 7%, and 50% of patients with severe disease are likely to reach that outcome.[5] According to the guidelines, there is no role of routine intravascular ultrasound (IVUS) surveillance or non-invasive computed tomography (CT)-based angiography for assessment of CAV. Immune-based markers, gene-based and protein-based biomarkers (B-type natriuretic peptide, cardiac-specific troponins, high-sensitivity C-reactive protein), microvascular function testing and stress-based imaging were not recommended for inclusion in the above nomenclature algorithm as markers for defining severity of CAV due to lack of standardisation.

Box 13.1 • ISHLT cardiac allograft vasculopathy nomenclature

ISHLT CAV0 (Not significant): No detectable angiographic lesion.

ISHLT CAV1 (Mild): Angiographic left main (LM) <50%, or primary vessel with maximum lesion of <70%, or any branch stenosis <70% (including diffuse narrowing) without allograft dysfunction.

ISHLT CAV2 (Moderate): Angiographic LM ≥50%;* a single primary vessel ≥70% or isolated branch stenosis ≥70% in branches of two systems, without allograft dysfunction.

ISHLT CAV3 (Severe): Angiographic LM ≥50%, or two or more primary vessels ≥70% stenosis, or isolated branch stenosis ≥70% in all three systems; or ISHLT CAV1 or CAV2 with allograft dysfunction (defined as left ventricular ejection fraction (LVEF) ≤45%) or evidence of significant restrictive physiology.

Definitions

(A) A 'primary vessel' denotes the proximal and middle 33% of the left anterior descending artery, the left circumflex, the ramus and the dominant or co-dominant right coronary artery with the posterior descending and posterolateral branches.

(B) A 'secondary branch vessel' includes the distal 33% of the primary vessels or any segment within a large septal perforator, diagonals and obtuse marginal branches or any portion of a non-dominant right coronary artery.

(C) Restrictive cardiac allograft physiology is defined as symptomatic heart failure with echocardiographic E to A velocity ratio >2 (>1.5 in children), shortened isovolumetric relaxation time (<60 ms), shortened deceleration time (<150 ms), or restrictive haemodynamic values (right atrial pressure >12 mmHg, pulmonary capillary wedge pressure >25 mmHg, cardiac index <2 L/min/m²).

* Normal graft function.

A key feature of these criteria is the lack of inclusion of biopsy histology. While biopsy criteria diagnostic for CAV have been developed, the findings have only limited sensitivity in detecting microvascular CAV; they were developed in small study populations and included non-specific findings. Moreover, normal coronary arteries may appear to have intimal thickening that is histologically characteristic of CAV. Thus the diagnostic criteria are now quite specific and may be useful in clinical trial design and interpretation.

While much focus has been placed on cellular immunity mediating this disorder, the demonstration of endothelial injury as a key feature has led to a renewed interest in anti-donor antibodies and antibody-mediated rejection (AMR). A considerable hurdle has been the lack of uniform diagnostic criteria for AMR in heart allografts. The histological criteria have recently been standardised and consensus obtained.[6] The Consensus Conference on Antibody Mediated Injury in Heart Transplantation performed a thorough review of the diagnostic and clinical considerations, recognising the strong relationship between AMR, CAV and recipient death.[7] Importantly, it was established that the detection of antibody within the allograft, even in the absence of cardiac dysfunction, is associated with a greater mortality and more likely development of CAV. The recognised spectrum of cardiac AMR includes a *latent phase* in which circulating antibody may be present, followed by a *silent* phase of deposition in the allograft without histological or clinical alterations, and progression to a *subclinical phase* with circulating antibody and histology, and finally *symptomatic* disease. This paradigm may be similar in other solid-organ injuries where antibody plays a role in the development of allograft failure.

Another recognised feature in the development of CAV is that antibody may develop not only to HLA determinants but also to structural proteins, resulting in autoantibodies. Antibodies directed to endothelial cell antigens have long been appreciated to have a connection with chronic injury and rejection, suggesting a link between endothelial injury and graft failure. Antibodies to vimentin, also present in leucocytes, fibroblasts and endothelial cells, have also been associated with the development of cardiac graft arteriopathy and the detection of these antibodies may identify those at risk. While anticardiac myosin and phospholipid antibodies have also been detected after heart transplantation, they have been predominantly associated with acute rejection episodes.

Recently, antibodies against the major histocompatibility class I-related chains A (MICA) and B (MICB), polymorphic cell surface proteins expressed by a wide variety of human cells including epithelial cells, endothelial cells and monocytes, have been associated with CAV. Current reports are inconclusive as to whether these antibodies to MICA and MICB are directly detrimental or whether they are biomarkers of high immunological risk recipients.[8,9]

Recommendations have been made for screening for donor-specific antibody (DSA) as well as timing for surveillance allograft biopsies on a serial basis. It is clear, however, that additional studies are needed to determine not only the most effective therapeutic interventions to minimise long-term CTD, but also to determine the effect of prophylactic therapy.[7]

Liver

Unlike the other solid organs, the liver may enjoy prolonged allograft survival, even with minimisation of immunosuppression. The contribution of cellular rejection episodes to long-term graft failure is lessened, perhaps in part due to the liver's tolerogenic capabilities.[10] Moreover, complications of immunosuppression such as nephrotoxicity and malignancy have a greater impact on recipient outcome. Similarly, recurrent disease is a key contributor to late graft failure and the development of newer therapies for hepatitis C may have a critical impact on the mortality and re-transplantation needs in this field. Thus significant efforts have been expended in the liver to identify those recipients that may be suitable candidates for immunosuppressive withdrawal as well as to identify more effective strategies to manage immunosuppression.[11] Because these studies are beyond the scope of this chapter, the reader is referred to other reviews on this topic.

Chronic allograft rejection, while a less common cause of late graft failure, is a recognised entity that is defined as an immunological injury to the allograft, usually as a result of persistent and unrelenting acute rejection, and results in irreversible damage to the bile ducts, veins and arteries.[12] The onset is months to years post-transplant and graft failure may occur within a year of transplantation. This may occur in about 3–5% of recipients, and risk factors include both immune-dependent and immune-independent factors. In the former, this includes the frequency and severity of acute cellular rejections, lower baseline immunosuppression and primary immune disease diagnosis; in the latter, risk factors are non-Caucasian race, younger recipient age and donor age greater than 40.

A critical component to diagnosis is histology, which is more complex than previously appreciated. Late allograft biopsy is typically performed due to abnormalities in routine lab testing for liver function. The use of terms such as 'vanishing bile duct syndrome' or 'ductopenic rejection' is no longer recommended, as bile duct loss is just one component of graft failure. Native disease recurrence is a critical issue, as already noted, and may confuse diagnostic interpretation.[13] These diagnoses include:

1. Infectious aetiologies (viral hepatitis A, B, C, D).
2. Dysregulated immunity (autoimmune hepatitis, primary biliary cirrhosis, primary sclerosing cholangitis, sarcoidosis).
3. Malignancies.
4. Toxicities (alcohol, drugs).
5. Metabolic disorders (including non-alcoholic steatohepatosis).
6. Other idiopathic disorders.

The minimum diagnostic criteria for chronic rejection are listed in Table 13.1.[12] Biopsies often include non-specific changes such as portal-based chronic inflammation. Interpretation should include an assessment of the adequacy (survey of at least six portal tracts), systematic examination of the tissue and through clinical correlation. Until recently, standard criteria have not been utilised and based on centre expertise. Thus, consensus criteria for common causes of late allograft failure have been developed and are discussed in depth.[13] This more structured analysis provides uniformity in diagnosis and highlights the common similarities in some disease features.

Lung

Bronchiolitis obliterans syndrome (BOS) is a major factor limiting long-term graft survival and is the clinical manifestation of CTD in the lung. Despite the potency of immunosuppression, BOS remains a difficult issue and nearly half of all lungs transplanted will develop this by 5 years after transplantation.[14] Once diagnosed, only 30–40% of recipients with BOS survive to 5 years and beyond its onset. Detection and grading of this disorder is primarily by measuring forced expiratory volume in 1 second (FEV_1) as opposed to histological or radiological findings (Table 13.2).[15]

> ✔✔ In 2001, a new classification system of BOS was proposed which included FEF_{25-75} (mid-expiratory flow rate) to recognise early airflow obstruction (Table 13.2).[15]

Other contributory factors that affect FEV_1 should be excluded, such as acute rejection, infection, excessive recipient weight gain, anastomotic dysfunction, respiratory muscle dysfunction and other technical problems. Immune-dependent risk factors for the development include degree of HLA mismatch, acute rejection episodes and autoimmune

Table 13.1 • Banff criteria for liver allograft chronic rejection (CR)

Structure	Early CR	Late CR
Small bile ducts (<60 mm)	Degenerative changes involving a majority of ducts: eosinophilic transformation of the cytoplasm; increased nuclear hyperchromasia; uneven nuclear spacing; ducts only partially lined by biliary epithelial cells	Degenerative changes in the remaining bile ducts Loss in ≥50% of portal tracts
Terminal hepatic venules and zone 3 hepatocytes	Intimal/luminal inflammation Lytic zone 3 necrosis and inflammation Mild perivenular fibrosis	Focal obliteration Variable inflammation Severe (bridging) fibrosis
Portal tract hepatic arterioles	Occasional loss involving <25% of portal tracts	Loss involving >25% of portal tracts
Other	So-called 'transition' hepatitis with spotty necrosis of hepatocytes	Sinusoidal foam cell accumulation; marked cholestasis
Large perihilar hepatic artery branches	Intimal inflammation, focal foam cell deposition without luminal compromise	Luminal narrowing by subintimal foam cells Fibrointimal proliferation
Large perihilar bile ducts	Inflammation damage and focal foam cell deposition	Mural fibrosis

Reproduced from Demetris A, Adams D, Bellamy C et al. Update of the International Banff Schema for Liver Allograft Rejection: working recommendations for the histopathologic staging and reporting of chronic rejection. An International Panel. Hepatology 2000; 31(3):792–9.

Table 13.2 • Proposed classifications of BOS

Grade	Finding/severity
BOS 0	FEV_1 >90% of baseline and FEF_{25-75} >75% of baseline
BOS 0-p	FEV_1 81–90% of baseline and/or FEF_{25-75} ≤75% of baseline
BOS 1	FEV_1 66–80% of baseline
BOS 2	FEV_1 51–65% of baseline
BOS 3	FEV_1 50% or less of baseline

BOS, bronchiolitis obliterans syndrome; FEF_{25-75}, mid-expiratory flow rate; FEV_1, forced expiratory volume in 1 second.

reactions to lung matrix components. Other antigen-independent factors include infections, gastro-oesophageal reflux, donor factors such as cigarette use, head injury as a cause of death, airway ischaemia and inhaled irritants.[16]

In BOS there is epithelial injury, mediated predominantly by cellular immune responses, although more recent data indicate both allo- and autoantibodies may contribute to injury.[16] Inflammation is associated with progressive airway damage and fibrosis, with eventual bronchial scarring and obstruction. Transbronchial biopsy histology may reveal inflammation and fibrosis of the cartilaginous airways and particularly within the smaller airways, with inflammation and fibrosis in the lamina propria and luminal surfaces of bronchioles, while larger bronchi may show peribronchial fibrosis and bronchiectasis. Surrounding alveoli and interstitium may appear normal.

Antibodies against non-HLA graft proteins have been associated with late graft failure in the lung. Analysis of serial serum samples from recipients with BOS has identified non-HLA antibodies in five of 16 recipients with BOS compared to none of the 11 without BOS.[17] The specificity of this anti-airway epithelial cell antibody is under investigation, but is associated with up-regulation of transforming growth factor (TGF)-β signalling in vitro. Complement activation is also seen in BOS biopsies, associated with anti-endothelial cell antibodies. Immune responses against collagen V epitopes have also been implicated in the pathology of graft failure in BOS.

Management

Management of these patients is complex. Intensification of immunosuppression may be needed if acute rejection is a key contributor, but in the setting of infection this may be ineffective and in fact harmful to infection clearance. A number of approaches have been attempted but there is no uniformly accepted management, and most are not highly effective.[18] Further investigation into the mechanisms of injury using preclinical models as well as human trials is a clear priority for this field.

Pancreas

Pancreas transplantation for type I diabetes mellitus has seen substantial improvements in success both in terms of patient and allograft survival. Graft survival varies based on whether transplantation is simultaneous with the kidney, with 10-year survival of 54% compared to only 27% in solitary pancreas transplantation.[19] CTD of the pancreas is known as chronic rejection. While the emphasis in the past has been on alloimmune injury to mediate chronic rejection, accumulating data suggest that recurrent autoimmune responses to islets may be a key contributor to graft loss, despite the use of potent immunosuppression.[20] Graft deterioration is associated with hyperglycaemia, although this is a non-specific finding and may also be seen in insulin resistance and beta-cell loss associated with tacrolimus therapy. Serum pancreatic enzyme elevations are similarly of limited value due to the lack of specificity. Loss of insulin expression following glucose or arginine stimulation or a decline and loss of C-peptide may also be seen, but when detected indicate irreversible loss of beta-cell function and, again, are non-specific findings. Thus there is no specific biomarker of CTD and allograft biopsy remains the primary technique to assess the aetiology of graft dysfunction. Histological features include septal (perivascular) fibrosis with mononuclear cell inflammation and progressive acinar loss. Vascular changes such as narrowing of arterial lumina and concentric fibroproliferative endarteritis are considered an integral part of the pattern of CTD. The extent of acinar inflammation during acute rejection episodes is recognised as a prognostic factor for the development of chronic rejection. Recently, standardised scoring was established by consensus at the Banff Meeting in 2007 (see Box 13.2) and provides a reproducible and reliable tool for assessing chronic rejection in allograft biopsies.[21] These criteria, based on data accrued from experienced pancreas transplant centres, suggest that biopsy may contribute useful information to patient and

Box 13.2 • Banff grading scheme for chronic rejection of the pancreas

Stage I (mild graft sclerosis)

Expansion of fibrous septa; the fibrosis occupies less than 30% of the core surface but the acinar lobules have eroded, irregular contours. The central lobular areas are normal.

Stage II (moderate graft sclerosis)

The fibrosis occupies 30–60% of the core surface. The exocrine atrophy affects the majority of the lobules in their periphery (irregular contours) and in their central areas (thin fibrous strands criss-cross between individual acini).

Stage III (severe graft sclerosis)

The fibrotic areas predominate and occupy more than 60% of the core surface, with only isolated areas of residual acinar tissue and/or islets present.

graft management. Therapeutic interventions have focused on glucose control and immunosuppression, and the latter may be ineffective due to the late detection of disease. Further investigations are needed in this area as well as the consideration of non-calcineurin therapies to ameliorate the contribution of islet toxicity for late graft failure.

Kidney

Even in this era of potent immunosuppression with superb short-term graft survival and minimal levels of acute rejection in the first 6 months of transplantation, progressive graft loss of the kidney remains a considerable issue.[22] Graft failure culminating in relisting for transplantation accounts for about 25–30% patients on the transplant waiting list. About half of kidney transplants are lost due to recipient death with a functioning graft due to cardiovascular disease, infection or malignancy. The remaining graft losses are due to failing function. In these recipients, chronic graft injury (CGI) is characterised by declining renal function with the histological features of progressive interstitial fibrosis and tubular atrophy (IF/TA), occurring months to years after transplantation, that may be accompanied by vascular and glomerular damage.[1] In the past, clinicians have described this disorder using various terms such as chronic allograft nephropathy (CAN)[23] and chronic rejection (CR). While these terms related to the characteristic histological features of IF/TA, they became a disease entity unto

themselves and were used as a cause of late graft failure even in the absence of tissue for histological diagnosis. Consequently, in current clinical practice, the term 'CAN' has been eliminated and specific pathological investigations into the causes of IF/TA and functional failure are emphasised.[24]

✔✔ The classification of chronic changes in kidney allografts was created in the Banff pathology meetings in the 1993–95 conferences and was revised in 2005 (Box 13.3).

More recent studies suggest that failing allografts have identifiable diagnoses for injury, suggesting specific treatments may be available to ameliorate declining function, discussed in more detail below. Adoption of serial protocol biopsies and newer laboratory techniques (C4d staining, molecular profiling and solid-phase antibody assays) has led to a better understanding into causes of CGI, and emphasises the role of the humoral immune response. Indeed, the assessment of kidney graft pathology was formed by consensus at the Banff Meeting in 2005 and emphasised new criteria to assess for antibody-mediated injury, discussed below.[24]

Why and how does IF/TA occur?
Clinical insights

IF/TA results as sequelae to a series of pathological insults to the kidney from the time of organ retrieval, which leads to incremental and cumulative damage to nephrons, and ultimate loss of graft function. Recent data from a number of studies now indicate that immune-mediated injury, especially related to alloantibodies, is a major threat to allografts even after the first year. In the recent cross-sectional analysis of failing kidney allografts from seven transplant centres in North America (the Deterioration of Kidney Allograft Function (DeKAF) study), the presence of IF/TA changes alone did not predict graft failure and allografts labelled as calcineurin inhibitor (CNI) toxicity fared no worse than other

Box 13.3 • Banff criteria for the severity of IF/TA

Grade I: Mild interstitial fibrosis and tubular atrophy – <25% of cortical area

Grade II: Moderate interstitial fibrosis and tubular atrophy – 26–50% of cortical area

Grade III: Severe interstitial fibrosis and tubular atrophy/loss – >50% of cortical area grafts in the absence of this diagnosis.[25] The preponderance of abnormalities in this study featured immunological injury including acute rejection[26] and antibody-mediated injury, occurring in about 57% of biopsies.[27] Moreover, the presence of inflammation in the allograft, in areas of fibrosis and tubular atrophy that are not included in the Banff analysis of chronic injury, was an independent negative feature of allograft failure.[28] Thus IF/TA is not an idiopathic and independent feature of a large proportion of failing allografts but identification of coincident pathology is important in defining outcome.

Additional single-centre data were published by El-Zoghby et al.[29] Three hundred and thirty kidney grafts were lost in 1317 conventional kidney recipients over a 10-year period. One hundred and fifty-three or 46% were lost due to graft failure. The causes of graft loss included glomerular disease such as recurrent disease, transplant glomerulopathy and de novo disease in 37%, acute rejection in 16%, other medical/surgical conditions in 16% and IF/TA in 31% of failed grafts. In this last group, an aetiology for IF/TA could be identified 81% of the time and CNI toxicity was rarely the cause, in only 0.7%, of failed allograft biopsies. These results demonstrate that glomerular damage is the most common cause of graft failure, as well as the paucity of true diagnoses of CNI toxicity.

With the enhanced capabilities to detect donor-specific antibody, it is not unexpected that diagnoses of antibody-mediated injury are more common. This includes the utilisation of C4d staining and consensus about grading and histological features of injury.[24,30,31] Moreover, there is now evidence that molecular analysis of allograft biopsies, even in the absence of diagnostic criteria for antibody-mediated rejection, may demonstrate endothelial cell activation indicative of active antibody-mediated damage and graft failure in patients with alloantibodies.[32] These and many other observational studies have led us to think that late graft loss is not always a result of CNI nephrotoxicity and emphasises the need to investigate the cause of IF/TA.

The aetiology of chronic graft injury

In understanding the development of CGI, a common paradigm is to classify these factors based on those that are antigen dependent (immunological) and those that are antigen independent (non-immunological). Note that this is an artificial partition and that non-immunological factors may ultimately mediate an immune response (Box 13.4).

An alternative paradigm is to consider the factors affecting long-term graft survival as defined by timing relative to transplantation:

• **Peri-transplant factors.** These include: *donor factors* of age, donor serum creatinine and comorbid conditions such as hypertension; *brain stem death* with the accompanying catecholamine storm; *preservation* and

Box 13.4 • Causes of allograft injury

Immunological (antigen dependent)
Cellular immunity
Direct versus indirect allorecognition
Donor–host HLA mismatch
Subclinical inflammation
Co-stimulatory signalling
Inadequacy of immunosuppression
Humoral immunity
Antibody-mediated rejection
Previous sensitisation
Infection
CMV
BK polyomavirus
Non-immunological (antigen independent)
Organ viability
Donor senescence
Donor age
Reduced renal mass
Donor brain injury
Living versus deceased donor
Prolonged cold ischaemic time
Delayed graft function/acute tubular necrosis
Treatment
Drug toxicity
Recipient factors
Lipid disorders
Diabetes
Recurrent disease
Adherence to medications
Hypertension
Urinary tract obstruction

Reproduced from Jevnikar AM, Mannon RB. Late kidney allograft loss: what we know about it, and what we can do about it. Clin J Am Soc Nephrol 2008; 3(Suppl 2):S56–67.

implantation injury, e.g. ischaemic damage and reperfusion injury, leading to *delayed graft function*.

- **Post-transplant factors.** These include immune response of *acute rejection*, both cellular and antibody mediated, and *infections* that may include urinary tract infection, donor derived infections and viral illnesses. Over time, *recipient factors* such as *hypertension*, *dyslipidaemia*, *diabetes* and *viral infections*, such as CMV and BK polyomavirus, play a more significant role in mediating renal tubular injury. In the past decade *immunosuppression* with CNIs was considered to be a significant contributor to late histological changes and allograft dysfunction; however, that paradigm has shifted, with evidence mounting in support of *alloimmune injury* being a major contributor of CGI.

Peri-transplant factors: beyond our control?

Donor age has a significant impact on graft survival and extremes of age are associated with worse long-term graft survival. With ageing, there is a reduction in nephron mass. Moreover, the ageing donor has attendant issues that affect long-term function. The concept of cellular senescence may limit the healing process in an organ allograft, due to a finite healing response in ageing tissue.[33] Additionally, recipient-based stresses such as hypertension and diabetes may similarly be poorly tolerated. Donation after **brain stem death** is also significantly associated with worse graft survival and increased incidences of delayed graft function and acute rejection compared to live donor organs. The systemic sequelae of brain death are not well understood and direct injury to the brain stem may result in labile blood pressure, alterations in thermal regulation, endocrine and biochemical derangements, and alterations in renal function. Surges in catecholamine release are experienced, with resultant physical and structural changes affecting the vital organs. It may also be the trigger for the systemic release of proinflammatory mediators, resulting in endothelial cell activation and thrombotic microangiopathy. These processes enhance the immunogenicity of the organ.

Delayed graft function (DGF) is a form of acute kidney injury seen following kidney transplantation, and may be defined as the need for dialysis support in the first 7 days post-transplantation. DGF incidence is rising, from 15% in 1985–1990 to 23% in 1998–2004,[34] based on data from the United States Renal Data System. This may be related to the rising use of expanded criteria donors (ECDs), and the use of donors after declaration of circulatory death (DCD). DGF is a considerable issue, with an estimated increase of 41% for graft failure in those with DGF as well as a higher rate of rejection of nearly 40%, compared to recipients without DGF. There is also a strong association with the development of CTD, although non-biopsy proven. This complex series of injuries is significantly detrimental to long-term success and has led to a substantial interest not only in donor management, but also in therapeutic strategies to ameliorate ischaemic injury.[35] Other strategies for improving outcomes include the use of perfusion of the kidney allograft; many centres have utilised this approach based on recent data demonstrating improved outcomes following pumping. Another opportunity may be graft protection through 'immuno-cloaking'; that is, blocking the preserved allograft from further immune injury and allowing appropriate reparative processes to occur unimpeded.[36] Finally, the kidney uniquely expresses TLR4 in mesangial cells, podocytes and tubular epithelium. As such, it is a focus of innate immune activation that triggers adaptive responses. Further therapies that may address this mechanism have potential to impact on DGF and thus CGI.

Post-transplant immunity: acute rejection

The low incidence of CGI in grafts from HLA-identical living-related donors supports the role for immunological factors in developing CGI. Indeed, there has been a long-standing recognised association between acute rejection and CGI. However, early rejection episodes in the first 6 months do not necessarily portend worse graft survival, while later graft rejection episodes from 6 to 12 months or repeated episodes are associated with a significantly higher risk of graft loss.

Importantly, if there is complete functional recovery with a late rejection episode, graft half-life is similar to recipients with no or early rejection episodes with impaired function.[37] A complicating feature of these late graft rejections may be the superimposed presence of antibody-mediated rejection (AMR). Indeed, many of the data in this context were from an era when AMR was not recognised in its presentation beyond the early acute setting and may thus indicate a continuum of injury that contributes to CGI.

Post-transplant immunity: antibody-mediated rejection

While the association of donor-specific antibodies with late graft failure has long been recognised, it has not been until the last decade that the negative impact of donor-specific antibodies has been recognised as a predictor of graft loss. Alloantibody has been correlated to chronic rejection and graft dysfunction. In a prospective multicentre trial of 2278 recipients, 500 recipients had HLA antibodies. In these recipients, 6.6% of grafts failed compared to 3.3% among the 1778 patients without antibodies; 8.6% of grafts failed in patients who made de novo antibodies as compared to 3.0% in patients who did not make any antibodies, showing a higher rate of graft failure in patients with HLA antibodies.[38] There are multiple studies correlating the development of donor-specific antibody (DSA) with allograft failure.[39]

Diagnosis of antibody-mediated rejection: acute and chronic

In 1993, Feucht et al. for the first time identified C4d as a marker of kidney injury and chronic rejection in human kidney allograft biopsies. Numerous studies have reported the association of presence of C4d positivity on the biopsy specimen with chronic rejection and graft failure. Thus, acute AMR is defined histologically by the features in Box 13.5.[40] Note that in the absence of detection of DSA, the diagnosis may be annotated as *suspicious* for AMR. Note that the presence of graft dysfunction is not required.

The routine use of biopsy staining for C4d has led to an increased acceptance of the role of antibody-mediated damage in CGI and biopsy criteria have been defined.[24]

Box 13.5 • Banff criteria for acute antibody-mediated injury

- The presence of C4d staining in peritubular capillaries
- Histological features of peritubular capillaritis, or acute tubular necrosis, or arterial/transmural inflammation with/without fibrinoid changes
- The detection of donor-specific antibody

Reproduced from Racusen LC, Colvin RB, Solez K et al. Antibody-mediated rejection criteria – an addition to the Banff 97 classification of renal allograft rejection. Am J Transplant 2003; 3(6):708–14.

✓✓ In 2005, criteria for chronic AMR were added to the Banff criteria for AMR. These criteria include:

1. Biopsy features including transplant glomerulopathy (TG; duplication or 'double contours' in glomerular basement membranes) and/or peritubular capillary basement membrane multilayering, and/or IF/TA with or without PTC loss, and/or fibrous intimal thickening in arteries without duplication of the internal elastica.
2. Diffuse C4d deposition in PTC.
3. Presence of donor-specific antibody (DSA).

Note that if only either C4d deposits (with no DSA) or DSA (with no C4d) are present, with documented morphological capillary changes, then the diagnosis of 'suggestive of chronic AMR' is made.

The entity of TG is now recognised as a phenomenon of chronic rejection with associated endothelial injury. This disorder is histologically characterised by widespread involvement of all glomeruli, with enlargement and duplication of the glomerular basement membrane, and endothelial cell activation. By electron microscopy, there is subendothelial accumulation of electron-lucent material, re-duplication of the basement membrane and interposition of mesangial cells into the capillary wall. Clinically, there is from 1 gram to greater than 3 grams of urinary protein excreted per day, progressive renal dysfunction and accelerated graft failure. The development of TG has now been recognised as an entity associated with anti-HLA antibodies and glomerular C4d staining. Detection of C4d in peritubular capillaries in otherwise morphologically normal biopsies is associated with subsequent development of this lesion. This antibody-associated immunity may also be a response to structural proteins in the kidney, rather than anti-HLA antibody: for example, the presence of circulating anti-glomerular basement membrane (anti-GBM) antibodies in the majority of recipients with TG, compared to recipients with typical chronic allograft nephropathy (11/16 compared to 3/16). These antibodies exhibit specificity to the GBM heparan sulphate proteoglycan agrin in patients with TG. The immune activation of this lesion is further supported by the observation that intraglomerular and periglomerular leucocytes express markers of T-cell activation CXCR3 and ICOS compared to their absence in biopsies with IF/TA alone. These studies support the need for further investigation into the prospective development of this lesion and the contributions of both cellular- and antibody-mediated components.

Associations of antibody and CGI

There is a particularly strong association between TG and anti-HLA class II antibodies. This combination has been associated with particularly poor survival. In one study, 26% of patients with pre-transplant anti-HLA II antibodies developed TG, compared to 8% without these antibodies.[41] A confounding factor in these observations is that the association between TG and C4d positivity is complex, suggesting a limitation of C4d staining. In one study, at the time of diagnosis of TG, C4d was positive in fewer than half of the cases.[42] This may be due to the existence of two distinct types of TG, C4d positive and negative, or it may be that not all antibody-mediated rejection episodes are associated with C4d positivity. Recognition of this phenomenon has been noted by the Banff working group in allograft pathology[30] and additional studies that correlate glomerulitis and peritubular capillaritis with donor-specific antibody and graft failure.[43] Moreover, data are accumulating for the determination of molecular activation of endothelial injury even when the histological criteria may not be entirely present.

The case for non-HLA antibodies contributing to CGI is also growing. In human kidney transplant recipients, antibodies directed against vascular endothelial cells have been associated with biopsy-proven chronic rejection and worsened graft outcome. Antibody against tubular basement membrane has also been rarely detected in a study from one transplant centre, but how it mediates chronic tubulointerstitial injury is not certain. In rodent models, TG may be associated with antibody against heparan sulphate proteoglycans. Recently, anti-angiotensin II type A receptor antibody has been detected in a subset of kidney transplant recipients with refractory vascular rejection episodes and malignant hypertension, suggesting a protective role for angiotensin receptor blockade.

Similar to cardiac transplants, antibodies against MICA and MICB are associated with poor kidney graft outcome. Terasaki et al. demonstrated that the existence of MICA antibody was associated with a risk of graft failure of nearly similar magnitude as anti-HLA antibody.[44] Sensitisation to MICA was associated with more frequent acute rejection episodes and worse graft survival, in spite of the extent of HLA matching between donor and recipient.[45] Moreover, these responses may be dependent on the specificity and intensity of the antibody produced.

It should be noted that not all the patients with anti-donor antibodies lose their allografts or develop CGI, suggesting that there may be other immunological triggers, differences in the properties of the anti-donor antibodies or other regulatory mechanisms at work. In a recently published prospective study of over 300 recipients at one centre with preoperative positive flow crossmatch at the time of transplant, two-thirds of the 69 patients showed complete elimination of the positive cytotoxic crossmatch and alloreactivity by single antigen bead assay by 1 year and demonstrated equivalent graft survival at 3 years when compared to the patients without antibodies. The other third who failed to eliminate the antibodies had inferior graft survival (67% at 3 years) secondary to chronic rejection but surprisingly, despite the persistence of alloantibodies, more than half the patients remained free of AMR or chronic rejection. There were no differences in the pre-transplant characteristics or the nature of the alloantibodies. The authors suggested that just the presence of alloantibodies is not enough to trigger an episode of rejection.[46]

Probably the most conclusive mechanistic studies of anti-donor antibody mediating CGI come from animal models of allograft rejection. For example, Russell et al. noted fibrous intimal thickening of coronary arteries in cardiac allograft at 1–2 months in immune-deficient scid mice after administration of repeated doses of anti-major histocompatibility complex (anti-MHC) class I alloantibody.[47] Moreover, the complete absence of donor MHC expression in mouse kidney allografts was associated with prolonged allograft survival, improved renal function and the absence of DSA in the recipient.[48] Further discussion about the initiation of injury and monitoring is given below.

Post-transplant factors: viral infections

Cytomegalovirus (CMV) infection

Cytomegalovirus (CMV) remains one of the most clinically significant organisms in solid-organ transplantation and viral replication can be detected in over 50% of allograft recipients. Risk factors include CMV-seronegative recipients receiving a CMV-seropositive transplant, older donor age, exposure to ciclosporin and/or antilymphocyte antibody, rejection episodes and impaired transplant function.[49] Management strategies include prophylactic antiviral therapy or pre-emptive monitoring in the context of viral replication. The latter is typically accomplished using polymerase chain reaction (PCR) detection in recipient lymphocytes.

Apart from its direct role in causing clinical manifestations of active disease, CMV has also been implicated in the development of CGI, as has latent infection. Experimental evidence supports this theory in animal models of cardiac, renal and lung transplantation.[50] Whether this is related to direct participation of the virus in kidney injury or the consequence of acute rejection coupled with infection remains uncertain. In cardiac transplants, CAV is much more common in those patients in the presence of ongoing CMV viraemia. Additionally, the progression of pathologies of late graft injury is further provoked by CMV infection, suggesting that CMV may aggravate an injury, leading to late graft failure.[51] Furthermore, treatment of CMV disease and CMV viraemia reduces the incidence and severity of CTD in experimental allografts. Limited data in human recipients from a recent trial of 148 recipients randomised to receive prophylactic versus pre-emptive therapy demonstrate that prophylactic treatment for CMV was strongly associated with better 4-year graft survival (92% vs. 73%).[52] Whether this is related to reduced infection or inflammatory responses to the allograft is not known.

Polyomavirus infection

Over the decade, there has been recognition of a serious quiescent virus that has a tropism to the genito-urinary epithelium that in the context of immunosuppression may be activated, and invasive, with rapid viral multiplication leading to renal graft injury and loss. The polyomavirus BK has been associated with nephropathy (BK PVN). The clinical presentation is progressive allograft dysfunction, and allograft biopsy demonstrates tubulointerstitial nephritis, and fibrosis and atrophy.[53] There are no systemic symptoms and signs such as fever or leucopenia that are seen with other viral infections. BK infection is encountered in the first year after transplantation, when immunosuppressive load is at its highest. Diagnosis is made by allograft biopsy showing characteristic features of interstitial nephritis, tubulitis, viral inclusions and positive immunostaining for the SV40 antigen. This is associated with detection of virus by real-time PCR of the urine and plasma. Indeed, the use of plasma viral testing has been adopted by many institutions as a monitoring strategy for early intervention.[54] This has led to systematic immunosuppressive therapy reductions with the hopes of allowing an appropriate antiviral response to occur.

A critical need is for highly effective non-toxic, antiviral therapy for BK virus infections.[55] While cidofovir has reactivity against BK, it is highly nephrotoxic, limiting its potential efficacy in this patient population. A recently identified oral congener with longer half-life and less nephrotoxicity is undergoing clinical trials.[56] Alternatives have included the use of intravenous immunoglobulin and DNA gyrase inhibitors such as ciprofloxacin, with varying success rates; leflunomide, an isoxazole derivative with modest antiviral effect and with anti-inflammatory properties, has also been used with varying reports of efficacy.[57,58] There is no cross-reactivity with other anti-herpes virus therapies. Consequently, clearance of infection is held to the development of an intrinsic antiviral response.

BK PVN has been detected with increasing frequency coincident with the use of tacrolimus and mycophenolate mofetil (MMF), as well as the more frequent use of lymphocyte depletional therapy, implicating the total burden of immunosuppression as opposed to a specific agent inciting the infection.[55] The long-term impact of BK PVN and its treatment on the development of CGI in kidney transplantation is considerable; with late detection and established fibrosis, the outcome of graft failure is frequent.

✓✓ The utility of the Banff Working Proposal 2009 for polyomavirus nephropathy derives from scoring of fibrosis and not extent of tubular injury or viral cytopathic effect.[59] Moreover, molecular studies of BK PVN demonstrate not only a strong cytotoxic T-cell response, similar to that of rejection, but a profibrotic response either directly mediated by the viral infection of tubular epithelial cells or as a response to inflammatory immune response and associated cytokines.[60] These intriguing results indicate the need for specific antiviral therapies in order to prevent long-term damage.

Post-transplant factors: immunosuppression

The use of the CNIs ciclosporin A (CsA) and tacrolimus has dramatically reduced first year graft rejection rates and facilitated improved graft survival in kidney transplantation. However, the considerable concern for the use of these agents is their nephrotoxicity. The histological findings include arteriolar hyalinosis, glomerulosclerosis, ischaemic glomerular collapse, interstitial fibrosis and tubular atrophy. This was demonstrated not only in the dose-dependent acute nephrotoxicity that was seen in kidney transplant recipients but also from the use of CsA in non-renal transplantation and autoimmune disease, where renal injury was progressive over time.[61] In more chronic injury, damage may be independent of drug levels or exposure to CNI.

A strong series of mechanistic studies using a rodent model of CNI nephrotoxicity demonstrated striped interstitial fibrosis and TA changes. These studies have identified several critical classes of mediators of CNI injury. These include angiotensin II, vasoconstrictive lipid mediators including eicosanoids, thromboxanes and leucotrienes, endothelin and nitric oxide. Other mechanisms implicated include the up-regulation of pro-apoptotic genes and the induction of endoplasmic reticulum (ER) stress in renal tubular epithelium.[62] Finally, the profibrogenic effects of CsA have been associated with the induction of platelet-derived growth factor (PDGF) and TGF-β within the kidney, as well as connective tissue growth factor (CTGF). The functional impact of TGF-β in this model has been further demonstrated by the mitigation of the CsA-induced fibrosis following treatment with pirfenidone, as well as anti-TGF-β antibodies. Furthermore, as angiotensin II expression has been linked with the induction of TGF-β, several studies have demonstrated a reduction in TGF-β when the angiotensin pathway is antagonised. While TGF-β is a unifying theme for the development of fibrosis in this model, antagonists of this pathway may have unintended consequences due to the immunomodulatory actions of TGF-β.

Provocative data using protocol biopsies of the kidney allograft in recipients on CNI-based immunosuppression demonstrated a near uniform development of arteriolar hyalinosis and IF/TA thought to be characteristic of CNI toxicity.[63] In this landmark study, Nankivell et al. described the findings of 961 protocol biopsies performed at intervals on 120 kidney and pancreas recipients over a period of 10 years with regards to the aetiology of late graft failure. Early changes of chronic damage were seen at 3 months, and were associated with ischaemic injury, prior severe rejection and subclinical rejection (SCR). Beyond 1 year, there was progressive high-grade hyalinosis with luminal narrowing, increasing glomerulosclerosis and additional tubulointerstitial damage was accompanied by the use of CNIs. By 10 years, severe evidence of chronic damage was seen in 58.4% of patients and glomerulosclerosis in about 38 % of patients. Thus the paradigm of CNI toxicity as the primary cause of late histological injury became widely accepted, and substantial efforts have been and are being directed to reduce or replace CNI therapy. This has led to the development of immunosuppressive protocols that minimise CNI and/or replace CNI.[64] Recent data, however, suggest that arteriolar hyalinosis may be a manifestation of endothelial injury from various stressors, especially from alloantibodies, and clinical data support the notion of antibody-mediated injury as a critical mediator of allograft failure and that the presence of CNI toxicity is not specifically associated with late graft failure.[26,27] However, we also should consider that chronic graft injury may be further provoked in the context of CNI therapy. Thus, the minimisation or conversion from CNI has been a consideration in the management of chronic allograft failure based on data from recent conversion trials.[65–67]

Post-transplant stressors

Hypertension

Hypertension is a common problem after kidney transplantation, seen in 60–80% of recipients.[68]

It is defined as a systolic blood pressure >140 mmHg, diastolic blood pressure >90 mmHg, or the need for antihypertensive therapy according to the *Seventh Report of the Joint National Committee on Prevention, Detection, Evaluation, and Treatment of High Blood Pressure* (JNC 7). It is a clear risk factor for graft failure and death; for every 10 mmHg of systolic blood pressure, there is a 5% increase in the risk of death in hypertensive transplant recipients.[69] Clinical management and assessment for kidney transplant recipients are elaborated in the Kidney Disease: Improving Global Outcomes (KDIGO) clinical practice guideline for the care of kidney transplant recipients,[70] endorsing the National Kidney Foundation's KDOQI (Kidney Disease Outcomes Quality Initiative) treatment targets of <130/80 in transplant recipients.[71] Control may include the use of a variety of agents, including diuretics, beta-blockers and vasodilators, and no specific agent has demonstrated a defined advantage. While the use of angiotensin-converting enzyme inhibitors and angiotensin receptor blockers slows progression of chronic kidney disease in non-transplanted recipients, definitive evidence for efficacy in providing renal protection or improved recipient survival is lacking.[72] Still, their use is advocated in adult recipients with greater than 1 gram of proteinuria, recognising the potential issues of alterations in glomerular filtration rate (GFR), hyperkalaemia and anaemia.[70]

Dyslipidaemia

Dyslipidaemia is defined as a total cholesterol level greater than 240 mg/dL, low-density lipoprotein (LDL) greater than 130 mg/dL, high-density lipoprotein (HDL) less than 35 mg/dL and/or triglycerides greater than 200 mg/dL. It is another fairly common issue, although rates vary from 40% up to as high as 80% of kidney recipients with a total cholesterol or LDL level above these values.[73] Contributory factors into these elevations include existing lipid disorders, genetic factors, as well as the use of immunosuppression, in particular steroids, CsA and mammalian target of rapamycin (mTOR) inhibitors, which have notable impact on triglyceride elevations. While dyslipidaemia is associated with an increased risk of cardiovascular disease in renal transplant patients, it is also an independent risk factor for chronic allograft dysfunction and graft failure. However, the impact of 3-hydroxy-3-methylglutaryl-coenzyme A (HMG-CoA) reductase inhibitors or statins on acute rejection rates has been equivocal. In transplant patients, the only randomised trial using fluvastatin, the ALERT trial, was associated with a significant reduction in non-fatal myocardial infarction or cardiac death, but no impact on renal function or graft loss.[74] This may in part be related to the power of these endpoints. Regardless, as cardiovascular disease is the leading cause of mortality after kidney transplantation, KDIGO guidelines[70] support the K/DOQI recommendations[75] for total cholesterol less than 200 mg/dL and LDL less than 100 mg/dL. Strategies include lifestyle modification, diet, and the use of statins and/or fibrates.[73]

Post-transplant diabetes mellitus

Post-transplant diabetes mellitus (PTDM), also known as new onset of diabetes mellitus after transplant (NODAT), is seen in kidney transplant recipients with reported incidence ranging from 2% to 53%. This variation is due to the definition of diagnosis, such as the use of anti-glycaemic agents versus the use of insulin. Diabetes is associated with worse patient survival and graft outcomes, in part due to the increase in cardiovascular and infectious morbidities. PTDM is typically characterised by insulin resistance, which may be compounded by weight gain after transplantation, even in the absence of steroid use. Risk factors for development include the use of steroids, older recipient age, African American and Hispanic race, history of hepatitis C, tacrolimus use, obesity and hypertension.[76] Other less consistent risk factors have included HLA matching, polycystic kidney disease and male recipient. Defined monitoring criteria following transplantation have been outlined by consensus.[70] The significant impact of treatment of PTDM is on patient survival. The role in preserving renal function is less clear. Data from three major trials in patients with type II diabetes without kidney transplants have demonstrated a positive impact of tight blood sugar control on preventing the development of nephropathy and microalbuminuria; however, these large randomised trials have not shown an impact in preventing the decline in kidney function, though there may be an effect in type I diabetes and this may result in significant hypoglycaemia. Management strategies have similarly been addressed and are beyond the scope of this chapter; they may include modification of immunosuppression in those with flagrant disease as well as those at high risk to develop PTDM.[76]

Anaemia

Anaemia, as defined by a haemoglobin concentration <13 mg/dL for men and <12 mg/dL for women,[13] is seen in up to 40% of post-kidney transplant recipients. The aetiology is multifactorial and includes iron deficiency, impaired allograft function, immunosuppressive therapy and other inflammatory processes leading to erythropoietin (EPO) resistance. In this patient population, it is unclear if there is a defined link to cardiovascular outcomes and a number of studies have demonstrated that EPO stimulating agent (ESA) use may be associated with poorer patient and graft outcomes.[77] There is a strong association with acute rejection episodes, but again this may relate not only to depressed GFR but also intensification of immunosuppression and inflammatory states. Data on ESA use have similarly been confusing in terms of preserving graft function, although quality of life is improved. With the lack of sufficient data, there have been no defined consensus guidelines so far regarding management[70] and, in those with impaired graft function, using K/DOQI guidelines would be most appropriate.[78]

Pathophysiology

One model of CGI has been elaborated utilising features characteristic of the progression of chronic native kidney disease[79] (**Fig. 13.1**). In the *initiation phase*, there is tissue injury mediated by any number or combination of antigen-dependent and -independent factors. Regardless of the type of insult, a *fibrogenesis phase* is engaged. There are two critical components of this phase: inflammation and proliferation. Both innate and adaptive immune responses may coalesce and are discussed further below. There is also a proliferative response, mediated by chemokines, cytokines and growth factors. In particular, TGF-β has long been the focus as a critical mediator of this fibrosis response, as well as the downstream effector CTGF. A number of studies have looked at the contribution of these and other growth factors, such as hepatocyte growth factor, and demonstrated an amelioration of chronic injury when these factors were inhibited.[79] However, with the overlap of multiple responses and stimulation by multiple

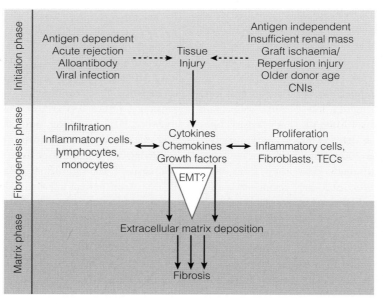

Figure 13.1 • The events that lead to fibrosis in chronic allograft injury are shown. Both immunological and non-immunological factors have been implicated in the pathogenesis of tissue injury. The resulting injury consists of an inflammatory and proliferative response, regulated by cytokines and growth factors. In particular, enhanced TGF-β has been associated with chronic allograft nephropathy. This cascade results in matrix accumulation, due to either increased production and/or reduced degradation of matrix, resulting in fibrosis. TEC, tubular epithelial cell.

injuries, it seems unlikely that just a single factor is playing a role here. In the *matrix phase*, there is deposition of collagen. This may be either over-production of matrix or reduced degradation, or a combination of both. Therapies targeted at this phase will be discussed below.

What are the targets that mediate chronic injury?

In the kidney, the primary cell considered to be under attack has been the tubular epithelial cell.[1] These cells are particularly vulnerable to ischaemic injuries, as well as direct toxicity due to CNIs. Histologically, they are the site of immune attack mediated by T cells (i.e. tubulitis), but also may engage each other once activated and promote cell death. A number of strategies have been under-taken, in preclinical models, to limit tubular injury and these therapies have had positive impact on re-nal function and transplant outcome.[1]

With the increasing focus on AMR, there is an ap-preciation that endothelial cell activation may also play a more definitive role in mediating graft failure. A primary mechanism by which alloantibody causes injury is via complement activation and subsequent cell death.[80] However, a number of investigators are identifying non-complement-mediated signal-ling pathways that initiate cell activation and pro-liferation. In CAV, for example, antibody binding mediates a signalling cascade mediating endothelial cell apoptosis and the production of profibrogenic extracellular matrix molecules that promote vascu-lar remodelling.[81] When endothelial cells (ECs) are cross-linked by anti-class I HLA antibody, signal transduction through Rho kinase initiates a cascade of downstream signals that promote actin contrac-tion and proliferation.[82] EC activation mediated by antibodies results in up-regulation of expression of leucocyte adhesion molecules such as vascular cell adhesion molecule 1 and intercellular adhesion molecule 1 expression, leading to increased leu-cocyte adhesion and inflammation. Finally, recent studies by Reed and colleagues have demonstrated that cross-linking of HLA determinants on endo-thelial cells initiates signalling through the mTOR signalling molecules mTORC1 and mTORC2, re-sulting in activation of the cells, mediates cell sur-vival signals and engages proliferative pathways.[83]

Phosphorylation of key signalling pathways in cell survival, activation and proliferation may also be seen with antibodies against class II determinants as well as non-HLA proteins. These exciting data point to several new targets to abrogate antibody-mediated chronic injury.

Recent studies also point to the microvasculature as a critical site for injury that may result in chronic allograft dysfunction. In the presence of inflamma-tion, revascularisation of a transplanted allograft is disrupted and is insufficient to sustain graft func-tion minimally. This 'inflammatory angiogenesis' response facilitates ongoing leucocyte recruitment and endothelial damage, eventually leading to isch-aemia. This creates a cycle of microvascular injury and hypoxia that limits tissue function, resulting in allograft fibrosis.[84] While these observations were made in tracheal allografts in mice, evidence for microvascular injury may be seen in the kidney in human recipients. Here, histological changes that are inflammatory such as glomerulitis and peritubu-lar capillaritis (**Fig. 13.2a**) and those with injury such as glomerulopathy (**Fig. 13.2b**) and peritubular cap-illary membrane multilayering are now recognised to be associated with donor-specific antibody and a significant phenotype of late allograft failure.[85]

What is the source of matrix?

Critical to our understanding of late graft failure is the understanding of how matrix is deposited into a failing allograft. Fibroblasts in the renal in-terstitium are responsible for matrix production. Activated fibroblasts, so-called myofibroblasts, express alpha-smooth muscle actin (α-SMA) or S100A4 (i.e. fibroblast-specific protein 1 or FSP-1). However, the origin of these cells remains uncertain. In hepatic fibrosis, myofibroblasts may be derived from bone marrow stem cells or fibrocytes (CD45 positive, CXCR4 positive, α-SMA positive).[86] Recent studies in a mouse tracheal transplant model dem-onstrate that disruption of specific chemotractant proteins limited fibrocyte migration into the allograft and ameliorated the fibro-obliterative response in the airways. In human lung transplant recipients, circulating fibrocyte levels correlated with the development of BOS, and correlated with BOS progression. In kidney transplants undergoing CGI, myofibroblasts present appeared to be of host

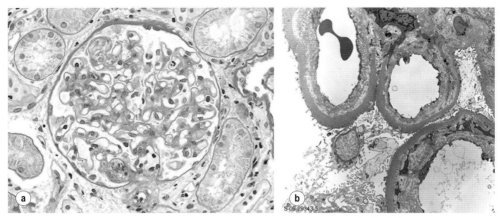

Figure 13.2 • **(a)** Periodic acid–Schiff staining of a human kidney biopsy showing the features of transplant glomerulopathy (×200). **(b)** Electron microscopy of a glomerulus with the characteristic basement membrane duplication seen in transplant glomerulopathy (×2500). These photos are courtesy of William J. Cook, MD, University of Alabama at Birmingham, Department of Pathology.

not donor origin, suggesting that a circulating precursor exists,[87] although the identity of these cells remains unknown.

A significant focus has been placed on the renal tubular epithelial cell and its potential for transformation into myofibroblasts. Such studies have been based on a large body of work demonstrating the ability of epithelial cells to transform and attain fibroblast-like characteristics in culture.[88] This process is known as epithelial mesenchymal transformation (EMT). In human transplantation, EMT markers were identified in a series of kidney allografts with IF/TA but were absent in stable functioning grafts, suggesting that tubular cell damage resulted in loss of epithelial features and expression of fibroblast features, leading to allograft fibrosis. In a study using surveillance (protocol) biopsies, the presence of EMT markers detected using immunohistochemistry at 3 months was 41%, more frequent in recipients with acute rejection and was further associated with later functional deterioration of progressive fibrosis of kidney allografts at 18 months. Similarly, in a series of patients on chronic CsA therapy, EMT marker expression advanced associated with a decline in allograft function and a progression in IF/TA changes, compared to biopsies in those withdrawn from CsA. However, the role of EMT in allograft fibrosis has been disputed by Nankivell and colleagues.[89] In this study of 24 recipients, markers of EMT at 1 and 3 months had no correlation to the development of IF/TA changes at 1 year post-transplant.

Additional mechanistic studies in rodent models of inflammatory renal disease have continued to call into question whether EMT actually occurs in vivo. While studies of cells in culture demonstrate phenotypic changes depending on the stimulus, fate tracing of fibroblasts shows no relationship to epithelial cells in mice following urinary outlet obstruction[90] and appears to reside in the perivascular space.[91] Further insights into the function of these fibroblast precursors should provide a new strategy for disruption of scar formation.

The contributions of the innate immune response

A number of components of the innate immune response have come under study as the focus has shifted from the adaptive or alloimmune response. We have typically considered these responses in the context of ischaemia–reperfusion injury (IRI) or in the context of other danger signals such as infections. Natural killer (NK) cells are large granular cytotoxic lymphocytes lacking the T-cell receptor, first identified by tumour cell killing that was not restricted by MHC expression. These cells are important components of the innate immune response that also are critical in killing virus-infected cells and mediating antibody-dependent cytotoxicity via the FcRIII (CD16). Recent studies have indicated that NK cells contribute to CGI; in these mouse studies, depletion or the genetic absence of NK cells mitigates chronic injury. In man, alterations in the number of NK cells are seen following depletional induction, and the numbers of NK cells in the periphery do return during repopulation, although they are only a small component of the peripheral compartment. They may make some contribution to antibody-mediated rejection as NK molecular signals are detected in allograft biopsies with AMR.[92] Thus, how these cells participate in the immune response remains uncertain.

Another component of the innate immune response receiving attention is the macrophage. These cells have been the focus of a number of studies of organ injury, not only in the context of organ transplantation. Macrophages are derived from peripheral blood mononuclear cells, and differentiate in response based on specific cytokine signals. Much like T cells, there are now recognised differentially functioning macrophages. These include M1 or classically activated and M2 or alternatively activated.[93] M1 macrophages differentiate when exposed to interferon (IFN)-γ produced by T cells or NK cells in concert with tumour necrosis factor (TNF)-γ produced by antigen-presenting cells (APCs) that have been activated through their Toll-like receptors (TLRs). Following activation, M1 cells produce interleukin (IL)-1, IL-6 and IL-23, potent proinflammatory cytokines that can induce tissue inflammation and activate Th17 cells. These macrophages are responsible for killing a variety of pathogens, including bacteria, viruses and parasites such as *Leishmania*. They are characterised phenotypically as F4/80 positive CD11c negative and mannose receptor (MR) negative. Alternatively, activated macrophages or M2 are activated by IL-4; this cytokine has a number of sources, including mast cells, basophils, Th2 T cells and chitin, a polysaccharide polymer found in some parasites and fungi. M2 macrophages may also be characterised by expression of mannose receptor and IL-10 production. Interestingly, IL-4 also stimulates arginase activity, which converts arginine to ornithine, leading to enhanced collagen production and wound healing. When undifferentiated macrophages are exposed in vitro to IL-4 and IL-13, extracellular matrix is produced and the intracellular pathogen killing is suppressed. Moreover, M2 cells produce chitinase and chitinase-like proteins whose roles may include matrix reorganisation. In contrast to M1, these cells tend to be F4/80 positive CD11c

negative MR positive. Finally, recent studies suggest a third phenotype of macrophages, the so-called regulatory macrophage (Mreg). These cells were identified following in vitro stimulation of mouse macrophages with high-density immune complexes plus TLR ligands, resulting in the production of IL-10 but not IL-12. Mregs appear to have biochemical and functional markers distinct from either M1 or M2 macrophages, including the expression of CCL1, lack of dependence of STAT 6 activation and lack of arginase expression. Interestingly, adoptive transfer of these cells suppresses inflammatory responses in some autoimmune models.

Based on animal studies, M1 and M2 cells may play a role in IRI as well as in unilateral urinary obstruction, a model of inflammatory renal disease. While the M1/M2 differentiation is intriguing, the relative contribution of these cells in organ transplantation is not known. Based on numerous animal studies, it is now recognised that macrophages participate in both acute and late allograft injury, not only in the kidney but also in heart allografts.[94] In humans, macrophages have long been identified in allograft biopsies of the kidney; as they arise as passengers in the donor organ, their presence declines over time in the early post-transplant period. However, in the setting of acute injury such as allograft rejection, macrophages may account for 38–60% of infiltrating leucocytes in rejecting kidney biopsies as detected by immunohistochemical staining. These cells may be actively recruited into the rejection organ by the chemokine MCP-1, a potent chemotractant. These cells are predominantly found in the interstitium, although tubulitis has been reported following T-cell depletion with alemtuzumab, as well as in the context of AMR in peritubular capillaritis. Transplant glomerulitis ('g'), a potential forerunner to glomerulopathy or chronic AMR, has also been associated with macrophage infiltrates in greater proportion than T cells. It should be noted that recent studies have demonstrated that monocyte infiltration, not lymphocyte infiltration, was quantitatively associated with this functional change as measured by serum creatinine.[95] Additionally, the presence of CX3CR1-positive macrophages in acute rejection biopsies is associated with poor steroid response and worse outcomes at 1 year.

The role of macrophages in CGI has been explored in a limited fashion. These cells may also accumulate in the interstitium in rodent models of IF/TA. In human recipients of kidney allografts, the presence of macrophages in an early biopsy was predictive of IF/TA development. Furthermore, targeting macrophage function or depletion of these cells ameliorates chronic injury in kidney and cardiac allograft CGI models.[94] Clearly, additional studies are needed to identify the exact mechanism of injury and determine if this may be an important therapeutic pathway in humans.

The management of chronic graft injury in the kidney

Principles of management

CGI is a clinical syndrome of gradually worsening renal function with associated hypertension and proteinuria. Diagnosis is assisted by allograft biopsy, as already noted above, with graded histological severity based on the extent of IF/TA changes. Careful investigation into the ethology is needed to provide not only diagnostic but therapeutic and prognostic implications. However, the prognostic significance of IF/TA changes alone is in and of itself limited. It is important to reiterate that simply relying on alterations of renal function and/or proteinuria can result in delayed diagnosis and usually the changes become irreversible. The multiple causes of CGI also indicate that a single treatment approach is not applicable, although there are some general principles to management based on the standards of chronic kidney disease. These include management of hypertension, hyperglycaemia in diabetic recipients, and lipid control.

A key consideration in patient management is that of immunosuppression. A number of studies have assessed the safety and efficacy of CNI avoidance using inhibitors of mTOR, demonstrating a positive impact on GFR in the early post-transplant course[96] but without significant impact in the long term.[97] Alternatively, removing CNI by conversion to an alternative agent may make biological sense, considering the ongoing toxicity of CNI therapy mediating a vasoconstrictive and ischaemic environment for the injured kidney. However, changing basal therapy must be made in the context of understanding the disorder mediating injury. For example, a biopsy indicating elements of acute and antibody-mediated rejection, with moderate fibrosis,

may suggest a strategy that includes the continued use of CNI therapy to effect the most potent immunosuppressive cocktail available. On the other hand, with more advanced graft failure (i.e. estimated glomerular filtration rate (eGFR) <30 mL/min), the use of full-dose therapy may not provide any useful improvement and, in fact, may mediate additional damage. For example, the conversion from CNI to rapamycin after 6 months of transplantation led to significantly worse outcomes in those with eGFR <40 mL/min, prompting the halt of that arm of the trial.

Because of the pleiotropic toxicities of available immunosuppressants, new approaches have employed agents that seek to mitigate nephrotoxicity. Belatacept is a selective co-stimulation blocker, a conjugate of cytotoxic lymphocyte antigen-4 (CTLA-4) and immunoglobulin (see Chapter 5). The use of this agent in the context of CNI conversion is also under investigation, and may provide a safe and effective alternative to chronic CNI use in the failing kidney.[98]

Finally, additional insight is available from a meta-analysis of CNI reduction trials from the time of transplantation that included 56 studies comprising data from 11 337 renal transplant recipients. There was a decrease in odds of overall graft failure with use of contemporary agents such as belatacept as well as tofacitinib, a JAK3 inhibitor under investigation, in combination with MMF. Similarly, CNI minimisation in combination with various induction and adjunctive agents reduced the odds of graft failure. Conversely, the use of mTOR inhibitors in combination with MMF increased the odds of graft failure.[99] Other promising agents for maintenance immunosuppression, used as monotherapy or synergistically, include monoclonal antibodies and fusion receptor proteins targeting the CD40–CD154 pathway (multiple anti-CD40 antibodies), the LFA3–CD2 pathway (i.e. alefacept) and small molecules such as tofacitinib.

Abrogating matrix deposition: a novel option for CGI management?

As discussed above, matrix deposition is mediated by either overexpression of matrix molecules, a reduction in matrix degradation or a combination of both.

While immunosuppressive management may reduce the chronic inflammatory state that stimulates this process, an adjunctive therapy in CGI may include targeted therapy to block fibrosis. The primary targets here include those growth factors and enzymes necessary for matrix synthesis.[79] In experimental models, a number of approaches have been addressed, including blocking prolyl-4-hydroxylase, a rate-limiting step in collagen synthesis, a strategy that reduced fibrosis and graft inflammation, and improved graft function in a murine model.[100] Inhibition of hepatocyte growth factor, the matrix metalloproteinase inhibitors, and TGF-β and its downstream effector CTGF has also shown some promise. However, a key consideration in the use of such agents in man includes appropriate timing of intervention. Due to the relatively unpredictable nature of IF/TA, initiating therapy in all patients at the time of transplant is neither practical nor safe. More advanced disease may be unaffected by any strategy once a 'point of no return' has been reached. Consequently, the design of trials in human kidney recipients has required the inclusion of surveillance biopsies to identify early IF/TA changes and to propose intervention in those subjects. Critical to such trials and to further our understanding of matrix abrogation are defined end-points, which should include biomarkers. This has been a key consideration of investigation during the current decade and is further elaborated below.

Diagnostic strategies in monitoring for CGI

A variety of methodologies have been examined with the potential for immune monitoring for CGI. These include genomics, proteomic and metabolomic platforms, not only for monitoring allograft injury but also to identify markers of graft failure that are more sensitive than serum creatinine and have potential for patient management.[101] There has been a considerable amount of research in kidney transplant recipients to identify potential biomarkers of CGI that may be useful in the monitoring of this developing injury. The most common method of monitoring the allograft function is by monitoring the serum creatinine or eGFR; however, these values are not specific since they are affected by other pre- and postrenal factors. Serum creatinine and eGFR

are not predictors of early histopathological changes and may result in delayed diagnosis. Screening for proteinuria, especially albuminuria, is also important since its presence is associated with poorer graft survival and can be a sign of TG or recurrent glomerular disease. KDIGO recommends monitoring for proteinuria at least once in the first month and then every 3 months for the first year and annually thereafter.[70] However, quarterly monitoring is the norm at many transplant centres.

Allograft biopsy

Renal allograft biopsy is the gold standard for identifying pathophysiological events that have a bearing on short- and long-term graft outcomes. Allograft biopsy is traditionally performed in the setting of acute or chronic deterioration in graft function. Recent consortium studies of failing kidney allografts and their biopsies demonstrate that while IF/TA may be uniformly present on biopsy, histological scoring by cluster analysis can identify groups of patients with varying outcomes.[26] Indeed, the presence of tubulitis ('t'), interstitial inflammation ('i') and vascular lesions ('v') is associated with worse prognosis. Similarly, a study of 234 biopsies for cause arranged Banff scoring patterns into patterns of disease including microcirculation change, IF and TA, suggesting that grouping of related lesions into diagnoses can explain the stress on various compartments in the kidney and may guide the interpretation of the biology of the lesion by acknowledging their relationships.

With the increasing recognition that a measurable decrease in renal function does not always accompany acute rejection or chronic changes, a number of transplant centres advocate the use of biopsy at set time points post-transplantation, so-called protocol or surveillance biopsies. This subject has been reviewed in depth by Nankivell and Chapman.[102] A number of studies have demonstrated an association of so-called subclinical rejection (SCR) with worsened graft outcomes. While initial studies at one centre supported therapeutic intervention, more recent data have been disappointing and may relate to the more potent immunosuppression currently in place in the early post-transplant course.[103] A cautionary note is that this was a small single-centre trial, albeit randomised, and that subclinical rejection findings were low in frequency, suggesting additional larger studies may provide further insight.

Moreover, the identification of subclinical findings is complex; the presence of 't' and 'i' is not specific and may be found not only in rejection but other inflammatory conditions. These findings may result due to multiple insults and may be non-specifically associated with late graft failure; interpretation of such biopsy findings should take into account the patient and transplant history and probabilities of specific disease entities based on these risks.

While the results of these studies suggest that intervention is ineffective in subclinical cellular rejection, protocol biopsies may be more useful in transplants involving highly sensitised patients and those who receive transplants against positive crossmatch kidneys, as these individuals are more likely to develop the presence of C4d on biopsies that may help detect the subclinical AMR, which may lead to early intervention with B-cell- or plasma-cell-depleting therapy. Another potential application of protocol biopsies is in their implementation in clinical trials designed to prevent CGI. An example is the phase II trial of belatacept in kidney transplantation, which demonstrated reduced IF/TA severity in the CNI-free belatacept arms.[104]

In addition to the histological analysis of biopsy tissue, the use of molecular analysis of biopsy pathology has been strongly advocated.[105] Using a series of allograft biopsies performed for change in renal function and/or proteinuria, a series of studies have identified and classified biopsies using pathogenesis-based transcript sets identifying the molecular heterogeneity of allograft rejection that is not evident by light microscopy alone. These studies have also pointed out the limitations in using Banff histological criteria alone,[106] but also demonstrate the potency of gene expression information in not only providing prognosis but also identifying key mechanisms of injury and potential for predicting late graft failure. While the focus of these studies has been with microarrays, other focused approaches using low-density arrays to analyse gene expression in tissue have similarly identified key insights into the disease pathogenesis of late graft failure. In an analysis of biopsies in recipients with PVN, Mannon et al. demonstrated that virally infected kidney tissue has a similar but more intense cytotoxic T-cell response within the allograft.[60] Moreover, PVN biopsies demonstrated a profibrotic gene profile compared to rejecting but uninfected tissue, indicating that there may be virally directed fibrosis responses. Further

integration of such strategies requires a methodology with rapid turnaround time, unequivocal interpretation and validation with clinical course.

Assays of whole blood: serum antibodies

Early detection of antibody-mediated injury has become a primary focus in post-transplant management. There have been various studies showing a strong association between development of alloantibodies and endothelial cell activation, TG and late allograft failure, as already noted above. Even though evidence linking alloantibodies with allograft failure continues to mount, the role of monitoring antibodies effectively in the post-transplant period is not well established. There are limited data to define the appropriate intervals at which to monitor, and the extent of the population to be monitored. Defined strategies of management once detected are not defined either, although many clinicians advocate allograft biopsy in spite of serum creatinine once detected. There is also no clear guidance regarding therapy once detected, but in part this may be assisted by allograft biopsy. Clearly, additional studies are needed in a broad clinical population to identify their cost-effectiveness and clinical utility.

Assays of whole blood: proteins

Previous studies implicated growth factors such as TGF-β as important molecules in the development of fibrosis in allografts. Other proteins such as advanced glycation end products, oxidative stress proteins, C-reactive proteins, SCD-30 and neopterin, metzincins and related proteins, tribbles-1 proteins expressed by endothelial cells and APCs have been shown to be up-regulated in recipients with IF/TA, but none of these markers have been validated in larger clinical studies.[101] Proteomic approaches have also been utilised, but to date there is no molecule specific in the identification of IF/TA, not surprising when considering the vast insults and aetiologies.

Assays of whole blood: gene expression

Gene transcript analysis using microarray or so-called low-density arrays has been investigated as a method for detecting and monitoring activity in peripheral blood mononuclear cells. Using such approaches, novel molecular transcripts have been identified in liver transplant recipients who have undergone conversion from CNI-based immunosuppression to rapamycin-based therapy, which may be a potential series of markers to follow for clinical graft stability. Studies in kidney transplant recipients have also identified a series of candidate biomarkers using a combined proteomic analysis with genomic analysis of peripheral blood mononuclear cells. The same group was able to map multiple sets of proteins to different functional pathways leading to IF/TA.[107] Further clinical studies are needed to validate these markers in the interpretation of kidney allograft pathology and severity of IF/TA.

Assays of whole blood: cellular functional analysis

Monitoring cellular alloreactivity has long been used to assess recipient immune response to donor tissue. Historical methods included mixed lymphocyte culture and assessment of CD4 cell proliferation or CD8 cell cytoxicity; these methods are limited by sensitivity, with the added nuisance of radionuclides. Recently, the enzyme-linked immunosorbent spot (ELISPOT) assay has replaced these methods as a more sensitive and quantitative assay. This test measures the frequency of peripheral blood lymphocytes producing IFN-γ in response to stimulator cells from the kidney donor or from third parties. Heeger et al. showed an independent correlation between early cellular alloreactivity and long-term renal function using this assay. Patients with low mean frequencies of IFN-γ-producing cells in the early post-transplant period were generally free from acute rejection and exhibited excellent renal function at 6 and 12 months post-transplant.[108] Serial monitoring after transplantation has also identified recipients at risk for acute rejection, with worse renal function in those with higher post-transplant frequencies of both donor and third-party responses. The ability to predict those more at risk for immune injury may provide an opportunity to intervene in the peri- and post-transplant periods, as well as determine a strategy of more intense clinical follow-up. Further studies are being undertaken to be able to use this test for serial immune monitoring.

Assays of urine: gene and proteomic approaches

A consideration in the above monitoring tests is their relative distance from the microenvironment of the affected organ. The opportunity exists to utilise urine much as a bronchoscopy and washings may help assess the intraparenchymal pathology of the lung allograft. A series of studies have utilised both genetic and proteomic approaches. These include examining urinary sediment and messenger RNA (mRNA) expression. Differential expression of angiotensin, epidermal growth factor receptor and TGF-β mRNA has been demonstrated in urine samples from recipients with IF/TA compared to those with stable function; the study population was, however, limited. The use of a combined expression panel of E-cadherin, vimentin, NKCC2 and 18S RNA was the most accurate in prediction of IF/TA in allograft biopsies.[109] The identification of inflammation may be even more useful to non-invasively monitor those with ongoing tubulitis that may have insufficient levels of immunosuppression.[110] Urine proteomics have similarly provided potential new candidates for monitoring, not only of IF/TA but also ongoing inflammation.[111] Ultimately, these studies that have predominantly correlated a marker with pathology must also be tested for their ability to predict later events.

Key points

- CTD remains a major cause of late graft loss following solid-organ transplantation.
- While fibrosis is a typical feature, non-specific histological changes are seen in different organs.
- The aetiology of CTD is multifactorial and reflects time-dependent changes that occur throughout the lifespan of the graft, and more than one factor may play a role at any given time.
- There is increasing evidence for the role of antibody-mediated rejection in CTD.
- The pathophysiology of CTD may involve endothelial cell activation, and ongoing inflammation in the allograft from both innate and adaptive pathways.
- Non-immunological factors such as hypertension, dyslipidaemia and hyperglycaemia may further aggravate failing allograft function.

- Treatment strategies include:
  - optimal management of risk factors such as hypertension and blood sugar;
  - alteration in maintenance immunosuppression to manage both antibody- and cellular-mediated injuries in the failing graft;
  - novel strategies such as inhibitors of matrix deposition may be potentially adjunctive.
- Immune monitoring assays capable of non-invasive diagnosis of CGI as well as for prediction of those at risk of CGI are under study.

References

1. Jevnikar AM, Mannon RB. Late kidney allograft loss: what we know about it, and what we can do about it. Clin J Am Soc Nephrol 2008;3(Suppl. 2):S56–67.

2. Taylor DO, Stehlik J, Edwards LB, et al. Registry of the International Society for Heart and Lung Transplantation: Twenty-sixth Official Adult Heart Transplant Report – 2009. J Heart Lung Transplant 2009;28(10):1007–22.

3. Colvin-Adams M, Agnihotri A. Cardiac allograft vasculopathy: current knowledge and future direction. Clin Transplant 2011;25(2):175–84.

4. Mehra MR, Crespo-Leiro MG, Dipchand A, et al. International Society for Heart and Lung Transplantation working formulation of a standardized nomenclature for cardiac allograft vasculopathy – 2010. J Heart Lung Transplant 2010;29(7):717–27.

5. Costanzo MR, Naftel DC, Pritzker MR, et al. Heart transplant coronary artery disease detected by coronary angiography: a multiinstitutional study of preoperative donor and recipient risk factors Cardiac Transplant Research Database. J Heart Lung Transplant 1998;17(8):744–53.

6. Berry GJ, Angelini A, Burke MM, et al. The ISHLT working formulation for pathologic diagnosis of antibody-mediated rejection in heart transplantation: evolution and current status (2005–2011). J Heart Lung Transplant 2011;30(6):601–11.

7. Kobashigawa J, Crespo-Leiro MG, Ensminger SM, et al. Report from a consensus conference on antibody-mediated rejection in heart transplantation. J Heart Lung Transplant 2011;30(3):252–69.

8. Smith JD, Brunner VM, Jigjidsuren S, et al. Lack of effect of MICA antibodies on graft survival following heart transplantation. Am J Transplant 2009;9(8):1912–9.

9. Suarez-Alvarez B, Lopez-Vazquez A, Gonzalez MZ, et al. The relationship of anti-MICA antibodies and MICA expression with heart allograft rejection. Am J Transplant 2007;7(7):1842–8.

10. Seyfert-Margolis V, Feng S. Tolerance: is it achievable in pediatric solid organ transplantation? Pediatr Clin North Am 2010;57(2):523–38.

11. Banff Working Group on Liver Allograft PathologyDemetris A. Importance of liver biopsy findings in immunosuppression management: biopsy monitoring and working criteria for patients with operational tolerance (OT). Liver Transpl 2012;18(10):1154–70.

12. Demetris A, Adams D, Bellamy C, et al. Update of the International Banff Schema for Liver Allograft Rejection: working recommendations for the histopathologic staging and reporting of chronic rejection An International Panel. Hepatology 2000;31(3):792–9.
   The current histological criteria for liver transplant rejection are presented here and provide a basis for tissue diagnosis.

13. Banff Working Group, Demetris AJ, Adeyi O, Bellamy CO, et al. Liver biopsy interpretation for causes of late liver allograft dysfunction. Hepatology 2006;44(2):489–501.

14. Christie JD, Edwards LB, Aurora P, et al. Registry of the International Society for Heart and Lung Transplantation: Twenty-fifth Official Adult Lung and Heart/lung Transplantation Report – 2008. J Heart Lung Transplant 2008;27(9):957–69.

15. Estenne M, Maurer JR, Boehler A, et al. Bronchiolitis obliterans syndrome 2001: an update of the diagnostic criteria. J Heart Lung Transplant 2002;21(3):297–310.
   The diagnostic criteria established for BOS are updated here based on consensus.

16. Todd JL, Palmer SM. Bronchiolitis obliterans syndrome: the final frontier for lung transplantation. Chest 2011;140(2):502–8.

17. Jaramillo A, Naziruddin B, Zhang L, et al. Activation of human airway epithelial cells by non-HLA antibodies developed after lung transplantation: a potential etiological factor for bronchiolitis obliterans syndrome. Transplantation 2001;71(7):966–76.

18. Hayes Jr D. A review of bronchiolitis obliterans syndrome and therapeutic strategies. J Cardiothorac Surg 2011;6:92.

19. Gruessner AC. 2011 update on pancreas transplantation: comprehensive trend analysis of 25,000 cases followed up over the course of twenty-four years at the International Pancreas Transplant Registry (IPTR). Rev Diab Stud 2011;8(1):6–16.

20. Pugliese A, Reijonen HK, Nepom J, et al. Recurrence of autoimmunity in pancreas transplant patients: research update. Diabetes Manag (Lond) 2011;1(2):229–38.

21. Drachenberg CB, Odorico J, Demetris AJ, et al. Banff schema for grading pancreas allograft rejection: working proposal by a multi-disciplinary international consensus panel. Am J Transplant 2008;8(6):1237–49.

22. Lamb KE, Lodhi S, Meier-Kriesche HU. Long-term renal allograft survival in the United States: a critical reappraisal. Am J Transplant 2011;11(3):450–62.

23. Racusen LC, Solez K, Colvin RB, et al. The Banff 97 working classification of renal allograft pathology. Kidney Int 1999;55(2):713–23.

24. Solez K, Colvin RB, Racusen LC, et al. Banff '05 Meeting Report: differential diagnosis of chronic allograft injury and elimination of chronic allograft nephropathy ('CAN'). Am J Transplant 2007;7(3):518–26.
Key update in Banff criteria establishing the current diagnosis for IF/TA.

25. Gourishankar S, Leduc R, Connett J, et al. Pathological and clinical characterization of the 'troubled transplant': data from the DeKAF study. Am J Transplant 2010;10(2):324–30.

26. Matas AJ, Leduc R, Rush D, et al. Histopathologic clusters differentiate subgroups within the non-specific diagnoses of CAN or CR: preliminary data from the DeKAF study. Am J Transplant 2010;10(2):315–23.

27. Gaston RS, Cecka JM, Kasiske BL, et al. Evidence for antibody-mediated injury as a major determinant of late kidney allograft failure. Transplantation 2010;90(1):68–74.

28. Mannon RB, Matas AJ, Grande J, et al. Inflammation in areas of tubular atrophy in kidney allograft biopsies: a potent predictor of allograft failure. Am J Transplant 2010;10(9):2066–73.

29. El-Zoghby ZM, Stegall MD, Lager DJ, et al. Identifying specific causes of kidney allograft loss. Am J Transplant 2009;9(3):527–35.

30. Mengel M, Sis B, Haas M, et al. Banff 2011 Meeting report: new concepts in antibody-mediated rejection. Am J Transplant 2012;12(3):563–70.

31. Sis B, Mengel M, Haas M, et al. Banff '09 meeting report: antibody mediated graft deterioration and implementation of Banff working groups. Am J Transplant 2010;10(3):464–71.

32. Sis B, Jhangri GS, Bunnag S, et al. Endothelial gene expression in kidney transplants with alloantibody indicates antibody-mediated damage despite lack of C4d staining. Am J Transplant 2009;9(10):2312–23.

33. Halloran PF, Melk A, Barth C. Rethinking chronic allograft nephropathy: the concept of accelerated senescence. J Am Soc Nephrol 1999;10(1):167–81.

34. Tapiawala SN, Tinckam KJ, Cardella CJ, et al. Delayed graft function and the risk for death with a functioning graft. J Am Soc Nephrol 2010;21(1):153–61.

35. Siedlecki A, Irish W, Brennan DC. Delayed graft function in the kidney transplant. Am J Transplant 2011;11(11):2279–96.

36. Hauet T, Eugene M. A new approach in organ preservation: potential role of new polymers. Kidney Int 2008;74(8):998–1003.

37. Opelz G, Dohler B. Influence of time of rejection on long-term graft survival in renal transplantation. Transplantation 2008;85(5):661–6.

38. Terasaki PI, Ozawa M. Predicting kidney graft failure by HLA antibodies: a prospective trial. Am J Transplant 2004;4(3):438–43.

39. Seveso M, Bosio E, Ancona E, et al. De novo anti-HLA antibody responses after renal transplantation: detection and clinical impact. Contrib Nephrol 2009;162:87–98.

40. Racusen LC, Colvin RB, Solez K, et al. Antibody-mediated rejection criteria – an addition to the Banff 97 classification of renal allograft rejection. Am J Transplant 2003;3(6):708–14.
Classic paper identifying the diagnostic criteria for antibody-mediated injury that led to the evolution of diagnosis of this disorder and provided a foundation for further clinical trials in the field.

41. Gloor JM, Sethi S, Stegall MD, et al. Transplant glomerulopathy: subclinical incidence and association with alloantibody. Am J Transplant 2007;7(9):2124–32.

42. Colvin RB. Antibody-mediated renal allograft rejection: diagnosis and pathogenesis. J Am Soc Nephrol 2007;18(4):1046–56.

43. Sis B, Jhangri GS, Riopel J, et al. A new diagnostic algorithm for antibody-mediated microcirculation inflammation in kidney transplants. Am J Transplant 2012;12(5):1168–79.

44. Terasaki PI, Ozawa M, Castro R. Four-year follow-up of a prospective trial of HLA and MICA antibodies on kidney graft survival. Am J Transplant 2007;7(2):408–15.

45. Zou Y, Stastny P, Susal C, et al. Antibodies against MICA antigens and kidney-transplant rejection. N Engl J Med 2007;357(13):1293–300.

46. Kimball PM, Baker MA, Wagner MB, et al. Surveillance of alloantibodies after transplantation identifies the risk of chronic rejection. Kidney Int 2011;79(10):1131–7.

47. Russell PS, Chase CM, Winn HJ, et al. Coronary atherosclerosis in transplanted mouse hearts I. Time course and immunogenetic and immunopathological considerations. Am J Pathol 1994;144(2):260–74.

48. Mannon RB, Griffiths R, Ruiz P, et al. Absence of donor MHC antigen expression ameliorates

chronic kidney allograft rejection. Kidney Int 2002;62(1):290–300.

49. De Keyzer K, Van Laecke S, Peeters P, et al. Human cytomegalovirus and kidney transplantation: a clinician's update. Am J Kidney Dis 2011;58(1):118–26.

50. Baron C, Forconi C, Lebranchu Y. Revisiting the effects of CMV on long-term transplant outcome. Curr Opin Organ Transplant 2010;15(4):492–8.

51. Streblow DN, Orloff SL, Nelson JA. Acceleration of allograft failure by cytomegalovirus. Curr Opin Immunol 2007;19(5):577–82.

52. Kliem V, Fricke L, Wollbrink T, et al. Improvement in long-term renal graft survival due to CMV prophylaxis with oral ganciclovir: results of a randomized clinical trial. Am J Transplant 2008;8(5):975–83.

53. Cannon RM, Ouseph R, Jones CM, et al. BK viral disease in renal transplantation. Curr Opin Organ Transplant 2011;16(6):576–9.

54. Chung BH, Hong YA, Kim HG, et al. Clinical usefulness of BK virus plasma quantitative PCR to prevent BK virus associated nephropathy. Transpl Int 2012;25(6):687–95.

55. Kuypers DR. Management of polyomavirus-associated nephropathy in renal transplant recipients. Nat Rev Nephrol 2012;8(7):390–402.

56. Clercq ED. Highlights in antiviral drug research: antivirals at the horizon. Med Res Rev 2012;May 2. Epub ahead of print.

57. Chon WJ, Josephson MA. Leflunomide in renal transplantation. Expert Rev Clin Immunol 2011;7(3):273–81.

58. Krisl JC, Taber DJ, Pilch N, et al. Leflunomide efficacy and pharmacodynamics for the treatment of BK viral infection. Clin J Am Soc Nephrol 2012;7(6):1003–9.

59. Masutani K, Shapiro R, Basu A, et al. The Banff 2009 Working Proposal for polyomavirus nephropathy: a critical evaluation of its utility as a determinant of clinical outcome. Am J Transplant 2012;12(4):907–18.
    Banff classification schema for BK PVN diagnosis with emphasis on prognosis and clinical management.

60. Mannon RB, Hoffmann SC, Kampen RL, et al. Molecular evaluation of BK polyomavirus nephropathy. Am J Transplant 2005;5(12):2883–93.

61. Andoh TF, Bennett WM. Chronic cyclosporine nephrotoxicity. Curr Opin Nephrol Hypertens 1998;7(3):265–70.

62. Pallet N, Rabant M, Xu-Dubois YC, et al. Response of human renal tubular cells to cyclosporine and sirolimus: a toxicogenomic study. Toxicol Appl Pharmacol 2008;229(2):184–96.

63. Nankivell BJ, Borrows RJ, Fung CL, et al. The natural history of chronic allograft nephropathy. N Engl J Med 2003;349(24):2326–33.

64. Casey MJ, Meier-Kriesche HU. Calcineurin inhibitors in kidney transplantation: friend or foe? Curr Opin Nephrol Hypertens 2011;20(6):610–5.

65. Albano L, Alamartine E, Toupance O, et al. Conversion from everolimus with low-exposure cyclosporine to everolimus with mycophenolate sodium maintenance therapy in kidney transplant recipients: a randomized, open-label multicenter study. Ann Transplant 2012;17(1):58–67.

66. Budde K, Lehner F, Sommerer C, et al. Conversion from cyclosporine to everolimus at 4.5 months posttransplant: 3-year results from the randomized ZEUS study. Am J Transplant 2012;12(6):1528–40.

67. Mjörnstedt L, Sørensen SS, von Zur Mühlen B, et al. Improved renal function after early conversion from a calcineurin inhibitor to everolimus: a randomized trial in kidney transplantation. Am J Transplant 2012;12(10):2744–53.

68. Mangray M, Vella JP. Hypertension after kidney transplant. Am J Kidney Dis 2011;57(2):331–41.

69. Kasiske BL, Anjum S, Shah R, et al. Hypertension after kidney transplantation. Am J Kidney Dis 2004;43(6):1071–81.

70. KDIGO. Clinical practice guideline for the care of kidney transplant recipients. Am J Transplant 2009;9(Suppl. 3):S1–155.

71. K/DOQI. Clinical practice guidelines on hypertension and antihypertensive agents in chronic kidney disease. Am J Kidney Dis 2004;43(5, Suppl. 1):S1–290.

72. Hiremath S, Fergusson D, Doucette S, et al. Renin angiotensin system blockade in kidney transplantation: a systematic review of the evidence. Am J Transplant 2007;7(10):2350–60.

73. Riella LV, Gabardi S, Chandraker A. Dyslipidemia and its therapeutic challenges in renal transplantation. Am J Transplant 2012;12(8):1975–82.

74. Holdaas H, Fellstrom B, Jardine AG, et al. Effect of fluvastatin on cardiac outcomes in renal transplant recipients: a multicentre, randomised, placebo-controlled trial. Lancet 2003;361(9374):2024–31.

75. Kasiske B, Cosio FG, Beto J, et al. Clinical practice guidelines for managing dyslipidemias in kidney transplant patients: a report from the Managing Dyslipidemias in Chronic Kidney Disease Work Group of the National Kidney Foundation Kidney Disease Outcomes Quality Initiative. Am J Transplant 2004;4(Suppl. 7):13–53.

76. Yates CJ, Fourlanos S, Hjelmesaeth J, et al. New-onset diabetes after kidney transplantation – changes and challenges. Am J Transplant 2012;12(4):820–8.

77. Yabu JM, Winkelmayer WC. Posttransplantation anemia: mechanisms and management. Clin J Am Soc Nephrol 2011;6(7):1794–801.

78. K/DOQI. Clinical practice guidelines for chronic kidney disease: evaluation, classification, and stratification. Am J Kidney Dis 2002;39(2, Suppl. 1):S1–266.

79. Mannon RB. Therapeutic targets in the treatment of allograft fibrosis. Am J Transplant 2006;6(5, Pt 1): 867–75.

80. Wehner J, Morrell CN, Reynolds T, et al. Antibody and complement in transplant vasculopathy. Circ Res 2007;100(2):191–203.

81. Cailhier JF, Laplante P, Hebert MJ. Endothelial apoptosis and chronic transplant vasculopathy: recent results, novel mechanisms. Am J Transplant 2006;6(2):247–53.

82. Jin YP, Korin Y, Zhang X, et al. RNA interference elucidates the role of focal adhesion kinase in HLA class I-mediated focal adhesion complex formation and proliferation in human endothelial cells. J Immunol 2007;178(12):7911–22.

83. Zhang X, Reed EF. Effect of antibodies on endothelium. Am J Transplant 2009;9(11):2459–65.

84. Babu AN, Murakawa T, Thurman JM, et al. Microvascular destruction identifies murine allografts that cannot be rescued from airway fibrosis. J Clin Invest 2007;117(12):3774–85.

85. Einecke G, Sis B, Reeve J, et al. Antibody-mediated microcirculation injury is the major cause of late kidney transplant failure. Am J Transplant 2009;9(11):2520–31.

86. Iredale JP. Models of liver fibrosis: exploring the dynamic nature of inflammation and repair in a solid organ. J Clin Invest 2007;117(3):539–48.

87. Grimm PC, Nickerson P, Jeffery J, et al. Neointimal and tubulointerstitial infiltration by recipient mesenchymal cells in chronic renal-allograft rejection. N Engl J Med 2001;345(2):93–7.

88. Zeisberg M, Neilson EG. Mechanisms of tubulointerstitial fibrosis. J Am Soc Nephrol 2010;21(11):1819–34.

89. Vitalone MJ, O'Connell PJ, Jimenez-Vera E, et al. Epithelial-to-mesenchymal transition in early transplant tubulointerstitial damage. J Am Soc Nephrol 2008;19(8):1571–83.

90. Humphreys BD, Lin SL, Kobayashi A, et al. Fate tracing reveals the pericyte and not epithelial origin of myofibroblasts in kidney fibrosis. Am J Pathol 2010;176(1):85–97.

91. Dulauroy S, Di Carlo SE, Langa F, et al. Lineage tracing and genetic ablation of ADAM12(+) perivascular cells identify a major source of profibrotic cells during acute tissue injury. Nat Med 2012; July 29. Epub ahead of print.

92. Hidalgo LG, Sis B, Sellares J, et al. NK cell transcripts and NK cells in kidney biopsies from patients with donor-specific antibodies: evidence for NK cell involvement in antibody-mediated rejection. Am J Transplant 2010;10(8):1812–22.

93. Mosser DM, Edwards JP. Exploring the full spectrum of macrophage activation. Nat Rev Immunol 2008;8(12):958–69.

94. Mannon RB. Macrophages: contributors to allograft dysfunction, repair, or innocent bystanders? Curr Opin Organ Transplant 2012;17(1):20–5.

95. Girlanda R, Kleiner DE, Duan Z, et al. Monocyte infiltration and kidney allograft dysfunction during acute rejection. Am J Transplant 2008;8(3): 600–7.

96. Budde K, Becker T, Arns W, et al. Everolimus-based, calcineurin-inhibitor-free regimen in recipients of de-novo kidney transplants: an open-label, randomised, controlled trial. Lancet 2011;377(9768):837–47.

97. Flechner SM, Glyda M, Cockfield S, et al. The ORION study: comparison of two sirolimus-based regimens versus tacrolimus and mycophenolate mofetil in renal allograft recipients. Am J Transplant 2011;11(8):1633–44.

98. Wojciechowski D, Vincenti F. How the development of new biological agents may help minimize immunosuppression in kidney transplantation: the impact of belatacept. Curr Opin Organ Transplant 2010;Oct 7. Epub ahead of print.

99. Sharif A, Shabir S, Chand S, et al. Meta-analysis of calcineurin-inhibitor-sparing regimens in kidney transplantation. J Am Soc Nephrol 2011;22(11):2107–18.

100. Franceschini N, Cheng O, Zhang X, et al. Inhibition of prolyl-4-hydroxylase ameliorates chronic rejection of mouse kidney allografts. Am J Transplant 2003;3(4):396–402.

101. Mannon RB. Immune monitoring and biomarkers to predict chronic allograft dysfunction. Kidney Int 2010;119(Suppl):S59–65.

102. Henderson LK, Nankivell BJ, Chapman JR. Surveillance protocol kidney transplant biopsies: their evolving role in clinical practice. Am J Transplant 2011;11(8):1570–5.

103. Rush D, Arlen D, Boucher A, et al. Lack of benefit of early protocol biopsies in renal transplant patients receiving TAC and MMF: a randomized study. Am J Transplant 2007;7(11):2538–45.

104. Vincenti F, Larsen C, Durrbach A, et al. Costimulation blockade with belatacept in renal transplantation. N Engl J Med 2005;353(8): 770–81.

105. Halloran PF, de Freitas DG, Einecke G, et al. An integrated view of molecular changes, histopathology and outcomes in kidney transplants. Am J Transplant 2010;10(10):2223–30.

106. Mengel M, Sis B, Halloran PF. SWOT analysis of Banff: strengths, weaknesses, opportunities and threats of the international Banff consensus process and classification system for renal allograft pathology. Am J Transplant 2007;7(10):2221–6.

107. Nakorchevsky A, Hewel JA, Kurian SM, et al. Molecular mechanisms of chronic kidney transplant rejection via large-scale proteogenomic

analysis of tissue biopsies. J Am Soc Nephrol 2010;21(2):362–73.

108. Hricik DE, Rodriguez V, Riley J, et al. Enzyme linked immunosorbent spot (ELISPOT) assay for interferon-gamma independently predicts renal function in kidney transplant recipients. Am J Transplant 2003;3(7):878–84.

109. Anglicheau D, Muthukumar T, Hummel A, et al. Discovery and validation of a molecular signature for the noninvasive diagnosis of human renal allograft fibrosis. Transplantation 2012;93(11):1136–46.

110. Sarwal MM, Benjamin J, Butte AJ, et al. Transplantomics and biomarkers in organ transplantation: a report from the first international conference. Transplantation 2011;91(4):379–82.

111. Ho J, Wiebe C, Gibson IW, et al. Immune monitoring of kidney allografts. Am J Kidney Dis 2012;60(4):629–40.

Index

NB: Page numbers followed by *f* indicate figures, *t* indicate tables and *b* indicate boxes.